The Real Vitamin and Mineral Book

The Real Vitamin and Mineral Book

A DEFINITIVE GUIDE

TO DESIGNING

YOUR PERSONAL

SUPPLEMENT

PROGRAM

THIRD EDITION

Shari Lieberman, Ph.D., CNS, FACN,
and Nancy Bruning

AVERY | a member of Penguin Group (USA) Inc.
New York

PUBLISHER'S NOTE

Every effort has been made to ensure that the information contained in this book is complete and accurate. However, neither the publisher nor the author is engaged in rendering professional advice or services to the individual reader. The ideas, procedures, and suggestions contained in this book are not intended as a substitute for consulting with your physician. All matters regarding your health require medical supervision. Neither the author nor the publisher shall be liable or responsible for any loss or damage allegedly arising from any information or suggestion in this book.

While the author has made every effort to provide accurate telephone numbers and Internet addresses at the time of publication, neither the publisher nor the author assumes any responsibility for errors, or for changes that occur after publication.

Most Avery books are available at special quantity discounts for bulk purchase for sales promotions, premiums, fund-raising, and educational needs. Special books or book excerpts also can be created to fit specific needs. For details, write Penguin Group (USA) Inc. Special Markets, 375 Hudson Street, New York, NY 10014.

a member of
Penguin Group (USA) Inc.
375 Hudson Street
New York, NY 10014
www.penguin.com

Library of Congress Cataloging-in-Publication Data

Lieberman, Shari.
The real vitamin and mineral book : a definitive guide to designing your personal supplement program / Shari Lieberman and Nancy Bruning.—3rd ed.
p.   cm.
Previous ed. published with the title: The real vitamin & mineral book
Includes bibliographical references and index.
ISBN 1-58333-152-2
1. Dietary supplements—Popular works.   2. Vitamins—Popular works.
3. Minerals in the body—Popular works.   I. Bruning, Nancy.   II. Lieberman, Shari.
Real vitamin & mineral book.   III. Title.

RM258.5 .L54   2003   2002043602
613.2'86—dc21

Printed in the United States of America
1   3   5   7   9   10   8   6   4   2

Book design by Tanya Maiboroda

SHARI LIEBERMAN
dedicates this book to the memory of her father and mother,
Mort and Sheila Lieberman.

NANCY BRUNING
dedicates this book to the memory of her mother,
and to her extended family of friends and colleagues,
who continue to nourish her in ways beyond comprehension.

Acknowledgments

DR. SHARI LIEBERMAN would like to thank Kirk Hamilton, for CP Currents, his superb monthly newsletter review of the scientific literature.

Contents

Part 5 Appendixes and Notes

Foreword

THE RELIABLE information concerning supplements given in *The Real Vitamin and Mineral Book* by Dr. Lieberman and Ms. Bruning is of paramount importance. Recently, the Pracon Study, commissioned by the Council for Responsible Nutrition, estimated that $8.7 billion could be saved on four major diseases if Americans consumed optimal levels of the antioxidants vitamin C, vitamin E, and beta-carotene. Diets optimal in vitamin C, vitamin E, and beta-carotene can lessen costs for breast, lung, and stomach cancer, and these same antioxidants could dramatically reduce the incidence and/or severity of cataracts in the older population. Although much benefit could be derived from diet alone, many individuals, for whatever reason, do not eat the five servings of fruits and vegetables suggested by the National Cancer Institute. A 1990 analysis by NHANES II found that less than 10 percent of Americans actually consume two servings of fruits and three of vegetables per day. Further analysis of data from this study revealed that 50 percent of Americans eat no vegetables, and 70 percent eat no fruits or vegetables rich in vitamin C.

The average American seeks means to attain a longer and healthier life. Many reasons exist to encourage the use of supplements to lengthen lifespan and reduce the severity of chronic diseases among the general population. To accomplish this, two broad concepts must be considered. The first concept is that genes play a significant role in the overall health and longevity of an individual. This is evident because people have a proclivity to develop maladies similar to those of their ancestors, e.g., early onset of cardiovascular disease. While much research has gone into discovering important genes involved in overall health and chronic diseases, suffice it to say that little can be done now to favorably alter genetic makeup. However, all is not lost when considering the second broad concept affecting long-term health. We can control our destiny to some extent, because environmental conditions, principally nutrition, also play a significant role in overall health. For example, the rapid increase in cardiovascular diseases found among Americans in the first half of the twentieth century was attributed to the "modern diet," which featured an increased intake of fats and sugars at the expense of complex carbohydrates and fibers. An inadequate intake of certain vitamins and minerals is also a feature of the modern diet. In turn, the more recent reversal of this same trend has been attributed to an awareness of the benefits of low-fat consumption and the use of vitamin and mineral supplements. Accordingly, genes may play a significant role in determining whether we live a long, healthy life. But within the constraints that genes impose on us, good nutritional practices can markedly influence health, as well.

Some years ago, my research led me into the field of nutrition. Although I initially focused on a small area of nutrition, in time I became aware that there was much more I needed to know. Following a conversation with Dr. Lieberman, she provided me with the first edition of *The Real Vitamin and Mineral Book*. I appreciated the brevity and clarity of each chapter on a specific topic. The book was highly informative and persuasive. Using what I learned, I started my own supplement plan after careful thought. As a long-time member of the Risk/Benefits Committee at Georgetown University Medical Center, I have examined human studies designed to evaluate therapeutic interventions. From reading the first edition of this book, I was impressed with the favorable risk/benefit ratios of many supplements. Although the evidence of therapeutic benefit may not be 100 percent conclusive in each case, there is often great potential to be gained from taking supplements with little risk involved.

Like the first and second editions, this edition of *The Real Vitamin and Mineral Book* is designed to provide maximal information in a concise fashion. After a brief but persuasive discussion supporting the use of supplementation, updated chapters follow on fat-soluble and water-soluble vitamins and minerals. The section concerning "other nutrients" has undergone extensive revisions to include information on DHEA, melatonin, and carnitine. No debate is necessary over the timeliness of these chapters. The appendix contains reference abstracts, allowing the reader to pursue in greater depth topics of interest. Accordingly, the setup of the book provides the reader with a guide to the nutritional supplements he or she really needs in their most effective dosages.

I believe that each individual should become acquainted with all aspects of supplements, good and bad. This book is an excellent starting point. With knowledge gained in reading this comprehensive guide and the good advice of a professional health-care provider, one can make wise decisions concerning supplementation, keeping in mind that individual programs should be updated as new information becomes available.

Harry G. Preuss, MD, FACN
Professor of Medicine and Pathology
Georgetown University Medical Center
Washington, DC

What's Your Real Vitamin and Mineral IQ?

IF YOU READ NEWSPAPERS, books, or magazines, if you listen to the radio or watch TV, you've been hearing a lot about vitamin and mineral supplements. Chances are, you've been hearing many contradictory statements and you are confused about the benefits that can actually be derived from each supplement. I don't blame you! Try this test, designed to find out what you really know. If you find your knowledge to be less clear than you thought—don't despair. This book will give you all the facts you need to separate the hype from reality.

1. If I eat well, I can get all the nutrients I need from food.
   A. True
   B. False

2. Vitamin E has been shown to:
   A. Improve your sex life
   B. Help prevent cancer
   C. Prevent baldness
   D. None of the above

3. Enriched white bread is just as nutritious as whole wheat bread.
   A. True
   B. False

4. Which drug(s) increases your need for certain vitamins and/or minerals?
   A. Antibiotics
   B. Aspirin
   C. Birth control pills
   D. All of the above

5. Who generally requires a higher intake of vitamins and minerals?
   A. Senior citizens
   B. Body builders
   C. Marathon runners
   D. All of the above

6. Which mineral(s) has been shown to protect against many forms of cancer?
   A. Calcium
   B. Magnesium
   C. Selenium
   D. None of the above

7. As long as you take supplements, you can eat whatever you want.
   A. True
   B. False

8. Vitamin C has been shown to _____ colds.
   A. Cure
   B. Prevent
   C. Shorten the duration of
   D. All of the above

9. Which nutrient(s) may be effective in preventing cardiovascular disease?
   A. Calcium
   B. Vitamin E
   C. Niacin
   D. All of the above

10. The more supplements you take, the better.
    A. True
    B. False

Answers

1. **B.** This may have been true for early humans, who lived physically active lives, ate wild, fresh, whole food, and breathed clean air. Today, we eat relatively few nutrient-dense fruits, nuts, and vegetables. Yet we are under physical and psychological stresses our ancestors never dreamed of, paradoxically raising our need for many nutrients. Even if we ate a "balanced" diet, our food has less nutrition to begin with because it is raised using synthetic chemicals, and then it is stored and processed to within an inch of its life. (For more information, see Chapter 2.)

2. **B.** Many studies have shown that vitamin E helps protect us against the harmful effects of a variety of carcinogens and toxins, including carbon tetrachloride, mercury, lead, benzene, ozone, and nitrous oxide. It prevents the formation of potent carcinogens called nitrosamines from the nitrates found in air pollution, cigarette smoke, and some foods. Vitamin E also prevents vitamins A and C, two other vitamins that protect us from carcinogens, from losing their potency in the body. Although severe vitamin E deficiency did cause infertility in experimental animals, no studies have shown this nutrient to improve the sex life of humans. Vitamin E does not prevent baldness. (For more information, see Chapter 8.)

3. **B.** The flour used to make white bread has been depleted of over twenty nutrients, including up to 40 percent of vitamin C, 85 percent of vitamin B_6, and 72 percent of zinc. The manufacturers then put back a handful of these nutrients (five, to be exact), and call the result "enriched"! Whole wheat bread and other whole grain breads are much higher in almost every vitamin and mineral, including trace minerals such as chromium, selenium, and manganese. They are also higher in protein and fiber. (For more information, see Chapter 2.)

4. **D.** It is widely recognized that many drugs interact with nutrients in the body, often causing nutrient depletion. Antibiotics have been shown to interfere with the B vitamins, vitamin C, and calcium. Antibiotics may also destroy useful bacteria in the colon, thus hinder-

ing vitamin K synthesis. Estrogen-containing medications, such as birth control pills, deplete the body of vitamin B_6, folic acid, and vitamin C. Even aspirin, if used over a long period of time, may deplete the body's stores of vitamin C and folic acid. (For more information, see Chapter 2.)

5. **D.** Because of their exercise regimens, marathoners and body-builders are under physical stress, which increases their need for many vitamins and minerals. In addition, people who exercise heavily tend to eat large amounts of carbohydrates, which increase the need for thiamin. Finally, sweating has been shown to increase the excretion of certain essential nutrients. Many studies have shown that because of reduced absorption and poor eating habits, the elderly are also at great risk for having low levels of nutrients, especially calcium; vitamins B_6, B_{12}, E, and D; folic acid; and zinc. (For more information, see Chapter 2.)

6. **C.** There is a higher incidence of cancer among people who live in geographical areas where the soil is lower in selenium. Studies have correlated many forms of cancer, but especially breast cancer, with a low selenium intake. There is some evidence that calcium may protect against colon cancer, but the data is too preliminary to draw any firm conclusions. (For more information, see Chapter 29.)

7. **B.** Supplements are just that—supplements. They should be taken in *addition* to an intelligent diet to make up for the nutrients lost in our food as a result of shipping, storage, processing, and other factors. Supplements are not meant to overcome a diet that is too high in fat and sugar and too low in fiber. They are designed to be part of a total health program that includes good fresh food, exercise, stress reduction, and avoidance of substances known to be harmful to the body. (For more information, see Chapter 5.)

8. **C.** Vitamin C has been shown to shorten the duration of colds and lessen the severity of the symptoms. Vitamin C is necessary for the optimum function of the immune system, but has never been conclusively proven to either prevent or cure the common cold. (For more information, see Chapter 20.)

9. **D.** Many studies correlate a higher calcium intake with lower blood pressure. Vitamin E may reduce cholesterol in the blood and increase levels of HDL (high-density lipoproteins, the "good" type of cholesterol). It may also help prevent platelets from clogging the arteries. Niacin has been shown to be effective in reducing cholesterol and triglycerides in the blood. In fact, two studies recommend niacin as the treatment of choice for these conditions. (For more information, see Chapters 8, 13, and 21.)

10. **B.** For each individual, there is an optimum amount of each nutrient beyond which the benefits are small or nonexistent. There is no reason to take, for example, 150 milligrams of the B vitamins if 50 milligrams will do the job. Although even very high doses of vitamin and mineral supplements are generally not harmful, it makes no sense economically or healthwise to take more than you really need. (For more information, see Chapter 4.)

Your Score

- 7–10 Correct: Excellent
- 4–6 Correct: Average
- 0–3 Correct: Poor

Back to Basics

WHAT DO I mean by the "Real" Vitamin and Mineral book? I mean several things. First of all, I mean that it is based on scientific research and not hype—real studies and data you can trust. Secondly, my recommendations are geared toward people who live in the real world of imperfect food and imperfect diets and various amounts of mental, emotional, and physical stress—not some nonexistent ideal world in which you can get everything you need from food. Third, it emphasizes the tried and true nutrients—vitamins and minerals—that form the basic foundation of a complete supplement program. So many people are being distracted and seduced by exotic supplements, and in the process are becoming confused and losing sight of the basic nutrients they really need for optimum health. Finally, the book incorporates the exciting and growing approach to health and medicine called "integrative medicine." This wonderful idea reflects the reality that when we combine so-called alternative or complementary therapies with conventional medicine, we often get a better result than when conventional medicine is used alone. I have been working with conventional physicians for years and have seen again and again that specific dietary supplementation can often make conventional treatment more effective, less toxic, and reduce the effective dose of a particular medication.

These concepts, which are at the heart of this book, are incredibly important information—information that could change your life. It has changed mine, it has changed my coauthor's, and it has changed that of the thousands of patients who have come to me for advice.

Initially, I wanted to be a medical doctor. I was interested in science, and I wanted to work with people, to help them. I thought that being a physician would allow me to do this.

However, as a premed student, I learned that traditional Western medicine takes quite a rigid and fragmented approach to health. It is primarily concerned with treating isolated symptoms and diseases, rather than promoting the health of the whole person. I realized that although conventional medicine has its place and can do a lot of good—even perform miracles—prevention is a far more potent tool in the larger scheme of things. In addition, it became clear to me that as long as an illness or condition is not life threatening, nutrition should be the first line of defense. Compared with modern Western medicine, the nutritional approach is a safe, nontoxic, effective alternative.

My coauthor, Nancy Bruning, came to nutrition and the writing of this book because of a very personal concern and involvement. Because she had heard that I work with cancer patients who are undergoing chemotherapy, she interviewed me for her book, *Coping With Chemotherapy.* A former cancer chemotherapy patient herself, Nancy was primarily interested in researching therapies that could be used to complement conventional chemotherapy to make it more comfortable, less damaging, and perhaps more effective. Although she learned firsthand the important role that nutrition plays in such circumstances, she also realized that disease prevention is a superior tactic, and that nutrition can have a tremendous impact on overall health. Twenty-two years postdiagnosis, and in excellent health, she specializes in writing about disease prevention and about the advantages of combining mainstream medicine with complementary approaches such as nutrition.

My research and clinical experience in working with a wide variety of people have shown me that in today's world, most people do not get all the nutrients they need from food. As a result, not only do they not enjoy optimum health, but they are setting the stage for poor health in the future.

When we first wrote this book, many people were concerned that they were not getting all they needed from food, but the average person was confused about what they should take, and how much. There were few books for the general public with clear guidelines based on scientific information. Today, almost the opposite is true. We are inundated with books on nutrition, often with single nutrients being touted as the latest cure-all. We are bombarded with article after article on vitamins and minerals, as the media jumps on the latest study, which it often misinterprets and misrepresents. Once again, people are confused. As a result, they either give up and take no supplements, or just take one or two single nutrients such as calcium or vitamin C. Still others jump on the latest fad bandwagon and start taking an exotic supplement such as an amino acid or evening primrose oil and completely forget about the basic vitamins and minerals that in reality will likely do much more to improve and protect their health.

Our purpose in writing this book is to clear away the confusion and clutter. It will help you get back to basics. We will provide you with the guidelines you need to create your own personalized basic supplement program. And we will also supply you with the scientific documentation that will help you feel confident that supplements have the potential to make a great difference in your health.

According to various polls and surveys, 35 to 50 percent of the American population takes vitamin and mineral supplements. But do people know what to take, or why they are taking it? As a clinician, as a teacher, as a researcher, and as a lecturer, I have found that people want to individualize and optimize their vitamin regimens to suit their own needs, in much the way they want to individualize and optimize their workouts and diets.

As a nutritionist, I've been seeing patients for over twenty years. They are generally referred to me by their physicians for a variety of problems and needs. Some are specific, such as acne, HIV/AIDS, psoriasis, menstrual and/or menopause problems, blood sugar problems, intestinal disorders, high blood pressure, high cholesterol, an inability to sleep, fatigue, depression, weight loss, chronic fatigue and immune dysfunction, and fibromyalgia. These people turn to nutrition as an adjunct or an alternative to the treatment offered by their physicians. But most people who come to me are not obviously sick—they are interested in nutrition as a means of improving their health and preventing illness. They want to live longer, healthier lives; to feel better, look better, have more energy, withstand stress better, and be able to avoid or minimize diseases that range from the common cold to cancer. They come to me because they are very confused about supplementation. In spite of all the books and articles they've read, they still don't know how to apply the available information to their own lives.

In all its subtleties, nutrition is a very complex subject—one that is challenging for even the qualified professional. Moreover, the field is growing and becoming full of self-styled experts who bombard you with contradictory advice and information almost daily. Many people deal with this confusion by going to a clinical nutritionist or to a physician whose practice is nutritionally oriented. But practitioners who are up-to-date and proficient in the field of nutrition and knowledgeable about nutritional supplementation are not available to everyone. This book was written so that you can intelligently design your own supplement program. It is also a useful tool for practitioners who were not trained in nutrition, and are interested in learning about the progressive approach to this subject. I am grateful to know that many professionals recommend this book to both their colleagues and their patients. In fact, this book has been used as a textbook in several universities.

It always amazes me when people say they either "believe" in taking vitamins, or they don't, as if this were some kind of religion, based on blind faith. I want to reassure you that the progressive nutritional approach to health is not a religion. It is a science that is taking its rightful place alongside other health sciences. This poses two basic problems that I hope to correct with this book.

The first problem is that because supplementation is a science, the language can get very technical. My education and professional experiences have taught me how to translate highly technical data into a language that the average person can understand.

The second problem is that because nutrition is no longer a new science, the scientific literature is filled with studies on diet and supplementation. In writing this book, I have searched the most up-to-date professional journals, including foreign research journals, as well as attending numerous scientific conferences and speaking with experts in the field of nutrition. I have interpreted the information and synthesized it to provide you with the most comprehensive, unified and scientifically sound picture of what vitamins, minerals, and other dietary supplements can—and cannot—do for you.

As you will see in this book, people are not getting the government-established Reference Daily Intakes (the RDIs, formerly called the Recommended Daily Allowances, or RDAs) from their diets. In addition, the RDIs are not high enough for many people. *The Real Vitamin and Mineral Book* focuses on optimizing your health, rather than meeting the RDIs to prevent deficiency diseases by providing merely adequate amounts of nutrients for "normal healthy people," as recommended by the United States Food and Nutrition Board. This book is written from the viewpoint that amounts in excess of the RDIs can be preventive, therapeutic, and safe. I have called these greater amounts the Optimum Daily Intakes (ODIs)—a dosage range within which nearly everyone can find his or her individual amount. Every recommendation in *The Real Vitamin and Mineral Book* is based on the latest reliable scientific data, including studies published in well-respected professional journals and at scientific conferences, as well as on my own and other clinicians' successes with patients. It is not based on hearsay or on highly questionable studies. When contradictory or inconclusive data exist, I make it clear that further studies are needed. For example, I would very much like to say that large doses of vitamin C cure cancer, but the evidence so far has not supported this statement. On the other hand, the evidence is strong enough to recommend taking vitamin C as a *preventive measure* against certain cancers and as an adjuvant to many forms of therapies.

Nutritionists, physicians, and researchers are in agreement that vitamins and minerals are essential for human health. Opinions differ only as far as specific uses and amounts are concerned. Clearly, some of the claims for "megavitamins" are not as well supported as others. As a result, people are taking the wrong supplements in the wrong amounts for the wrong reasons. Many of them are wasting their time and money, either on multivitamins, which can be hit-or-miss, or on dosages that are either unnecessarily high or too low to have an appreciable effect. Other people would like to take supplements, but are confused, and so have never begun a supplement regimen.

If you, like many of my patients, have looked through or read other nutrition books but found them too technical, not specific enough, or just plain overwhelming, this book is for you. *The Real Vitamin and Mineral Book* dispels the confusion caused by medical jargon and conflicting information, taking the guesswork out of taking supplements. Moreover, this book deals only with supplements that are generally available to the public. This does not mean that you are getting *less* information, just *less distracting* information. You get clarity, not clutter. The information is presented in a straightforward, usable form, providing—in simple, honest, realistic terms—exactly the foundation you need to create a workable supplement plan for yourself.

Part One of *The Real Vitamin and Mineral Book* explains the RDIs and the ODIs, and guides you in using the remainder of the book. These introductory chapters give you a basic grasp of the concepts, goals, and guidelines of vitamin and mineral supplementation.

Part Two consists of individual chapters on each vitamin, including the doses I recommend to my patients both for general optimum health and for specific problems.

Part Three consists of individual chapters on minerals.

Part Four goes beyond the basics and consists of chapters on nutrients that are not vitamins or minerals, but may have specific health benefits.

Part Five provides handy reference tables and sample worksheets to help you apply what you have learned to the custom design of your individual supplement program. I have also included reference abstracts for each nutrient chapter—summaries of the most recent scientific studies for anyone who wishes to research the subject further.

With the help of this book, you will find it easy to create a personal supplement plan. To get an overall picture of what supplements can do for you, I recommend that you first read through Part Two, "The Vitamins"; Part Three, "The Minerals"; and Part Four, "Beyond Vitamins and Minerals." Then tear out or photocopy the worksheet on pages 280 and 281 and, pen in hand, go through the book again, chapter by chapter, filling in your individual Optimum Daily Intake for each nutrient.

If you have any medical condition, please consult your physician before taking any vitamin or mineral supplements. If he or she is not versed in nutrition, bring this book to the office. The ODIs are not meant to be a substitute for any medications, therapies, or medical treatments. In most cases, they may be used in addition to the recommended medical treatment. However, once again, consult your physician first.

Part 1

The Case for Supplementation

1 | What Are Vitamins and Minerals?

VITAMINS AND MINERALS are nutrients that are essential to life. They are often called micronutrients because, in comparison with the four major nutrients—carbohydrates, proteins, fats, and water—they are needed in relatively small amounts.

Vitamins are organic compounds, meaning that they occur naturally in plants and animals. By and large, vitamins function as coenzymes. Enzymes are catalysts or activators in the chemical reactions that are continually taking place in our bodies. Vitamins are a fundamental part of the enzymes, much the way your muscles are a fundamental part of your arms and legs.

Most people are aware that our enzymes help us digest our food. But enzymes do more than digest food. They are at the very foundation of all our bodily functions. Enzymes are what make things happen, and happen faster. Without enzymes, you can't breathe, blink, or walk. Your body can't break down proteins into essential amino acids, electrons can't flow, and nerve transmissions can't occur. You can't pull your hand out of the fire (or put it there in the first place), smell a rose, see a sunset, or taste an apple. And without vitamins, the enzymes can't do their job. For example, consider a particular enzyme that is needed to transmit nerve impulses to your fingers. No matter how plentiful this enzyme is in your body, if you are deficient in B_6, this enzyme cannot be activated. As a result, you might feel some numbness in your fingers.

Minerals are inorganic elements, meaning that they are not produced by plants and animals. Like vitamins, many minerals function as coenzymes, enabling chemical reactions to occur throughout the body.

In addition to their role as coenzymes, some micronutrients have other functions. For example, vitamin E acts as an antioxidant; calcium, magnesium, and phosphorus form our bones; iron enables the transport of oxygen from the lungs to the body cells; and active vitamin D functions as a hormone.

After they have been absorbed, vitamins and minerals actually become part of the structure of the body—of the cells, enzymes, hormones, muscles, blood, and bones. As part of the body pool, these substances remain in the body for varying amounts of time. Some are utilized immediately and some are stored and utilized over a period of time.

The vitamins that stay in the body for a short period of time—two to four days—are called water-soluble vitamins. The B vitamins and vitamin C belong to this group. Utilization of water-soluble vitamins begins the minute they are absorbed through your digestive system. Thus, these nutrients must be replenished regularly. Since they are not stored but are quickly excreted from the body, toxicities are virtually unknown. Fat-soluble vitamins, on the other hand, stay in the body for a longer period of time. Vitamins A, D, E, and K belong to this group. Although these vitamins are usually stored in fat (lipid) tissue, some may also be stored in some organs, especially the liver. Therefore, you can have toxicity problems with some of the fat-soluble vitamins, but only when you take very large doses.

Minerals also belong to two groups: the macro, or bulk, minerals; and the micro, or trace, minerals. Macrominerals are needed in larger amounts than microminerals. The macrominerals include calcium, magnesium, and phosphorus. The microminerals include zinc, iron, copper, manganese, chromium, selenium, iodine, potassium, and boron. Minerals are stored in various parts of the body—primarily in bone and muscle tissue. Therefore, it is also possible to overdose on minerals if you take extremely large amounts.

If you are concerned about toxicity, you must remember that there is no vitamin or mineral that is as toxic as are most of the drugs you can buy over the counter, including aspirin. Did you know that 2,500 people die each year from aspirin, and that 100 die each year from acetaminophen, the main ingredient in Tylenol? To reach toxicity with vitamin and mineral supplements, you must go out of your way to abuse supplements by taking massive quantities, usually for a prolonged period of time. The dose ranges I suggest for vitamin and mineral supplements are completely safe and have been used in human clinical studies with no evidence of toxicity.

Other nutrients, while not considered essential for overall health, appear to be essential for certain conditions and situations. For example, CoQ_{10} supplementation can prevent heart damage from Adriamycin (a drug used in cancer chemotherapy). It can also prevent the depletion of CoQ_{10} from heart muscles, when patients are given certain blood pressure and cholesterol-lowering medications, thus reducing the risk of death. I discuss these nutrients in the section called "Beyond Vitamins and Minerals" because ongoing studies have thus far yielded promising results and have shown that they are safe when taken in the recommended amounts. Unlike the basic vitamins and minerals, though, these nutrients either have not yet been proven to be needed by everyone or may be obtained by most people in sufficient quantities from their diets. Because of this, and the fact that they tend to be costly, there are no ODIs for these nutrients, and I generally recommend that their use be limited to the treatment and prevention of specific disorders.

2 | The RDIs—The Minimum Wages of Nutrition

CLEARLY, vitamins and minerals are essential to good health, and even to life itself. But how do we know whether we are getting sufficient nutrients to ensure our well-being? For approximately fifty years, the Recommended Daily Allowances (RDAs) were our guidelines. They were the United States Food and Nutrition Board's estimates of the amounts of nutrients required by most people to prevent overt deficiency symptoms. Most statements such as, "We can get everything we need from a well-balanced diet," and "Vitamin and mineral supplements are a waste of money," are based on a widespread acceptance of these guidelines. However, while the RDAs were a significant first step in understanding nutrition, we are beginning to realize that the RDAs—as well as their successors, the RDIs—have very important limitations.

After their creation, the RDAs were periodically evaluated and updated based on a continuing analysis of our rapidly expanding knowledge of nutrition. But in 1985, there was such widespread disagreement among the scientists involved that the National Research Council was unable to issue its scheduled new edition of the RDAs until 1989. This near inability of even the most conservative nutrition experts to agree illustrates some of the reservations about the RDAs that I and other nutritionists, physicians, and researchers expressed for some time.

The RDAs were fairly complex. For each nutrient, separate recommendations were made based on gender, age, and other factors. In an effort to provide simpler standards, the final version of the Nutrition Labeling and Education Act of 1993 replaced the RDAs with the RDIs (Reference Daily Intakes), which represent an average need. Since January 1997, the RDA nomenclature has no longer been used. The official term is now RDI. The term RDI is used throughout this book except in discussions of studies that based their doses on the RDAs. In those cases, the term RDA has been retained.

It should be noted that the RDI values are for children and adults of four or more years of age. The RDAs and RDIs are essentially the same values. In some cases, the RDIs are lower than the former RDAs; in some cases, they are higher. RDIs are still generally lower than the ODIs.

Just like the RDAs, the RDIs have three basic problems: (1) you cannot get all of the nutrients you need from today's food; (2) the RDIs reflect amounts that are adequate to prevent nutrient-deficiency diseases and are not tailored for individual needs; and (3) the RDIs do not address or consider optimum health or the prevention of degenerative diseases such as cancer and heart disease. In addition, they are not adequate for treating certain conditions. This chapter examines each of these problems in turn.

Problem 1: Can You Really Get Everything You Need from Food?

The RDIs are intended to be met solely through diet. However, it is virtually impossible to meet the RDIs by eating the food available to us today. As a clinician who sees real people, I know how impractical and misleading the typical well-balanced diet explained in nutrition handbooks can be. Such a diet does not take into consideration people's individual lifestyles, food preferences, and habits; nutrient bioavailability; the inaccuracy of the food value tables; or the loss of nutrients that occurs during storage, shipping, processing, and cooking.

THE MYTH OF THE WELL-BALANCED DIET

Most people simply do not eat a well-balanced diet, which, according to the latest recommendations of the Dietary Guidelines Committee, should resemble what is called the U.S. "Food Pyramid." Many of you have seen this pyramid, in which foods are divided into groups to comprise sections of a pyramid. The largest food group is at the base of the pyramid—this group consists of grains such as breads, cereals, rice, and pasta, and the government recommends six to eleven servings per day. The next largest group is fruits and vegetables, and the recommendation is for three to five vegetables and two to four fruits per day. Then comes the "protein" group—milk, dairy eggs, meat, fish, poultry—of which you should have a total of four to six servings. At the tip of the pyramid is the smallest group, the types of foods you should go easy on—the oils, fats, and sweets. While the pyramid goes a long way in simplifying the dietary guidelines, how many people think about pyramids at six A.M. when a Pop-Tart is in the toaster, or at 7 P.M. after a long day of work? Does a student eat five fruits and vegetables every day? Does even the most health-conscious marathon runner eat a perfect diet every day? Of course not.

In addition, there is the calorie problem. Most popular weight-loss diets allow 1,800 calories a day or less. However, you must consume 2,500 calories of wholesome, nutrient-rich foods to even approach the RDI. It seems that there's a new miracle diet every year, but they all essentially translate into fewer nutrients. Not only do these diets not work over the long term, but they may be setting you up for nutrition-related health problems for the future. What's more, low levels of certain nutrients may actually sabotage weight-loss efforts. Some plans, like the Atkins diet, remove most of the major food groups such as carbohydrates, making it impossible to get RDIs without supplementation. But very low-fat diets aren't the answer, either. For example, preliminary reports suggest that lipotropic (fat-loving) nutrients, such as chromium, L-carnitine, and choline, may enhance fat loss, provided an individual is eating a low-fat diet and engaging in regular aerobic exercise. Someone who is dieting may not be getting enough of these nutrients through food, theoretically making it more difficult to burn body fat and lose weight.

The danger of large-scale deficiencies is not just theory. Many published reports in the United States, Great Britain, and Europe show that portions of even affluent societies may be highly deficient in certain nutrients. Women are especially at risk for deficiencies. For example, one American study found that women generally consume 60 percent as many calories as men and therefore obtain about 60 percent as much of each nutrient as men do.

Although overt vitamin deficiency, evidenced by conditions such as scurvy, is rare in the United States, cancer and heart disease are not. And study after study has linked the growing incidence of such disorders with diets that are typically too high in fat and too low in the vitamins, minerals, and other nutrients needed for good health.

We have now reached that critical mass of evidence that is too large for the medical establishment to ignore. More and more respected physicians and scientists from world-famous medical institutions are supporting the addition of vitamin and mineral supplements to a healthy overall lifestyle. For example, Dr. Walter Willett of Harvard recommends multiple vitamins for most people. Dr. David Haber of UCLA also recommends a basic multivitamin/mineral supplement, plus extra single supplements of vitamin E, C, and calcium. Even the conservative *Journal of the American Medical Association* is now recommending vitamins for most people. (See "RIP: The 'We Don't Need Supplements' Myth" below). In an article commenting on the *JAMA* findings, Annette Dickinson, Ph.D., of the Council for Responsible Nutrition, stated, "There is no question that the amount of scientific evidence in favor of consistent use of vitamins, particularly multivitamins, is formidable and must be taken seriously."

I have found it especially interesting—and, frankly, amusing—that a survey of over six hundred dieticians found that nearly 60 percent of them use nutritional supplements. Add to this the fact that a show of hands at a 1994 conference of the American College of Cardiology revealed that approximately two-thirds of the seven hundred physicians in

RIP: The "We Don't Need Supplements" Myth

In 2002, the notion that most people don't need or benefit from vitamin and mineral supplements was finally laid to rest. In June of that year, the prestigious *Journal of the American Medical Association* published an article by two Harvard researchers. After reviewing thirty years of English language articles about the relationship between vitamins and chronic disease, they recommended that "all adults take one multivitamin daily." In their summary, they state that a large proportion of the general population has less-than-optimal intakes of a number of vitamins, putting them at increased risk for cardiovascular disease, cancer, and osteoporosis.

attendance took daily doses of antioxidants. Apparently, a majority of the food experts who have traditionally espoused the view that a balanced diet provides all the nutrients you need—as well as a number of other health-care practitioners—now realize how unrealistic this view is, at least when it comes to safeguarding their own health.

THE CASE OF THE MISSING NUTRIENTS

Evidence shows that the food tables that supposedly tell us the nutrient content of the foods we eat probably overstate nutritional value. As a result, the orange you just bought is probably not nearly as full of vitamin C as you may have been led to believe.

What's more, the nutrient content of foods, especially regarding minerals, fluctuates widely, depending on the growing conditions. Our soil is depleted of selenium in most parts of the country and often has only marginal levels of zinc, magnesium, calcium, and other minerals. Without mineral-rich soils, it is impossible for fruits and vegetables to contain a rich supply of nutrients.

Artificial fertilizers are widely used to increase crop yields, but, as is often the case, quantity does not necessarily equal quality. Of the twenty-six elements that have thus far been established as essential for human life, only sixteen are essential for plants. Plants contain elements they themselves don't require because they are part of the food chain: they philanthropically provide plant-eating animals, and thus meat-eating animals, with the nutrients those animals require. Artificial fertilizers that are based solely on plant needs overlook human requirements and could be creating more problems than they solve.

Fruits and vegetables begin to lose nutrients from the moment they are picked. Most of the fresh fruits and vegetables we buy have actually been picked, then stored, then shipped, and then stored again—possibly for weeks or months. After we buy them, we store them some more. Then we may cook them, or at least cut or slice them. Or a food may be processed before we buy it. Each of these steps causes further nutrient loss.

For example, the vitamin C content of apples may fall by two-thirds after only two or three months. Potatoes may have 30 milligrams of vitamin C per 100 grams when they are freshly harvested in the fall; but by springtime, they have only 8 milligrams per 100 grams; and by summer, they have practically none. Green vegetables suffer even more—they lose almost all their vitamin C after a few days of being stored at room temperature. Everyone knows that orange juice is high in vitamin C. But few people realize that an orange loses 30 percent of its vitamin C soon after it is squeezed. Nonfortified commercial orange juice has almost no natural vitamin C left.

Most people aren't aware that a surprising amount of the total nutrient content in many foods exists in a form that is not bioavailable, meaning that our bodies can't absorb and use it. About 40 percent of the vitamin C that is left in fresh-squeezed orange juice is biologically inactive. According to the food value tables, one cup of green cabbage has 33 milligrams of vitamin C—over half the RDI. What the food table doesn't tell you is that it is present in a form that is very poorly absorbed.

Next, we must consider how the heat, light, water, and chemicals used to process foods further deplete their nutrients. Blanching, a process that vegetables undergo before they are canned or frozen, can destroy up to 60 percent of the vitamin C content, 40 percent of the riboflavin, and 30 percent of the thiamin. The sterilization process used to can foods further destroys vitamins. For example, 39 percent of the vitamin A may be destroyed, and 69 percent of the remaining thiamin. While freezing itself seems preferable to canning, vitamin C may be depleted by about 25 percent. After they are processed, foods are stored and continue to lose their nutrients.

Even the simple act of cutting fruits and vegetables, which exposes the food to oxygen, encourages both vitamin and mineral losses. Cooking methods generally deplete about 50 percent of the less stable vitamins, especially vitamin C. By the time you put cooked peas on the table, only 44 percent (for fresh peas), 17 percent (for frozen peas), or as little as 6 percent (for canned peas) of the original vitamin C may be left.

Perhaps one of the greatest injustices inflicted upon foods occurs during the milling of grains. When wheat is processed into white flour, up to 40 percent of the vitamin C, and from 65 to 85 percent of various B vitamins, are depleted. In addition, many minerals are lost, including 59 percent of the magnesium and 72 percent of the zinc. Also lost are significant amounts of other vitamins, protein, and fiber. All in all, an appalling twenty-six essential nutrients are removed. The food industry then puts back a few cents' worth of iron, calcium, niacin, thiamin, and riboflavin—and calls its bread enriched!

As might be expected, our meats, which come from animals raised on some of the same nutrient-depleted foods that are available to us, are also

Food Isn't What It Used to Be

Today, our food is both less (nutritionally speaking) and more (chemically contaminated) than in the past. No wonder organic foods are growing in popularity.

- Food in the United States travels 1,300 miles from farm to market shelf, on average.
- Nearly every state buys 90 percent of its food from outside the state.
- Ten calories of fossil fuel are used to produce one calorie of food energy.
- Our food is bombarded with the equivalent of up to 233 billion chest X rays to kill bacteria and lengthen shelf life.
- Thirty percent of American dairy animals are fed genetically engineered bovine growth hormone.
- Only 9 cents of every food dollar goes to farmers; 10 cents goes to Philip Morris, who is a major player in agribusiness, and ConAgra, who supplies chemicals used in agriculture.
- Sixty-three percent of Americans buy organic foods and beverages, and 40 percent plan to buy more in the future.

— from "The Ethics of Eating," *National Catholic Reporter,* May 24, 2002.

lower in vitamins and minerals than indicated in food tables. The nutrient levels in our factory-farm livestock, which are fed artificial diets, also differ from those of animals that enjoy a more natural existence. And, of course, cooking robs meat of even more nutrients—up to half of its thiamin, B_6, and pantothenic acid.

Problem 2: Are the RDIs Really for Everyone?

The RDIs are one size fits all. They are designed to satisfy the needs of a mythical average healthy person, not individual needs. Unfortunately, this person does not exist in reality, just as the average American family, with its 2.2 children, never really existed. For instance, the RDIs do not take into account the twenty-five documented inborn errors of metabolism, some of which can increase an individual's vitamin requirements by a factor of 10 to 1,000. In Wilson's disease, for example, abnormal copper metabolism greatly increases the body's need for zinc, which is necessary to regulate copper absorption. Experiments have shown that it is highly probable that many individuals have more subtle difficulties with specific nutrients. While these problems may be harder to diagnose, they can diminish our quality of life and lead to future problems as serious as cancer and heart disease.

In addition to the individual biological blueprint with which each of us comes into the world, throughout life we each continue to change and undergo different experiences, such as environmental pollution, stress, disease, drug therapy, and aging. Each of these has the potential to increase our body's use of specific nutrients, interfere with nutrient metabolism, or otherwise affect our nutritional needs.

ENVIRONMENTAL POLLUTION

Today, there are an unprecedented number of chemicals all around us—in our food, our water, and the very air we breathe. The Environmental Protection Agency has estimated that sixty thousand chemicals have been buried or dumped throughout the United States over the years and are now penetrating our water supply. Automobiles and industry spew millions of pounds of pollutants into the atmosphere every year. Our food has become a chemical feast that is sprayed with pesticides, injected with hormones, fed with antibiotics, and adulterated with over three thousand chemicals in the form of artificial colors, flavors, textures, and preservatives. Cigarette smokers not only pollute their own lungs, but also endanger the health of others through secondhand smoke. Living or working with smokers can be equivalent to smoking several cigarettes a day. Many of the chemicals now in our environment have been proven to pose hazards to human health. Others may be potentially hazardous.

Fortunately, it has been found that certain vitamins and minerals are protective against some of these toxic substances. For example, vitamins C and E have been shown to be protective against nitrosamine, a carcinogen your body forms from the nitrates and nitrites found in processed meats such as hot dogs, bacon, ham, and bologna. These same carcinogens form from pollutants in the air and in cigarette smoke.

In addition to being cancer-causing agents, toxic chemicals have become a prime suspect in male infertility. Sperm counts all over the world are half what they were in the late 1930s, and of low quality. But sperm counts of men who eat organically grown food are twice as high as average. And vitamin C and glutathione have been shown to increase the percentage of normal sperm, sperm motility, and sperm viability in infertile men with lowered sperm count. Whether the chemicals deplete nutrients or increase your requirements, I feel it's wise to superfortify your body so that you can withstand these chemical insults.

MENTAL AND PHYSICAL STRESS

It has been well documented that when you are under any sort of stress, you deplete your store of certain vitamins and minerals more rapidly. Whether the stress is physical, such as strenuous exercise, or emotional, such as changing jobs, such a situation generally calls for higher intakes of vitamins and minerals. For example, female athletes appear to be at risk for iron deficiency. Athletic performance was enhanced in women who were anemic when they were supplemented with iron. Some male athletes may require iron as well, provided a diagnosis of iron deficiency anemia has been confirmed. There have been conflicting reports on the use of vitamins and minerals as ergogenic aids—substances that enhance exercise performance. However, some recent research focusing on the effect of oxidative stress on muscle soreness after exercise has shown that antioxidant supplementation both reduces oxidative stress and speeds muscle recovery.

DISEASE AND DISORDERS

There are many diseases that interfere with the ingestion, digestion, absorption, and requirement of nutrients. Diseases that affect the digestive system—such as celiac disease, Crohn's disease, irritable bowel syndrome, lactose intolerance, and bacterial, viral, and parasitic infections—are the most obvious. But infections in any part of the body can rapidly deplete stores of most vitamins and minerals. In addition, your appetite usually decreases during times of illness, which further depletes nutrient supplies. During the recuperation process following an illness, trauma, burns, or surgery, the body's stores of nutrients need to be replenished and the injured tissues repaired. Nutrients are also important for building up our immune systems, especially at critical times. Ironically, a downward spiral often occurs, in which illness depletes the body of nutrients, which lowers the resistance to infection, which in turn lowers the nutrient levels even more, and so on. The results of several studies have indicated that hospital patients as a group are some of the most mal-nourished people in the world. In one study, only 12 percent of the pa-tients tested had normal levels of vitamins in their bodies. Yet most of them had been eating a typical American diet while in the hospital.

As you will see in the upcoming chapters on individual vitamins and minerals, people with overt diagnosed medical conditions or diseases of-ten have low levels of one or more vitamins or minerals in their bodies. This occurs even when these conditions are not usually associated with nutritional deficiencies. This may indicate either that nutrient deficiencies play a previously unacknowledged role in the development of a particu-lar disease or condition, or that deficiencies are a direct or indirect result of the condition. Whatever the relationship between the illness and the deficiency, supplementation can often be an effective means of treatment and prevention. The therapeutic potential of supplementation has been particularly apparent in the accumulating reports on patients with HIV infection, AIDS, multiple sclerosis, rheumatoid arthritis, multiple chemi-cal sensitivities, and chronic fatigue. For these patients, who have few treatment options, nutritional supplementation has often been not only beneficial, but also safe. Certainly, your present and past physical condi-tion, as well as your family's health history, should always be considered when planning a nutritional regimen.

DRUGS

It is widely recognized that many drugs interact with nutrients in the body, often causing depletion. Tetracycline, a widely used antibiotic, inter-feres with the absorption of calcium, magnesium, potassium, zinc, and iron. Many other antibiotics are known to interfere with the B-complex vita-mins. Hormones in medications such as oral contraceptives appear to re-duce the levels of some of the water-soluble vitamins. Antacids, which coat the walls of the intestines to protect them from stomach acid, also prevent several nutrients—most notably, calcium—from being absorbed. Questran, a commonly prescribed drug used to lower cholesterol, limits the absorption of vitamins A, B_{12}, D, E, K, and folic acid. (For details on a number of drug-nutrient interactions, see pages 269 to 275). Statin drugs used to lower cholesterol seriously lower CoQ_{10} levels in the heart.

Alcohol is another drug that can interfere with nutrient absorption. Alcoholics have multiple nutritional deficiencies both for this reason and because they use alcohol as a substitute for food.

AGING

Studies have shown that your body changes throughout life. As you age, your organs generally tend to function less efficiently, your digestion may be affected, and you decrease your ability to absorb and utilize nutrients. Moreover, as your level of physical activity diminishes and your metabolism slows, your overall food intake lessens, too, so as you age you are at particular risk for suboptimal nutrition.

Many studies of older people have shown that they are simply not getting enough nutrients from their diets. It may come as no surprise to learn that a survey of fourteen nursing homes found that not one of them provided meals that met the RDAs for all nutrients. But another study—this one of 270 healthy elderly people living in the area of Albuquerque, New Mexico—provided truly startling results. Although the subjects were Caucasian and highly educated, had higher-than-average incomes, and were considered to be health conscious, it was found that up to 86 percent of the women and 85 percent of the men were getting less than the RDAs for vitamins B_6, B_{12}, E, and D; folic acid; calcium; and zinc.

As we age, we do require more nutrients—particularly calcium and magnesium. In addition, many diseases associated with aging, such as cancer, high blood pressure, heart disease, and diabetes, as well as the aging process itself, may raise our requirements for certain antioxidant nutrients. These effects are more fully discussed in Chapter 3 and in chapters on the individual antioxidant nutrients. For example, several studies—including work done at the Human Nutrition Research Center on Aging at Tufts University—have shown that supplementation with single nutrients, such as vitamin E, or with multivitamin and mineral supplements at levels above the RDA, result in improved immune responses. Two Canadian studies showed lower rates of infectious disease and cataracts among elderly people who took antioxidant vitamins. In the United States, a large-scale ongoing study of 87,000 nurses, ages forty-five to sixty-seven, has found that vitamin C supplementation, which continues for over ten years, reduces the risk of cataracts by 45 percent. Those subjects with the highest intake of vitamin A and beta-carotene had a 39 percent lower risk of cataracts. In another study, beta-carotene and related compounds also significantly reduced the risk of macular degeneration, a major cause of blindness in the elderly.

In a one hundred–page report prepared by the Council for Responsible Nutrition, Dr. Annette Dickinson notes that we usually accept frequent illness as part of growing old, but that adding nutritional supplements can *potentially cut these sick days in half.* She found strong evidence that when older people consistently take certain supplements this can improve the immune system, help protect eye and brain function, and maintain bone mass. As many as 80 percent of the elderly subjects she studied were not getting enough of four or more key nutrients. It's also likely that what we mistake for normal signs of aging are really signs of inadequate vitamins and minerals, according to the Senate Special Committee on Aging. This group recognized that although the elderly are often victims of useless remedies, they also acknowledged that "essential nutrient inadequacies can lead to adverse effects on nearly all organ systems" and we should consider deficiencies as contributing factors to many of the physical and mental complications seen in nursing homes.

We might not like to admit it, but we baby boomers are now middle-aged and at higher risk for degenerative, nutrition-related disease every day. As Dickinson points out, supplements can fill the nutrition gap left by poor eating and diminished absorption and utilization, reduce the risk of cardiovascular disease and stroke, and maintain eye function, memory, thinking, and our bones.

Problem 3: Do the RDIs Ensure Optimum Health?

The RDIs are designed to prevent only overt deficiency symptoms. Prolonged deficiency of a certain vitamin or mineral generally results in severe disease with easily observable signs. For example, vitamin A deficiency leads to night blindness and other eye problems; niacin deficiency causes pellagra, characterized by diarrhea, dermatitis, and dementia; and iron or B_{12} deficiency results in anemia. There is no question that the estimated RDIs are sufficient to prevent severe deficiency disorders in most people. But are they high enough to maintain optimum health? And is looking at severe, overt deficiency symptoms an accurate way of determining what you need? Maybe there are subtle changes that occur in the cells before the deficiency manifests itself in overt symptoms such as skin sores, mental disturbances, or crippling bone loss. Chapter 3, which is devoted to this issue, explains how the alternative to the RDIs, the ODIs, may help to ensure optimal health, not just the absence of disease.

As it currently stands, the RDI is a limited concept, the meaning and usefulness of which are being questioned even by the experts who are responsible for establishing and maintaining it. In today's world, the RDIs are, with a few exceptions, the nutritional equivalent of the minimum wage. They are probably high enough to keep you alive—although even this is open to question. But they do not appear high enough to allow you to enjoy the best quality of life. And why should you not strive for the best?

3 | The Optimum Daily Intakes (ODIs)

ECENT EVIDENCE INDICATES that most of the RDIs are far too low. Why? Because vitamins and minerals do more than just prevent the severe, overt symptoms that are traditionally associated with deficiencies. Remember: Vitamins and minerals are used in every process of the body. We now know, for example, that vitamin A does more than prevent night blindness, that thiamin prevents more than beriberi, and that vitamin C does much more than prevent scurvy. By optimizing our daily intake of nutrients, we don't simply prevent disease. We help ensure a state of optimal health.

Subclinical Deficiencies

State-of-the-art biochemistry shows that classic, overt deficiency symptoms, like those of beriberi, are merely the last event in a long chain of reactions in the body, the way an erupting volcano or earthquake is the last dramatic step in a series of underground processes. That we are not always aware of these processes does not mean that they do not exist, or that they will not eventually cause an explosion of ill health at some point in the future. When we do not get enough of a specific vitamin, the initial reactions occur on the molecular level. The first thing that happens is a depletion of the vitamin stores in the body. Then the enzymes, of which the vitamin is a part, become depleted. This, in turn, brings about changes on the cellular level: Some of the cells of the body, which depend upon these enzymes, can no longer carry out their normal functions. It is not until the depletion is prolonged and severe that the classic clinical signs of deficiency appear.

Such cellular changes are also known as subclinical deficiencies because they are not the kind of deficiencies that your doctor would necessarily discover through a routine physical exam and blood tests. But while they may not be obvious, easily definable, or immediately debilitating, these deficiencies do have an effect on the body's well-being. For example, volunteers who were depleted of vitamin B_1 showed no detectable body changes for the first five to ten days. After ten days, there was evidence of changes in the cells' metabolism. Classic anatomical signs of B_1 deficiency became obvious only after about two hundred days. However, during that time, the subjects experienced a gradual decline in their health with nonspecific symptoms of loss of weight, loss of appetite, general malaise, insomnia, and irritability.

The subtle, subclinical changes due to poor nutrition may be responsible for a broad range of diffuse, nonspecific conditions that can at first be merely annoying and reduce our overall health and quality of life. These conditions can include chronic fatigue, skin problems, recurrent or lingering infections and colds, digestive problems, sleep problems, headaches, hormonal problems, depression, and nervousness. Poor nutrient intake may also leave us more vulnerable to genetically predisposed diseases and conditions such as cardiovascular disease, diabetes, and cancer. The role that the other nutrients, such as fat and carbohydrates, play in these diseases is becoming more and more solidly documented. Why should we be surprised by the accumulating evidence that vitamins and minerals also play a part?

Nutrition—Nature's Protector

As already discussed, nutrients do far more than protect the body against deficiency diseases. By buttressing our immune system, they protect us from foreign invaders and therefore help fight infection. By guarding us from the ravages of oxidative stress, they prevent or slow the progress of a variety of degenerative illnesses, including cancer. And by helping regulate the balance of fats in the body, they fight heart disease. A brief look at each of these functions will provide a clearer idea of the importance of optimum nutrient intake to good health.

NUTRIENTS AND THE IMMUNE SYSTEM

Our immune system is a complex system of blood cells and special proteins acting together to defend us from harm. Improving our immune defense system is the main thrust behind modern preventive medicine because it protects us in so many important ways. For example, the immune system has the ability to engulf and kill bacteria and viruses. It can also repair or destroy a damaged cell before it grows into a cancerous tumor. This system, though powerful, is extremely delicate, its parts exquisitely interdependent upon one another. If any one aspect is compromised, we may become more susceptible to infections; degenerative diseases such as cancer and diabetes; and, perhaps, cardiovascular disease and certain forms of arthritis.

In many studies, inadequate nutrition has been shown to weaken one or more of the components of our defense system. Insufficient protein, too little fiber, and too much fat have all been implicated in impaired immunity, as have vitamin and mineral deficiencies. On the other hand, excesses of the RDIs of almost all vitamins and minerals have been shown to enhance immunity. Those that seem to exert the most profound effect are the antioxidants, vitamins C and E, beta-carotene, and selenium; minerals such as zinc; and specific B vitamins, such as vitamin B_{12}.

NUTRIENTS AND OXIDATIVE STRESS

A free radical is an atom or group of atoms that has at least one unpaired electron. An electron is a negatively charged particle that usually occurs in pairs, forming a chemically stable arrangement. When an electron is unpaired, another atom or molecule can then easily bond with it, causing a chemical reaction. Because they join so readily with other compounds, free radicals can effect dramatic changes in the body, causing a great deal of damage—damage often referred to as oxidative stress. Oxidative stress, which can accumulate over time, has been associated with the signs of aging and with debilitating and life-threatening degenerative diseases, including arthritis, hardening of the arteries, and heart and kidney ailments. It has also been implicated in the development of cancer. In fact, there's accumulating evidence that damage from out-of-control free radicals may lead to over sixty degenerative diseases.

Free radicals are formed by exposure to toxic chemicals in our food, water, and air; by radiation; by excessive sunlight; and, in part, by normal bodily processes. When the body obtains nutrients through the diet, it uses both these nutrients and oxygen to create energy. In this process, oxygen molecules containing unpaired electrons are released. These oxygen free radicals can cause damage to the body when produced in extremely large amounts. A diet that is high in fat, and particularly polyunsaturated fat, is especially associated with increased free-radical activity because oxidation more readily occurs in fat molecules than it does in protein and carbohydrate molecules.

Although the formation of free radicals is taking place all the time, our body has certain defense mechanisms that keep these processes under control. One of the body's defense mechanisms is to repair the cell damage caused by free radicals. Another such mechanism is interception of the free radicals before they do any harm. This is where antioxidants come in. Antioxidants—which include vitamins C and E, beta-carotene, and selenium—either help the body protect itself, or are themselves protective. For example, in one study, 400 milligrams of vitamin C a day reduced the lipid (fat) peroxide level—a measurement of oxidative stress—by 13 percent in one year. Supplements of both vitamins E and C reduced the level by 25 percent. This is just one of the many studies that combined several antioxidant nutrients and highlights the fact that antioxidants very often work synergistically with one another or with other nutrients in the body's defense. For example, vitamin E, which is known as a scavenger of free radicals formed by the oxidation of fats, works synergistically with selenium. It also protects vitamin C from oxidation, thus preserving the potency of another antioxidant. This is why you'll find many "antioxidant formulas" among the nutritional supplements, and suggests that we should be taking at least a full-spectrum antioxidant supplement, especially if we are not eating at least five fruits and vegetables everyday.

Studies show that if our bodies become overwhelmed by free radicals, or if we are not getting enough of the protective vitamins and minerals from our diets, antioxidant supplements can help protect us against oxidative stress. One study published in 1993 focused on Linxian, China, which has one of the highest rates of esophageal stomach cancer and a persistently low intake of micronutrients. In this study, approximately thirty thousand adults who were given supplements of beta-carotene, vitamin E, and selenium showed a 42 percent reduction in esophageal cancer and a reduced risk of death from cancer. The China study confirmed the work of Dr. Gladys Block, a respected epidemiologist who has written comprehensive reviews of the available scientific literature on antioxidants in food and supplements. She found, for example, that of approximately 130 studies in which subjects either took supplemental vitamin C, beta-carotene, or vitamin E, or ate antioxidant-rich foods, 120 studies showed statistically significant reduced risks of many, many cancers, including cancers of the lung, larynx, esophagus, oral cavity, pancreas, stomach, cervix, rectum, colon, ovary, endometrium, breast, and bladder.

Bruce Ames, a prominent researcher, has found that deficiencies in certain nutrients can damage DNA in a way that is very similar to that of exposure to radiation. Up to 20 percent of the U.S. population gets less than 50 percent of the RDI for many of these nutrients. He feels this could help explain why the almost quarter of the population that eats the fewest fruits and vegetables have double the cancer rate compared with the quarter that eats the most fruits and vegetables.

NUTRIENTS AND HEART DISEASE

Until recently, blood fats have gotten the most attention as risk factors for heart disease. But as you'll see, there's a new kid on the block, called homocysteine, that appears to be just as important. Nutrition also plays an important role in the balance of fats and homocysteine.

Our blood contains a variety of fats (lipids) and fatlike substances. Although our body requires a certain amount of fat to function well, an excess of some types of fats has been implicated in cardiovascular disease. These bad fats include serum cholesterol; low-density lipoproteins (LDLs), often called bad cholesterol; and triglycerides. On the other hand, good fats—high-density lipoproteins (HDLs), often called good cholesterol—are actually associated with a lowered risk of heart disease.

The balance between good and bad fats is determined by several factors, including diet (nutrition), exercise, and heredity. Fortunately, we can manipulate two out of three of these factors to create a more desirable balance. For example, there is evidence that levels of both triglycerides—a type of fat that may increase the risk of heart disease—and cholesterol can be lowered by the consumption of certain supplements. These supplements, which include niacin, vitamins C and E, chromium, EPA (eicosapentaenoic acid), and coenzyme Q_{10}, may also lower LDL and raise HDL cholesterol. Moreover, antioxidants such as vitamin E, beta-carotene, garlic, and coenzyme Q_{10} have been shown to protect LDLs from oxidizing and causing havoc in our arteries. Aerobic exercise and a very low-fat, high-fiber diet have also proven effective in this regard. Be aware that simply reducing the amount of cholesterol in your diet is a rather ineffective way of changing your blood cholesterol levels. The most effective plan for lowering blood cholesterol includes all of these measures. And unlike the drugs commonly used to lower cholesterol, this plan is safe.

Two large-scale, ongoing, Harvard-based studies have already demonstrated the power that nutrients can have in the prevention of heart disease. One, the Health Professionals Follow-up Study, involves forty thousand male physicians; the other, the Nurses' Health Study, involves eighty-seven thousand female nurses. These studies have found that vitamin E supplementation reduces the rate of heart disease in both men and women by 40 percent; that high intakes of beta-carotene reduce the rate of stroke in women by 40 percent; and that beta-carotene supplementation reduces heart attack, stroke, and death rates by half in men with heart disease.

But fats are only half the picture. Your body's cells all go through a metabolic cycle called methylation. In this process, an amino acid called methionine functions as the carrier for units of carbon that are used to build other compounds. This process generates another amino acid, called homocysteine, as a by-product, which is also crucial in the methylation process. When all is working well and you have enough of vitamin B_6, B_{12}, and folic acid, your body continually creates and transforms homocysteine into something else in a constant cycle of use and re-use. However, as is the case with free radicals (see earlier discussion) homocysteine can accumulate and become toxic. Uncontrolled, excess homocysteine is now thought to be a primary risk factor in heart disease and many other conditions, including cancer, arthritis, depression, and Alzheimer's disease and other forms of cognitive decline. For example, in the ongoing Physicians' Health Study, it was found that physicians who had the highest homocysteine levels had 3.4 times the risk of those with lower or normal levels. (For more information about homocysteine, see *The Methylation Miracle*, by Paul Frankel, Ph.D., and Nancy Bruning.)

The Changing View of Nutritional Supplements

Traditionally, the medical community has been very skeptical of the use of vitamin supplements. However, this is starting to change, especially regarding antioxidant nutrients. That's because of the overwhelming evidence that antioxidants may help prevent, slow, and even reverse serious diseases and conditions such as atherosclerosis, cancer, and cataracts.

Two large-scale, ongoing Harvard-based studies—the Health Professionals Follow-up Study and the Nurses' Health Study—stand out as the turning point for many health professionals. These studies, which were discussed above, are demonstrating the beneficial effects of antioxidants in the prevention of coronary disease. Research such as this is gradually providing consistent enough evidence to convince many former skeptics that supplementation with reasonable amounts of vitamins and minerals provides us with the optimum protection we need. At a recent American College of Cardiology meeting, two-thirds of the audience of approximately seven hundred physicians acknowledged that they themselves took antioxidant supplements daily.

Dr. Anthony J. Verlangieri, director of the Atherosclerosis Research Laboratories and professor of Pharmacology and Toxicology at the University of Mississippi School of Pharmacy, states, "Yes, absolutely, everyone should take supplementary vitamins." Based on twenty-five years of his research, he recommends that everyone take 200 international units of natural vitamin E, 4,000 milligrams of vitamin C, and either 2,500 international units of vitamin A or 15 to 25 milligrams of beta-carotene daily, in divided doses. He states, "It is a myth that we all get the vitamins we need in our daily diets." In addition, he points out that there are absolutely no toxicities associated with these levels of antioxidant supplementation.

While it is not a rule that more is always better, some experiments have shown that amounts of nutrients in excess of the RDIs, whether from food or supplements, do have a more positive effect than lower amounts. Some doctors have claimed that any excess micronutrients are a waste—that they simply end up in the urine. Although excess vitamins and minerals are eliminated from the body, research indicates that even this may not be a waste. For example, studies in which animals or humans were given substantially higher doses than the RDA for vitamin C

If We All Took Supplements

The Council of Responsible Nutrition evaluated ten years of the best scientific studies relating to the health benefits of vitamins and mineral supplements. They found that consistently taking supplements for a long period of time provides the strongest benefits, for people of all ages. Some highlights:

- percentage by which neural tube birth defects could be reduced: 70
- savings per year in health-care costs by delaying cardiovascular disease, stroke, and hip fractiure: $89 billion
- percentage by which sick days could be reduced in the elderly: 50

have suggested that any excess vitamin C that spills into the urine may have a protective effect against urinary and bladder cancer.

One factor that may be persuading some clinicians of the benefits of supplementation is that of cost. Several economists have estimated that by increasing our intake of vitamins and minerals, we would reduce health-care costs by 25 percent for cardiovascular disease, 16 to 30 percent for a variety of cancers, and 50 percent for cataracts. Another example of cost-effectiveness relates to carpal tunnel syndrome. When vitamin B_6 is used to treat this problem, it costs about $5 for a three-month supply. Compare this amount with that of surgery, and the savings are clear.

The ODIs—A Redefinition of Health

We have gradually expanded our knowledge and our thinking to include the notion that health should no longer be negatively defined as the absence of disease. Our current concept of real health is not one of mere survival, but one of a positive state of total mental and physical well-being. We have drawn a distinction between maintaining minimum or adequate health—which is what the RDIs appear to do—and attaining and maintaining optimum health—which the RDIs do not ensure. We want to be as healthy as we can be in our daily lives. This includes taking advantage of the most current research on the prevention of disease and the integration of nutritional therapies with appropriate medical care during the early, most treatable stage of disease.

WHY DO WE NEED THE ODIs?

In order to attain a state of optimum health and disease prevention, we must take into our bodies optimum—not minimum—amounts of vitamins and minerals. To distinguish them from the lesser amounts characteristic of the RDIs, I have called these amounts the Optimum Daily Intakes, or ODIs. The need for ODIs is based on six factors:

1. The RDIs are generally based on an amount that simply prevents overt deficiency diseases.
2. The RDIs do not take into account preventive or therapeutic levels of nutrients.
3. We cannot meet the RDIs even if we eat the perfect diet.
4. Because of many factors, including loss of nutrients through shipping, storage, and processing, the foods available to us do not contain the amounts of vitamins and minerals they should contain.
5. The vitamins and minerals in foods and supplements are never 100 percent absorbed.
6. Owing to the constant bombardment of stress factors, from pollution to emotional stress, we require higher levels of vitamins and minerals than originally thought.

In acknowledgment of the fact that people are individuals, and so require differing amounts of nutrients, each of the ODIs in this book is presented as a range of doses. Although a few ODIs are close to or the same as the RDIs, they are generally in excess of the RDIs and are often many times that amount. However, they are not megadoses—a term that is not only limiting, but totally inaccurate. Mega has come to mean ten times in popular usage and in some scientific articles; however, the term literally means million. In The Real Vitamin and Mineral Book, the ODI is often much more than ten times the RDI. However, it is never a million times the RDI.

WHAT IS THE BASIS FOR THE ODIs?

The ODIs are based on data from three sources: the most up-to-date research studies published in highly respected American and foreign professional journals, my own clinical experience, and the experiences of other well-known clinicians in the field. It should be noted that it is often difficult to draw firm conclusions when there is no uniform standard that allows us to compare study results fairly. Among various studies:

- Different amounts of supplements are used.
- Different forms of supplements are used—e.g., d-alpha (natural vitamin E) versus d,l-alpha tocopherol (synthetic vitamin E).
- Different study designs are used—e.g., supplements are given for varying amounts of time, and diet and daily habits may or may not be considered.
- Different study populations are used. That is, the study may test if something lowered the cholesterol levels in people who do not have elevated cholesterol; the study may test for a blood pressure–lowering effect on people who do not have hypertension; study subjects may be male or female; or studies may involve people in different age groups.

EVALUATING THE STUDIES

It has been estimated that our knowledge of the biological sciences is doubling every five to ten years, and human nutrition is an especially fast-growing field. Many practitioners, including myself, are interested in new findings and new ideas. We prefer to look forward, rather than backward. This means that we are sometimes in the position of having to take sketchy, somewhat experimental data and apply it to real-life situations, perhaps before the data is completely understood. So in many instances, I have had to take the research studies a step further. But I consider case studies to be "clinical pearls"; and applying the results of preliminary and pilot studies published in peer-reviewed journals has no downside because there are virtually no adverse effects with natural supplements. So why would you not try something if you were ill?

One example of this regards the stated uses of vitamin C. It has been shown that vitamin C blocks the formation of nitrosamine from the nitrates in food. Therefore, it stands to reason that the same would hold true for nitrosamines formed from air pollution in our lungs.

Another example of extrapolation regards animal studies. Wherever feasible, my recommendations have been based on human studies. However, sometimes animal studies are all that is available, in part because it would be unethical to use similar methods on humans. For instance, tumors are often induced in animals, after which supplements are given to assess their efficacy in suppressing tumor growth. The animals are usually killed after the experiment is completed to measure the effects of nutrition on various parts of the body.

According to the American Medical Association, the extrapolation from animal studies to humans is widely accepted in the medical profession. Many major breakthroughs in medicine, in fact, have occurred as a consequence of animal research. The efficacy and toxicity of almost all the drugs used in medical practice were originally based on animal research. Animal studies have also been generally accepted as sufficient proof that certain substances, such as cyclamates and red dye number 2, may be cancer-producing in humans. It is logical to conclude that in many cases, extrapolation of data from animal studies with respect to human nutrition is just as valid. For instance, as mentioned earlier, the ODIs reflect the fact that individual needs for nutrients vary. This is based not only on our knowledge of human beings, but also on our knowledge of animals. Nobel Prize winner Linus Pauling found that the vitamin requirements of individual animals within the same species vary by as much as 2,000 percent. He inferred that the same is probably true of humans.

A third example of extrapolation regards epidemiological studies—studies of the causes, distribution, and control of disease in populations. For instance, researchers may measure the level of a certain vitamin in the diet or blood of groups of people. They then see whether there is any correlation between vitamin levels and state of health. Many of the studies linking a higher level of vitamin A or carotenoids with a lower risk of cancer are of this type.

THE GOLD STANDARD OR DOUBLE STANDARD?

Some nutritionists and physicians have disputed many of the findings of these types of studies and have demanded stronger experimental proof. They want to see the same kind of placebo-controlled double-blind studies that are required to evaluate drugs. In this type of study, subjects are divided into two groups, one of which gets the drug, while the other gets a placebo (a dummy or sugar pill). Both the subjects and investigators are "blind"; that is, neither one knows which group of subjects is getting the drug or the placebo until the study is over and the code is broken. The Food and Drug Administration requires that two such studies be multi-center trials and show efficacy before a new medication is approved.

There are a number of problems with requiring that nutrients be evaluated using this so-called "gold standard" of testing. First of all, these studies cost millions of dollars to conduct. Pharmaceutical companies, which may profit handsomely from a patentable drug, are better able to fund such studies than nutritional supplement companies, because nutrients are rarely patentable. Second—and, actually, more important—this type of study is usually based on the magic bullet approach, in which a single specific drug is used to cure or relieve the symptoms of a disease. This approach makes less sense in nutrition. Nutrients are not single magic bullets. They do not work alone. They work synergistically, and their effects cannot be adequately appreciated when they are studied as isolated substances.

So although the medical community is accustomed to seeing double-blind placebo-controlled studies, many experts believe that these studies may not be applicable in the evaluation of nutrients. Researcher and educator Jeffrey Bland, Ph.D., doesn't believe that we'll ever have unequivocal proof that supplements work—nor that we need it in the same way we do for drugs. He argues, "You can't hold people on controlled diets with nutritional supplements for thirty years, with a placebo group, to find answers to these questions about something that at its worst does no harm."

In the Harvard School of Public Health's December 1985 issue of *Nutrition Reviews*, Dr. D. M. Hegsted addressed this issue, pointing out the inconsistency in the skeptics' reasoning. He notes, "There is a large body of science, as valid as any other science, which rests upon observation and deduction rather than experimentation—such as astronomy, geology, and archeology. Indeed, the crowning achievement of biology—the theory of evolution—is based upon observation and deduction."

There's another problem with the gold standard. Recently, it has come to light that even drug testing itself does not come up to its own avowed level of scientific testing. People generally assume that there must be evidence that a drug or procedure is safe and effective or it would not be legal or ethical to use it. This is not the case—it has been estimated that up to 90 percent of conventional medical practices are not based on scientifically conducted studies! This includes such serious "life-saving" surgical procedures as angioplasty and bypass surgery, as well as the insertion of breast implants for cosmetic purposes.

And even when a drug or procedure has undergone testing and the results have been published in peer-reviewed medical journals—you can't always trust the information. To find out why, we need only to follow the money.

It costs an estimated 300 to 600 million dollars to develop a new drug—money that must be recouped if the pharmaceutical company is to survive and please its stockholders. Today, the pharmaceutical companies—not an impartial institution or our government—pay for 70 percent of the studies. This situation creates both pressure (to prove a drug works and make back the investment) and control (over the studies that supposedly evaluate the drug). If you think this just might create a conflict of interest—you're right. To its credit, the medical establishment is beginning to recognize the scope of the problem within its own ranks. In 2000, Thomas Boderheimer wrote an article that was published in the *New England Journal of Medicine*. He concludes that drug companies that pay for research have been suppressing unfavorable results and manipulating the results to look better than they really are. This conclusion was based on a review of articles in the medical literature and interviews with thirty-nine participants in the drug development and testing process. The evidence must have been very strong to be published in the conservative *NEJM*, a journal that publishes the very types of articles the author was condemning.

There are many ways in which this power is abused. Trials may be speeded up and drugs not tested long enough for adverse effects to show up. Studies are designed in ways that improve the likelihood of positive results; for example, they may use a younger and healthier population than would actually be receiving the drug, or they may compare it with a low dose or ineffective form of a competing drug. In addition, they may report only a portion of the data and leave out the less favorable data. And they may outright suppress publication of negative studies. Often, a professional medical writer employed by the drug company writes the article, not the scientist "authors" listed. Or a clinical investigator may appear as the author but has neither analyzed the data nor written a word of the article. No one knows how often these abuses occur. However, in one article, 5 percent of industry-sponsored cancer drugs reached negative conclusions (the drug did not work or was too toxic), compared with 38 percent of non-industry funded studies. Another study published in the *NEJM* in 1998 found that 96 percent of the scientists involved in peer-reviewed articles had financial ties to the drug being studied. Is it any wonder that drugs are being taken off the market left and right because of adverse effects? Is it any surprise that many of my medical doctor colleagues will not prescribe a new drug and would rather stay with the older drug that they know?

Of course, not all studies are dishonest and there are signs that the medical establishment is trying to restore its tarnished reputation. In September 2002, eight of the world's top medical journals jointly unveiled uniform requirements for studies they publish. The new policy is an attempt to make sure that investigators have substantial input into the trial design, access to raw data, full participation in interpreting the data, and control over the decision to publish. Now all we have to do is make sure that the Food and Drug Administration's expert panels, who advise the agency on whether to approve a drug for market, do not consist of people with ties to the very industry that they are supposed to be judging.

So, when you consider whether to take supplements, bear this in mind. The amounts of nutritional supplements I recommend in this book have been proven safe—not only do they not have adverse effects, but they have a multitude of beneficial effects, unlike the magic bullet mentality in conventional drugs. Our bodies have the remarkable ability to adapt and protect us from the ever-increasing abuses of life. Some people can tolerate a good deal of these insults, while others are much more sensitive and need optimal nutritional protection. However, we have no way of knowing for sure who falls into which category. Taking the Optimal Daily Intakes recommended in this book means that you are joining the legions of nutritionally aware people who would rather be safe than sorry.

4 How to Design Your Own Nutritional Supplement Program

To DESIGN a nutritional supplement program that is suited to your particular needs, I recommend that you first read through Part 2, "The Vitamins"; Part 3, "The Minerals"; and Part 4, "Beyond Vitamins and Minerals." This will give you an overall picture of what the various supplements can do. Then tear out or photocopy the Sample Worksheet on pages 280 to 281 in Part 5, and go through the book again, chapter by chapter, filling in your Optimum Daily Intake for each nutrient.

Remember: You must never take just one nutritional supplement or just a select few. Although each has its own biochemical function in the body, nutrients tend to work together synergistically. They help one another. You must take appropriate amounts of them all, and in proportion to one another, to get the most out of them. For example, vitamin C can regenerate vitamin E in our bodies and make it more effective. In addition, because supplements compete for absorption in the body, supplementation of a single nutrient may put you at risk for developing a deficiency of those nutrients that are not being supplemented.

Step 1: Determine Your Basic ODI

Notice that in each nutrient chapter, I have provided a basic Optimum Daily Intake. This is a safe dose range for general optimum health and will help prevent illnesses in most people. Using the basic ODI program given in the Sample Worksheet on pages 280 to 281 as a guide, your first step is to fill in your basic ODI for each nutrient. If you are in good health, with no particular health concerns, and are primarily interested in all-round disease prevention, I advise you to start at the lower end of this basic ODI range. If you continue to feel well, this is probably all you will need to take. If you are generally not feeling well, I recommend that you start at the low end and gradually increase the dose until you notice an improvement.

Step 2: Individualize Your ODI

Some people are at higher risk for illness owing to personal or family health history, environmental pollution, or other forms of stress. That is why in each chapter I also provide specific examples of amounts that I have found useful for preventing specific conditions and concerns. These ODIs for specific uses generally go higher than the basic ODIs because, based on both research and my experience, certain circumstances require higher amounts. Although they are higher than the basic ODIs, they are still nontoxic and will not result in any adverse effects. In some cases, these higher amounts have also been effective as the primary treatment for an already existing condition, or have proven valuable as an adjunct to appropriate medical treatment, and perhaps for those who have not been helped by medical treatment.

However, large doses of certain supplements may have undesirable effects in some individuals with medical conditions, or may reduce or enhance the effectiveness of any medication being taken. I cannot emphasize too strongly that if you have a suspected or diagnosed medical condition, for your own protection, you must check with your physician before taking any nutritional supplement. In general, pregnant women may safely take the low end of the basic ODI; but again, please check with your physician.

If you are at high risk for a particular disease, your next step is to decide how much more than the basic ODI you want to take of specific nutrients. For example, if cancer runs in your family, I recommend that you take higher amounts of vitamins A, B complex, C, D, and E; the minerals zinc, chromium, and selenium; and the essential fatty acids GLA and EPA—all nutrients that have been shown to be protective against cancer.

If you smoke, live or work with a smoker, or live in a polluted city environment, you also might want to take higher amounts of certain nutrients. The same holds true if you have a tendency toward high blood pressure or other forms of coronary disease, diabetes, premenstrual syndrome, fibrocystic breast disease, and so on. [To serve as a guide, the worksheet includes programs for some of the most common specific concerns, such as emotional stress, immunity enhancement, cancer prevention, cardiovascular disease prevention, skin problems, and diabetes prevention.] You might also want to consider the higher amounts if you already have a disorder and are under a doctor's care.

In addition, you can use the examples on the following pages to get an idea of how supplement programs can be individualized for people in a variety of circumstances. When reading through the examples, keep in mind that, as mentioned earlier, I generally reserve the supplements discussed in the section called "Beyond Vitamins and Minerals" for certain specific conditions, or for situations in which other supplements have failed to achieve the desired results—but these are always taken in addition to the basic program of vitamins and minerals.

I'll start with myself. I'm in my forties, and I live and run my practice in New York City. I am under a lot of stress, both from my polluted environment and from business pressures. I play tennis, lift weights, and get regular aerobic exercise. My diet is optimal (low fat, low sugar, high fiber), but there is a strong family propensity toward heart disease, high cholesterol, and high triglycerides. More recently, several family members were diagnosed with cancer. My basic supplement program looks like this:

SUPPLEMENT	DAILY DOSAGE
Vitamin A	5,000 IU
Carotenoids	100,000 IU
B complex	50 mg
Vitamin C	4,000 mg
Vitamin D	800 IU
Vitamin E	800 IU
Quercetin	2,000 mg
Boron	3 mg
Calcium	1,200 mg
Copper	Obtained from food sources

Chromium	200 mcg
Iodine	150 mcg
Magnesium	600 mg
Manganese	25 mg
Phosphorus	Obtained from food sources
Selenium	400 mcg
Zinc	50 mg

In addition, I also take:

Coenzyme Q_{10}	400 mg
Fish oil	3,000 mg
Glutathione	400 mg
Alphalipoic acid	300 mg

My co-author, Nancy Bruning, is in her fifties and is a professional with her own business. She lives in New York City and so is exposed to a fair amount of urban pollution. As a freelance writer, she is also subject to a fair amount of stress. Twenty-two years ago, she was treated with surgery and chemotherapy for breast cancer and now has no evidence of the disease. She tends to have allergies and is postmenopausal. Her basic program is:

SUPPLEMENT	DAILY DOSAGE
Vitamin A	10,000 IU
Carotenoids	75,000 IU
B complex	50 mg
Vitamin B_6	100 mg
Vitamin C	4,000–5,000 mg
Vitamin D	400 IU
Vitamin E	800 IU
Calcium	1,000 mg
Copper	Obtained from food sources
Chromium	200 mcg
Iodine	150 mcg
Iron	25 mg
Magnesium	500 mg

Manganese	30 mg
Phosphorus	Obtained from food sources
Selenium	400 mcg
Zinc	50 mg

In addition, she also takes:

Fish oil	3,000 mg
Coenzyme Q$_{10}$	300 mg
Quercetin	3,000 mg
NAC	1,200 mg
Glutathione	500 mg

R. M. is a twenty-five-year-old woman who lives and works as a secretary in the suburbs. She gets very little exercise and is overweight. She has no health complaints and does not feel particularly stressed about anything other than her weight and her craving for sweets. Her basic program is:

SUPPLEMENT	DAILY DOSAGE
Vitamin A	5,000 IU
Carotenoids	10,000 IU
B complex	25 mg
Vitamin C	1,000 mg
Vitamin D	400 IU
Vitamin E	400 IU
Calcium	1,000 mg
Copper	2 mg
Chromium	600 mcg
Iodine	300 mcg
Iron	25 mg
Magnesium	500 mg
Manganese	15 mg
Phosphorus	Obtained from food sources
Selenium	100 mcg
Zinc	22.5 mg

She also takes:

GLA	140–240 mg

J. S. is a thirty-five-year-old businessman who lives and works in Los Angeles. His brother and father have a history of bowel cancer, and he is quite worried that he will get it, too, especially since he has a history of spastic colitis. He does not eat an optimal diet or get regular exercise. However, he is willing to make changes. His basic program is:

SUPPLEMENT	DAILY DOSAGE
Vitamin A	10,000 IU
Carotenoids	50,000 IU
B complex	50 mg
Vitamin C	5,000 mg
Vitamin D	400 IU
Vitamin E	800 IU
Quercetin	3,000 mg
Calcium	1,000 mg
Copper	2 mg
Chromium	200 mcg
Iodine	50 mcg
Magnesium	500 mg
Manganese	15 mg
Phosphorus	Obtained from food sources
Selenium	300 mcg
Zinc	50 mg

He also takes:

Fish oil	3,000 mg

S. S. is a sixty-seven-year-old retired teacher with osteoporosis and arthritis. She has become interested in nutrition over the years, and her diet is good. However, she cannot eat more than 1,200 calories a day because she is sedentary and is worried about gaining weight. She refuses to take drugs. Her basic program is:

SUPPLEMENT	DAILY DOSAGE
Vitamin A	10,000 IU
Carotenoids	11,000 IU
B complex	100 mg
Vitamin C	5,000 mg
Vitamin D	800 IU
Vitamin E	1,200 IU
Quercetin	2,000 mg
Boron	6 mg
Calcium	2,000 mg
Copper	2 mg
Chromium	600 mcg
Iodine	300 mcg
Iron	25 mg
Magnesium	1,000 mg
Manganese	30 mg
Phosphorus	400 mg
Selenium	200 mcg
Zinc	50 mg

She also takes:

Fish oil	3,000 mg

E. B. is a sixteen-year-old high school student. In addition to his school-work, he has daily practice and training for the basketball team. He is very stressed, always feels rushed, and often feels tired. His physician has diagnosed iron deficiency anemia. He also feels that E. B. is underweight. E. B. skips breakfast and eats school lunches. Dinner is the only good meal he eats, since his mother cooks it. His basic program is:

SUPPLEMENT	DAILY DOSAGE
Vitamin A	5,000 IU
Carotenoids	10,000 IU
B complex	50 mg
Vitamin C	3,000 mg
Vitamin D	400 IU

Vitamin E	400 IU
Calcium	1,500 mg
Copper	2 mg
Chromium	400 mcg
Iodine	50 mcg
Iron	30 mg
Magnesium	750 mg
Manganese	15 mg
Phosphorus	400 mg
Selenium	100 mcg
Zinc	30 mg

M. R. is a thirty-eight-year-old man who lives and works in Chicago. His job as a postal worker means he has irregular hours. This has affected his eating habits, leaving him underweight. He worries about his blood pressure, which is slightly elevated. In addition to advising M. R. to reduce dietary sodium, I would recommend the following basic program:

SUPPLEMENT	DAILY DOSAGE
Vitamin A	5,000 IU
Carotenoids	25,000 IU
B complex	200 mg
Vitamin C	3,000 mg
Vitamin D	400 IU
Vitamin E	400 IU
Calcium	1,500 mg
Copper	2 mg
Chromium	200 mcg
Iodine	150 mcg
Iron	15 mg
Magnesium	750 mg
Manganese	15 mg
Phosphorus	Obtained from food sources
Potassium	Obtained from food sources
Selenium	100 mcg
Zinc	25 mg

I might also recommend that he add:

Fish oil	3,000 mg
Garlic	1,000 mg
Coenzyme Q_{10}	200 mg

J. K. is seventeen years old and lives away from home at a college in the country. Her diet is poor, and she must rely mostly on cafeteria food. Since beginning to take birth control pills, she has noticed some water retention, mild anxiety and depression, and cramps during menstruation. Her basic program is:

SUPPLEMENT	DAILY DOSAGE
Vitamin A	5,000 IU
Carotenoids	10,000 IU
B complex	100 mg
Vitamin C	3,000 mg
Vitamin D	400 IU
Vitamin E	400 IU
Calcium	1,500 mg
Copper	Obtained from food sources
Chromium	400 mcg
Iodine	150 mcg
Iron	25 mg
Magnesium	750 mg
Manganese	30 mg
Phosphorus	Obtained from food sources
Selenium	200 mcg
Zinc	50 mg

I would also recommend that she take:

GLA	140–240 mg

R. S., who lives in the suburbs, has become sedentary since his recent retirement from the police force. He is feeling depressed and complains of joint and lower-back pain. He smokes cigarettes. His basic program is:

SUPPLEMENT	DAILY DOSAGE
Vitamin A	10,000 IU
Carotenoids	50,000 IU
B complex	150 mg
Vitamin C	3,000 mg
Vitamin D	400 IU
Vitamin E	800 IU
Quercetin	3,000 mg
Boron	3 mg
Calcium	1,200 mg
Copper	2 mg
Chromium	200 mcg
Iodine	150 mcg
Iron	15 mg
Magnesium	750 mg
Manganese	30 mg
Phosphorus	Obtained from food sources
Selenium	400 mcg
Zinc	50 mg

He also takes:

Fish oil	3,000 mg

L. L. is a thirty-five-year-old unemployed female with chronic fatigue and immune dysfunction (CFIDS). She often feels as though she is about to get the flu. Her PMS symptoms have become more intense over the past year. L. L. also has mild fibromyalgia, which causes muscle pain and weakness. Her basic program is:

SUPPLEMENT	DAILY DOSAGE
Vitamin A	10,000 IU
Carotenoids	100,000 IU
B complex	100 mg
Vitamin C	6,000 mg
Vitamin D	400 IU
Vitamin E	800 IU

Calcium	800 mg
Chromium	400 mcg
Iodine	150 mcg
Iron	25 mg
Magnesium malate	1,200 mg
Malic acid	400 mg
Manganese	20 mg
Quercetin	3,000 mg
Selenium	200 mcg
Zinc	50 mg

She also takes:

Coenzyme Q$_{10}$	200 mg
GLA	500 mg
Alpha-lipoic acid	600 mg
L-carnitine	2 g
Fish oil	3,000 mg

M. M. is a thirty-eight-year-old HIV-positive male. He has no symptoms and no history of infections. He refuses to take any antiviral prophylactic medications. His program includes a large amount of vitamin C, the specific dose of which was individually determined according to bowel tolerance. M. M. added 1,000 milligrams of vitamin C to his program each week, until he reached a dosage that caused loose stools. He then cut back on the dose slightly to normalize bowel movements. This is his basic program:

SUPPLEMENT	DAILY DOSAGE
Vitamin A	25,000 IU
Carotenoids	300,000 IU
B complex	50 mg
Vitamin C	15,000 mg (to bowel tolerance)
Vitamin D	400 IU
Vitamin E	800 IU
Calcium	800 mg
Chromium	200 mcg

Iodine	150 mcg
Iron	30 mg
Magnesium	400 mg
Quercetin	4,000 mg
Selenium	400 mcg
Zinc	50 mg
Manganese	20 mg

He also takes:

Coenzyme Q_{10}	200 mg
Fish oil	3,000 mg
Garlic	1,500 mg
Alpha-lipoic Acid	600 mg
Glutathione	500 mg
NAC	1,200 mg

R. S. is a forty-five-year-old woman recently diagnosed with systemic lupus erythematosus.* She is feeling very fatigued and has joint pains and some characteristic skin lesions on her face. Her basic program is:

SUPPLEMENT	DAILY DOSAGE
Vitamin A	15,000 IU
Carotenoids	100,000 IU
B complex	100 mg
Vitamin C	6,000 mg
Vitamin D	400 IU
Vitamin E	1,200 IU
Calcium	800 mg
Chromium	400 mcg
Iodine	150 mcg
Magnesium	400 mg
Manganese	20 mg

*Programs for multiple sclerosis (MS) or similar autoimmune disorder would be similar. Some people with MS respond better to GLA (1,000 mg) or a combination of fish oil and GLA.

Selenium	200 mcg
Zinc	50 mg

She also takes:

Coenzyme Q$_{10}$	200 mg
Fish oil	4,500 mg
Quercetin	3,000 mg

Step 3: Match Your ODIs with Your Supplements

A simple way to obtain your own ODI is to start with a good multivitamin-mineral formula that contains all the basic vitamins and minerals. When shopping for a multiformula, look for preparations that imply high potency—for example, "extra potency," "megavitamins," or "therapeutic" formula. This type of supplement will take care of most of the nutrients covered in this book. Usually you will need to take four to six tablets per day—unfortunately, it is impossible to design a single pill that contains optimum amounts of everything you need while keeping it small enough to swallow.

Having settled on your basic formula, you can further customize your program by adding to the basic formula those individual nutrients you feel you need more of. For example, your multiformula may contain 25,000 international units of vitamin A. If you want to take a total of 50,000 international units because you have acne, you can add 25,000 international units of vitamin A. If your multiformula supplement has 200 micrograms of chromium and you have diabetes, you might want to add 400 micrograms of chromium for a total of 600 micrograms per day. If you have a family history of heart disease, you may want to add 1,500 milligrams of EPA.

Working with Your Health-Care Practitioner

If you prefer to work with a nutritionist, it is important that you ask about his or her educational experience. In 1977, the National Nutrition Consortium—five nationally recognized organizations that included the American Dietetic Association and the American Institute of Nutrition—

issued their report *Qualifications, Standards, and Competence in Nutrition.* According to this report, the definition of a nutritionist is one trained by education and experience in the science and practice of nutrition. This education involves a graduate program that includes basic science and professional courses designed to develop at least minimum competence in nutrition and allied sciences. In contrast, the definition of a dietitian is one who has earned a baccalaureate degree and has met the basic academic and experience requirements needed to write the qualifying examination for professional registration in dietetics offered by the American Dietetic Association. Since entry level for the RD (Registered Dietitian) examination is an undergraduate (baccalaureate) degree, having this credential does not ensure that the individual is a nutritionist. State licensing and certification programs have further blurred the educational distinction between a dietitian and a nutritionist by lumping the two titles together or by credentialing dietitians as nutritionists. The only nationally recognized graduate-level certification program for nutritionists is offered by the Certification Board for Nutrition Specialists. Candidates who pass the examination receive the CNS (Certified Nutrition Specialist) credential. There are also physicians who have passed the exam and hold the CNS credential.

Unfortunately, most physicians are still not well versed in nutrition. Although this is lamentable, it is completely understandable and is in large part due to inadequate nutritional education in medical school. Nutrition is generally offered as an elective to medical students, and the entire course usually consists of a grand total of three hours of basic nutrition. Also, medical training emphasizes the diagnosis and treatment of disease, rather than its prevention through nutrition or another means. While the situation is improving, if you have a nutritionally oriented physician, you should consider yourself lucky. Some medical schools are now teaching "integrative medicine," which includes such factors as diet, herbs, vitamins, minerals, exercise, and stress reduction. There are also several medical organizations that have as their members practitioners who are up to date in this new type of medicine.

If you do not find a holistic physician or one who practices integrative medicine, the ideal situation is to have your physician and nutritionist work together, particularly if you have a medical problem. Many of my patients have this arrangement, and it can work out beautifully. You can't expect your physician to know and do everything. When health professionals read medical literature, we tend to read what is most relevant to our specialty. Even though much of the research in this book is from widely read and respected medical journals, your physician may not be familiar with the studies. For example, when I read *The Journal of the American Medical Association*, I naturally read the research pertaining to nutrition, rather than the latest surgical developments. There simply isn't the time to read all the research about every specialty. However, it is reasonable to expect your physician to be open-minded about the nutritional approach, since nutritional research is widespread throughout medical literature.

How and When to Take Supplements

Your body can absorb and use only so much of a vitamin or mineral at one time. So to increase the utilization of these nutrients, try to divide the dosage over the course of the day, especially if you are working with higher doses. For example, if you are taking a total of 3,000 milligrams of vitamin C daily, take 1,000 milligrams three times a day. In addition, supplements are best taken at mealtime, along with your food. This increases absorption and prevents the indigestion that sometimes occurs when supplements are taken on an empty stomach. You may take supplements a few minutes before a meal, or up to a half hour after a meal.

There has been a lot of confusing information published about the interference of certain nutrients with the absorption of others. In my opinion, the evidence is not strong enough for me to advise not taking certain vitamins and minerals together, or with certain foods. As I say to my patients, nature supplies us with a variety of nutrients in each meal, so why should taking supplements together pose a problem? Life is complicated enough without your having to worry about whether your bran muffin is interfering with your absorption of calcium. In addition, studies indicate that this problem generally occurs only when you are taking a large amount of one or a few nutrients, as opposed to the full spectrum of nutrients.

How Will You Know If Your Supplements Are Working?

When people begin taking supplements for general good health and disease prevention, they usually just feel better. They feel calmer, get fewer colds, have more energy, and enjoy a general sense of well-being. Even my patients who were resistant to the idea of taking supplements have confessed this to me. These people sometimes go off their vitamins and minerals for a while, and then come back to me and say, "You know, skeptical as I was, I must admit that the supplements did make a difference in the way I felt."

If you are taking supplements to prevent a specific condition, and the condition fails to materialize, there is, of course, no way of knowing for sure whether the supplements worked, or whether you would have remained healthy anyway. For people who take vitamins and minerals as a kind of health insurance, no news is good news.

When you are taking supplements for a specific condition, you will know whether they are working because you will have tangible confirmation—your condition will improve. Let's suppose that you have a skin problem and you take extra vitamin A. If your skin clears up, you will know the vitamin is working. If you have high blood pressure, you might take extra calcium and magnesium—and, hopefully, modify your diet. Then, if your blood pressure improves, again, you will know that the nutrients are working in your favor.

Vitamins and minerals do not work overnight! If you are nervous and irritable today and take a B-complex vitamin tonight, do not expect to feel calm and serene tomorrow. You must give it time—but do not wait forever. In general, you should begin to notice beneficial effects in three to four weeks. One exception is treatment for premenstrual syndrome. In this case, you will need at least two menstrual cycles to determine if supplementation is effective.

If you begin at the lower end of the ODI range and you see no results at this dose, you may increase the dose and give it another few weeks. Keep raising the dose, if necessary, until you reach the highest range of the ODI. Give that another month or so, unless you start noticing some adverse effects. For example, if you are taking carotenoids for acne, you might start at 50,000 international units per day. If after a couple of weeks you see some improvement, but nothing spectacular, you may try going up to 75,000 international units for a while. If your skin clears up more, you might want to go up to 100,000 international units to see if this will improve it even further. If your skin begins to look slightly yellow or orange and this bothers you (some people like the tan look)—the only adverse effect of certain carotenoids—you should then cut back to 75,000 international units. If you have gone up to the maximum safe dose and have stayed there for a month or two, but have seen no results, I would suggest you cut back gradually to a more moderate level. Obviously, large doses do not work in your case, and you should investigate other means of controlling your condition.

Vitamin and mineral supplementation is an ongoing, evolving process. As your body changes with time, your need for supplements may change, too. You might, for instance, want to increase your Optimum Daily Intake of the B-complex vitamins and/or vitamin C during times of illness or extreme stress. Evaluate how you feel; see if any condition you've been treating has improved. Obviously, you want to take the smallest amount needed to correct a particular problem. Why take 75,000 international units of vitamin A if 50,000 or 25,000 works fine, or if you can get similar results with carotenoids? Generally, you can take a supplement for a specific problem for six months. After that, try lowering the dose. If the condition returns, your body is telling you to return to the higher dose.

Can Nutritional Supplements Cause Harm?

Some people are afraid that they will overdose on vitamins, minerals, or other nutritional supplements and cause their bodies harm. Such caveats fall especially from the lips of nutritionally unsophisticated practitioners and are then passed on to the public by the media. The fact is that only a few vitamins and minerals have any known toxicity level. Statistics gathered from the Centers for Disease Control and the National Capitol Poison Control Center over a period of seven years (1983 to 1989) revealed a total of 2,069 reported drug fatalities compared with absolutely no vitamin fatalities. These statistics, which appeared in a 1991 issue of the *American Journal of Emergency Medicine*, suggest that vitamins are 2,000 times safer than drugs.

The Food and Drug Administration's web site includes unconfirmed reports of adverse effects due to dietary supplements. When some of these reports were investigated, it was discovered that people were also taking drugs, which were in all likelihood the cause of the adverse effect. Drugs are the fourth leading cause of deaths in hospitals. There are hundreds and thousands of deaths due to prescription and nonprescription drugs collectively. Even aspirin is estimated to be responsible for 2,500 deaths per year, in addition to causing gastric bleeding ulcer. Does that mean aspirin should be taken off the market or that no one should take it? Certainly not—there is wonderful research that taking a small amount of aspirin daily protects against cardiovascular disease.

Anything—even pure water—can be harmful if you take enough of it. But vitamins and minerals are among the safest substances on earth. The amounts needed to reach toxic levels are enormous. According to all available studies, none of the ODIs in this book will create any toxicity in a normally healthy adult. By this, I mean that you are not on any medication and do not have a medical condition, as these factors can influence your vitamin and mineral requirements, making them higher or lower. I have included some data about these requirements. However, you should consult your physician for specifics if you have any questions.

You may fear that your body will grow dependent on large amounts of vitamins or minerals after a while. There is very little convincing evidence of this. There is some indication that certain individuals who take very high doses of vitamin C and then suddenly stop run the risk of having symptoms of rebound scurvy. While this has not been proven, common sense dictates that it is not wise to stop anything cold turkey if you have been ingesting it for a prolonged period of time. This holds true both for drugs—Valium, hormones such as cortisone, and many psychiatric drugs—and for vitamins. If your body has been finely tuned and is accustomed to having an optimal amount of a certain nutrient, it naturally will have to adjust when you change the way you are feeding it.

Therefore, if you want to cut back for any reason, it is logical to wean yourself away from supplements gradually. I generally recommend stepping down every two weeks until you reach your desired new level. For instance, many people increase their intake of vitamin C during the cold and flu season. If you have been taking 5,000 milligrams of vitamin C every day during the winter, you may cut down to 4,000 milligrams for two weeks, then to 3,000 milligrams for the next two weeks, then to 2,000 milligrams, and so on.

If you're traveling and want to reduce your dosages because of the inconvenience, it is generally safe to cut your doses in half during this time. Nothing dramatic will happen if you forget to take your vitamins for a day every once in a while, either. Even the water-soluble vitamins remain in the body for about two days, so you do have a margin of safety.

A Guide to Buying Supplements

One of the most common questions my patients ask me is: "Should I buy 'natural' or 'synthetic' vitamins?" As far as I know, there doesn't seem to be much difference between a vitamin found in food and one made in the laboratory. They are essentially the same chemical, made of the same molecules. The fat-soluble vitamins may be the exception: Studies have shown that the naturally occurring form of vitamin E is more absorbable and biologically active than its synthetic counterpart.

However, the word natural on the label does not necessarily mean that all the vitamins in the bottle are simply extracted from a natural food source. In fact, most so-called natural vitamins actually contain a large amount of synthetic vitamins. The reason for this is primarily economic: If vitamin C supplements, for example, were derived solely from rose hips, the cost would be enormous.

The term natural really refers to the fact that the supplement does not contain other unnatural ingredients. Here, there is a difference. Supplements that are not labeled natural may also include coal tars, artificial coloring, preservatives, sugars, starch, and sometimes other additives. This is why I generally recommend natural vitamins. Why take potentially harmful substances into the body when you don't have to?

Mineral supplements may be chelated, meaning that they are surrounded by a carrier protein that transports the mineral to the bloodstream in an attempt to enhance absorption. Because studies on the absorbability of the various forms of mineral supplements are rather sparse at this time, I cannot recommend chelated minerals across the board. However, some combinations have been shown to be more absorbable. Unfortunately, they are often more expensive and may not be cost-effective. If the difference in price is not enormous, you may prefer to buy chelated minerals for possible enhanced absorption. Keep in mind, though, that if you take supplements with a meal, they are usually automatically chelated in your stomach during digestion.

Some supplements are offered in a time-release formula in an attempt to release the nutrients gradually. While this sounds fine in theory, in practice, it may actually decrease absorption. Studies have shown, for instance, that time-release or sustained-release vitamin C does not raise blood levels of vitamin C as effectively as nontime-release supplements. Some newer technology for gradual release formulas may have improved absorption. But the research is still lacking. However, I have patients and colleagues that have reported excellent results with certain time-released formulas.

In the following chapters, I have listed the most common forms of supplements available. New and innovative forms are being created all the time in an effort to find a form that is easily absorbed by the body, bioavailable (usable by the body once it has been absorbed), and able to enter the enzyme system more quickly. But without good studies, it's difficult to decide whether these claims are valid. Check with your health-food store or your nutritional professional to see if there is any literature about the new forms of any nutrient you are considering taking. Some practitioners feel that certain forms are more preferable than others. Oftentimes this is based on their clinical experience and observation of hundreds or thousands of patients, rather than on published research.

A Guide to Storing Supplements

Supplements do not last forever; their potency gradually diminishes over a period of time. Unopened, vitamins generally last for two to three years. Opened, they generally last for about one year. Mineral supplements last longer, and usually it is not the minerals themselves that go bad—it is the other substances in the supplement, such as the chelating agents, that spoil. As a safeguard, it's best to buy supplements with an expiration date. Supplements should be stored in a cool, dry, dark place. The refrigerator usually has a lot of moisture in it and is quite cold, which could affect certain vitamins, so I don't recommend this as a storage place except for supplements that are oils—vitamin E, fish oil, primrose oil, and flaxseed and borage oil. Many people keep their supplements on top of the refrigerator; however, this location is generally too warm. A room-temperature closet is usually fine.

Many people transfer their supplements to smaller, more convenient containers for work and travel. If the container is opaque and closes tightly, supplements can be stored in them for several months without losing much of their potency.

5 | Your Total Health Plan

TAKING SUPPLEMENTS does not give you carte blanche to eat and drink anything you want, nor is it a panacea for all your ills. Nutritional supplements are just that—supplements. They work best when they are part of a well-rounded plan for optimum health. Along with your supplements, it is important for you to also eat wholesome foods, get a reasonable amount of exercise, and maintain a healthy, wholesome lifestyle that includes no smoking, a minimum of alcohol and other drugs, and stress management.

The Basic Intelligent Diet

For all their value, nutritional supplements do not take the place of good, fresh food. In the first place, you still need a balanced amount of carbohydrates, fats, and proteins—nutrients not found in supplement capsules. In the second place, by eating nutritious foods, you are assured of getting at least some vitamins and minerals in their natural form. This is important, because when nutrients are ingested as part of the food in which they are naturally found, they are generally absorbed and utilized better. Then, by taking supplements along with nutritious foods, you will enhance the absorption of the nutrients contained in the supplements, as well. Taking supplements after eating a bowl of low-fat yogurt mixed with fresh fruit would probably result in better nutrient absorption than would taking them after a snack of potato chips or cookies.

Finally, there is so much we still don't know about the many beneficial components of certain foods. Plants—fruits, vegetables, and herbs—contain an enormous number of compounds, collectively known as phytochemicals (phyto means plant). Unlike vitamins and minerals, phytochemicals are not classified as essential nutrients; yet they appear to have many benefits. Those that protect against cancer have been the most studied, but there are many other biological actions that may prove helpful as well and that may or may not be due to antioxidant properties. For instance, diidoylmethane (DIM) or indole-3-carbinole, found in vegetables in the cabbage family, appears to deter the growth of blood vessels that nourish cancerous tumors. Indoles—substances found in cabbage, Brussels sprouts, and kale—also seem to protect against cancer. Carotenoids, present in the same foods that contain beta-carotenes, are antioxidants and thus protect against many diseases and conditions associated with aging. Quercetin, found in citrus fruits, has antioxidant, antihistamine, anticancer, antiviral, and antiinflammatory activities. Phytosterols like beta-sitosterol, contained in plants such as yams and alfalfa sprouts, play a role in maintaining the hormone balance in the body. We can only guess at the many other undiscovered substances, let alone put them in a pill.

My Basic Intelligent Diet, which I recommend for most of my patients in addition to their Optimum Daily Intake of vitamins and minerals, is high in fiber, low in fat and sugar, and moderate in protein. Below, you will find some dietary guidelines designed to help you choose and prepare the foods on this diet. Following this, you'll find two Daily Food Guides and two sample menus—customized for men and women—that illustrate how these guidelines can be followed to make meals that are wholesome and enjoyable.

HEALTHY EATING GUIDELINES

Eating wisely involves the selection of healthful foods and the avoidance of foods that are low in nutrients and high in harmful substances like salt and sugar. The following tips should help you choose the best possible foods and prepare them in a way that maximizes their nutritional value.

- Avoid processed foods such as white flour and sugar.
- Eat an abundant amount of vegetables and a moderate amount of fruits.

- Minimize grains, but if you do eat grains, make sure they are whole grains such as barley, buckwheat, and oats. Most other grains such as rice—even brown rice—have relatively high glycemic levels, meaning they raise your blood sugar relatively quickly, which has many detrimental health effects—including overweight.
- Eat whole fresh foods rather than canned, frozen, or commercially prepared foods. Try to use organic foods whenever possible.
- Use low-fat or fat-free dairy products, soymilk, rice milk, tofu, or soy cheese.
- Minimize your consumption of high-fat meats such as pork, lamb, and beef. If you choose to eat red meat, use leaner cuts. Preferable to beef and pork are white meat chicken and turkey, seafood, fish, and organic eggs. Choose smaller fish and salmon, which are lowest in mercury.
- Use butter and oil very sparingly. Do not use margarine, which contains oil that has been hydrogenated. Hydrogenated vegetable oils contain transfatty acids, which may increase low-density lipoproteins (LDLs, often referred to as bad cholesterol) as much as saturated fats do and also decrease high-density lipoproteins (HDLs, often referred to as good cholesterol), which saturated fats do not do. Instead, use vegetable or chicken broth or apple juice for sautéing and flavoring dishes.
- Minimize your use of salt. Many foods naturally contain some salt, so try not to add any extra. Substitute salt-free spices and herbs such as garlic, ginger, oregano, rosemary, pepper, and lemon juice.
- Avoid using sugar and even try to avoid using honey, maple syrup, or other sweeteners. Many people also consume too much fruit juice—some drink a gallon of orange juice a day. Fruit juice is a major source of sugar and raises blood sugar and insulin too quickly for optimum health.
- Minimize your consumption of coffee, tea, sodas, other caffeine- and sugar-containing beverages, and chocolate. Club soda or seltzer, herbal teas, grain-type coffee substitute, and filtered or bottled water are preferable. Natural fruit juices are good, too, but drink them only in moderation. Remember that one glass of natural, unsweetened juice contains the equivalent of three to four fruits. Try mixing juice with salt-free club soda or water to make it less sweet and concentrated.
- To preserve as many nutrients as possible, cook food quickly, using a

minimum of fat or water. Eat vegetables raw, steamed, or quickly stir-fried in a small amount of oil, apple juice, or vegetable broth.

- Eat slowly and enjoy your food! The slower you eat, the less you eat.

DAILY FOOD GUIDES AND MENUS

The Basic Intelligent Diet is both well-balanced and satisfying and will help you maintain or achieve a lower, healthier, more attractive level of body fat. Below you will find Daily Food Guides for men and women. Each guide shows exactly how much of each type of food should be eaten each day. For specific menus, see pages 70 and 71. If you are at all concerned about your weight (and who isn't?), our book *Dare to Lose* has more information about the healthy way to eat to keep your weight under control.

THE DAILY FOOD GUIDE FOR WOMEN The following Daily Food Guide is for women five feet three inches to five feet nine inches tall. If you are over five feet nine inches, add one portion each of vegetables and fiber foods. If you are under five feet three inches, subtract one portion each of vegetables and low to moderate glycemic index foods.

- 8 ounces of nonfat milk or yogurt, or ½ cup nonfat cottage cheese. (If you have a problem digesting dairy products, substitute soy products such as low-fat or nonfat soymilk, soy yogurt, and tofu, or try rice milk. Do not use nut milks, which are generally high in fat, unless you can find low-fat—1-percent fat—or fat-free products.)
- 6 or more cups of salad/vegetables: lettuce, zucchini, tomatoes, broccoli, cucumber, cabbage, etc.
- 2 fresh fruits or 1–2 cups of diced fresh fruit.
- 2–4 moderate and low-glycemic index food servings. (For low to moderate glycemic index foods, equivalents, see Table 5.1.)
- Use potatoes, brown rice, and other low-fiber grains and starchy foods sparingly, especially if you are trying to control your weight or blood sugar.
- 4–6 ounces of lean protein for at least two meals per day: seafood, eggs, fat-free cheese, nonfat yogurt, nonfat milk, chicken, turkey, fat-free or low-fat soy products, or other vegetable-protein products, such as veggie-burgers.

Table 5.1. Low-to-Moderate Glycemic Index of Carbohydrate Foods

One Low-to-Moderate Carbohydrate Serving

½ cup high protein pasta or other grain

1 slice whole-grain bread (high fiber)

1 ear of corn

½ cup low-fat, sugar-free granola

½ cup squash (spaghetti, winter, summer, etc.)

½ yam, sweet potato

½ cup cooked peas, beans, or lentils

1½ tablespoons nut butter, or 20 nuts*

2 potato skins

1 tablespoon oat bran

1 tablespoon wheat germ

*Have no more than one serving per day. Omit if you want to reduce body fat.

THE DAILY FOOD GUIDE FOR MEN The following Daily Food Guide is for men five feet ten inches tall and up. If you are under five feet ten inches tall, subtract one serving each of vegetables and low and moderate glycemic index foods.

- 8 ounces of nonfat milk or yogurt or ½ cup nonfat cottage cheese. (If you have a problem digesting dairy products, substitute soy products such as low-fat or nonfat soymilk, soy yogurt, and tofu, or try rice milk. Do not use nut milks, which are generally high in fat, unless you can find low-fat—1-percent fat—or fat-free products.)
- 6 or more cups of salad/vegetables: lettuce, zucchini, tomatoes, broccoli, etc.
- 3–4 fresh fruits or 2–3 cups diced fresh fruit.
- 4–6 low to moderate glycemic index foods servings. (For low to moderate glycemic index foods, see Table 5.1.)
- 6–8 ounces of lean protein food at each meal: seafood, eggs, fat-free cheese, nonfat yogurt, nonfat milk, chicken, turkey, fat-free or low-fat soy products, or other vegetable-protein products, such as veggie-burgers.

- Use potatoes, brown rice, and other low-fiber grains and starchy foods sparingly, especially if you are trying to control your weight or blood sugar.

THE SAMPLE MENUS The following sample menus show you how the Daily Food Guides translate into a typical day's meals. If you are physically active, you may eat more by increasing your intake of nonfat or low-fat protein and low to moderate glycemic index foods by two to three servings. If butter, oil, or dressings are used, remember to add them only sparingly. I recommend putting the oil in a spray bottle and using only one or two squirts. You may also have additional fruit juice diluted with water or club soda. But don't drink too much juice! Women should not exceed one cup per day, and men should not exceed two cups.

SAMPLE MENU 1

Women: 1,200 Calories	Men: 1,800 Calories
BREAKFAST:	
• ½ cup no-sugar granola	• 1 cup no-sugar granola
• ½ banana	• 1 banana
• ½ cup nonfat milk or yogurt	• 1 cup low-fat milk or yogurt
LUNCH:	
• 2–3 cups salad or fresh vegetables	• 3–4 cups salad or fresh vegetables
• 4–6 ounces chicken	• 6–8 ounces chicken
• ½ yam	• 1 yam
	• 1 cup lentil soup
DINNER:	
• ½ cup high-protein pasta with tomato sauce	• 1 cup high-protein pasta with tomato sauce
• 4–6 ounces broiled filet of sole	• 6–8 ounces broiled filet of sole
• 2–3 cups salad or fresh vegetables	• 3–4 cups salad or fresh vegetables
SNACK:	
• ½–1 cup nonfat yogurt	• 1–2 cups low-fat yogurt
• 1 medium apple	• 1 medium apple
• 1 teaspoon oat bran	• 1 tablespoon oat bran

SAMPLE MENU 2

Women: 1,200 Calories	Men: 1,800 Calories
BREAKFAST:	
• 1 slice whole wheat bread • 4–6 ounces low-fat cottage cheese • 2 slices tomato	• 2 slices whole wheat bread • 6–8 ounces nonfat soy Jarlsberg cheese • 3 slices tomato
LUNCH:	
• 2–3 cups salad or fresh vegetables • 4–6 ounces baked fish • 1 medium baked potato	• 3–4 cups salad or fresh vegetables • 6–8 ounces baked fish • 1 medium baked potato or yam • 1 ear of corn
DINNER:	
• 4–6 ounces broiled chicken • 2–3 cups salad or vegetables • ½ cup beans • 1 baked or fresh apple	• 6–8 ounces broiled chicken • 2 cups salad or vegetables • 1 cup beans • 1 baked or fresh apple
SNACK:	
• ½–1 cup low-fat cottage cheese • 1 medium pear • 1 teaspoon oat bran or wheat germ	• 1 cup low-fat cottage cheese • 1 medium pear • 1 tablespoon oat bran or wheat germ

The Exercise Prescription

The benefits of exercise are almost endless. Exercise lowers your risk of heart disease, diabetes, osteoporosis, colon cancer, and breast cancer. Cancer patients who exercise live longer, as do heart patients who exercise. Patients with Chronic Fatigue Immune Deficiency Syndrome (CFIDS), fibromyalgia, diabetes, rheumatoid arthritis—just about any illness or disability—improve with regular exercise. It enhances energy, helps you handle stress better, and gives you a psychological lift and a general sense of well-being. And it helps you normalize your weight by burning calories, speeding up your metabolism, and controlling appetite. As if these aren't enough reasons to exercise, in 1996, the continuing Aerobics Center Longitudinal Study, designed to examine the effects of different fitness levels, showed that low fitness may actually pose as great a risk to health as smoking, and a greater risk than high cholesterol, high blood pressure, and obesity. This report, published in the *Journal of the American Medical Association*, underscores the importance of exercise in a healthy lifestyle.

Aerobic exercise is the best form of activity for your cardiovascular system. It enhances circulation and exercises your heart, lungs, and major muscles. To reap the greatest rewards from your aerobic exercise sessions, move at an intensity sufficient to raise your heart rate, exercise continuously for at least twenty to thirty minutes, and exercise at least three times a week. Examples of aerobic exercise include brisk walking, jogging, running, stair climbing, bicycling, aerobic dancing, skating, swimming, jumping rope, rowing, and cross-country skiing—either the actual sports or use of a rowing or skiing machine.

For many people, walking is the easiest way to begin and maintain a more active lifestyle. If you are out of shape, start with just five minutes. Then add one minute each week until you can sustain twenty to thirty minutes of continuous walking.

By varying your exercises, you will ensure that you exercise all parts of your body, reduce your chance of injury, and help keep boredom at bay. I recommend that you add at least a light weight-training program to your aerobic sessions to condition and strengthen many different muscle groups. Be sure to also include some stretching exercises, such as yoga, to keep your joints limber and your muscles long and lithe.

At least initially, I suggest that you work with a professional who can design a program for you and make sure you are doing the exercises properly. Most health clubs have such trainers. There are many books and videotapes that can assist you, as well. Also, look for ways to add more activity to your daily life. For instance, whenever possible, walk instead of drive and take the stairs instead of the elevator.

A word of caution is in order. If you are over thirty-five, have been sedentary for some time, or have any health problems, it is important to consult with your health-care provider before starting any exercise program.

While even a well-rounded diet cannot provide you with everything you need to be at your best, it is a vital first step toward optimal nutrition. Couple it with the proper supplement program and adequate exercise, as well as other wholesome lifestyle choices, and you have the perfect formula for good health.

Part 2

The Vitamins

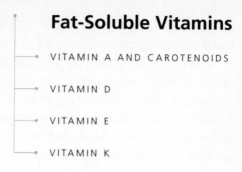

Fat-Soluble Vitamins

- VITAMIN A AND CAROTENOIDS
- VITAMIN D
- VITAMIN E
- VITAMIN K

6 | Vitamin A and Carotenoids

VITAMIN A, also called retinol, has a number of important functions in the body. It plays an important role in immune system function, it helps protect the body from cardiovascular disease and cancer, it is needed for the growth and maintenance of the skin, and it is essential for the proper function of the eye.

Beta-carotene belongs to a group of compounds called carotenoids. Historically, beta-carotene has been lumped together with vitamin A because it is readily converted into vitamin A in the body and, unlike the preformed vitamin, it is nontoxic. For these reasons, researchers began using beta-carotene as a supplement many years ago and today it is therefore the most well-known and most researched carotenoid. However, things have not remained this simple. We now know that beta-carotene has its own unique antioxidant actions beyond its role as a vitamin A precursor. And we also know that research on other carotenoids indicates that they each have their own unique biological effects—and that antioxidant activity may be only one such effect. The carotenoids include lycopene, lutein, alpha-carotene, and zeaxanthin, and recent research is proving them to be as important as beta-carotene for optimum health and disease prevention—and even treatment.

As of this writing, most of the research on the other carotenoids has focused on lycopene and lutein, but other studies on these remarkable compounds are sure to follow, and in the next edition of this book, we will probably need to devote a separate chapter to them. I hope that we will also see more studies that include beta-carotene. Many of the earlier studies with beta-carotene supplements are conflicting or have negative results. But to my knowledge, these studies used synthetic beta-carotene and we now realize that synthetic beta-carotene is not the same as the natural form. Dr. Kedar Prasad, one of the foremost experts on antioxidants and their relationship to cancer randomly analyzed synthetic beta-carotene supplements. He found that all of the supplements he studied had virtually no beta-carotene activity! Furthermore, it is feasible that whatever was in the synthetic supplements actually interfered with the absorption of natural beta-carotene and carotenoids in the diet. It's also possible that instead of having an antioxidant effect, it had a pro-oxidant effect. It's easy to understand why synthetic beta-carotene was used alone: Synthetic beta-carotene is cheap but natural beta-carotene is not, and scientists prefer to study one compound at a time. But if future studies are going to be valid scientifically and ethically, we need to use natural beta-carotene supplements that include a mixture of other carotenoids as well.

Functions and Uses

INFECTIONS AND IMMUNITY

In many animal studies, vitamin A has been shown to improve resistance to infections and to be especially useful in preventing both infectious and noninfectious diseases of the respiratory system. In my clinical experience, I have found that vitamin A supplementation is a safe and effective immune system booster. Chronic infections and illnesses can reduce the body's levels of vitamin A, thereby weakening the mucous membranes and making them more susceptible to viral infection. Patients who get frequent sore throats, colds, flu, sinusitis, or bronchitis have experienced a marked decrease in the frequency and severity of these respiratory infections when given optimal amounts of vitamin A. I have also found that vitamin A supplementation is effective in decreasing the symptoms associated with allergic reactions, emphysema, and asthma.

CARDIOVASCULAR DISEASE

While most of the research on the prevention of coronary heart disease has focused on vitamin E (see Chapter 8), human studies have shown that carotenoids may have various protective and therapeutic effects regarding cardiovascular disease.

Like vitamin E, beta-carotene is incorporated into low-density lipoproteins (LDLs) and may work synergistically with other nutrients, including vitamin A, to prevent LDL oxidation, a major culprit in the development of coronary heart disease. In the ongoing Physicians' Health Study, Harvard researchers have been studying a total of over twenty-two thousand male physicians over the long term. Ten years into this study, the researchers evaluated a subgroup of 333 men who had histories of cardiovascular disease. The data showed that the physicians in this group who took 50 milligrams (approximately 85,000 international units) of beta-carotene every other day had half as many heart attacks, strokes, and deaths due to heart disease as those who did not take the supplements. The beneficial effects of the supplements did not appear until the second year of the study. Interestingly, the reduction of all aspects of cardiovascular disease appeared to be greater with beta-carotene than with aspirin, which is commonly recommended to prevent heart attacks. Remember, researchers got these positive results even though they were using synthetic beta-carotene, which has very little beta-carotene activity. In addition, when participants in studies such as this one know that the study is about beta-carotene, they actually start eating foods rich in natural beta-carotene. This always confounds the results to some degree. Imagine what the results would be if they used natural beta-carotene supplements in therapeutic doses.

Yet another study conducted in India looked at the effects of a combined antioxidant treatment, including 50,000 international units of vitamin A, 1,000 milligrams of vitamin C, 400 international units of vitamin E, and 25 milligrams of beta-carotene. In this double-blind study, sixty-three patients received the supplements, while sixty-two received the placebo. All subjects were suspected of having acute myocardial infarction (heart attack). The results of this study reveal that such a combined antioxidant treatment in patients with recent heart attacks may be protective against cardiac necrosis (tissue death) and oxidative stress and could be beneficial in preventing complication and future heart attacks. In another study of about five hundred men and women, published in

2001, researchers looked at the blood levels of several nutrients including beta-carotene. Men who had low blood concentrations of beta-carotene (or vitamin E) were 2.5 times as likely to have narrowing of the carotid artery of more than 30 percent, compared with men who had the highest blood concentrations. This opens up another possibility of action for beta-carotene, and perhaps other carotenoids, as we see in some preliminary research.

As the above studies suggest, most of the research has looked at beta-carotene, but studies also show that lycopene may prevent cardiovascular disease. For example, individuals with the highest blood levels of this carotenoid also had the lowest risk of atherosclerosis. And people with high lycopene intakes had a lower risk of myocardial infarction (heart attack).

CANCER PREVENTION

There is growing evidence that vitamin A and carotenoids can provide some protection against certain forms of cancer. In many countries of the world, investigations of dietary intake and blood levels of beta-carotene and vitamin A have generally found that lower levels of the nutrients are associated with an increased incidence of certain cancers, including cancers of the bronchus, mouth, larynx, esophagus, endometrium, bladder, breast, prostate, cervix, colon, rectum, and stomach, as well as melanoma, a deadly form of skin cancer. On the other hand, increased levels of beta-carotene and vitamin A have been correlated with a lower risk of cancer, with results including a threefold decrease in lung cancer and an 80-percent decrease in cancer of the cervix. There is also evidence that these nutrients may offer protection from gastrointestinal ulcers. Since people with ulcers are more prone to gastrointestinal cancer, it is possible that this nutrient may also protect against the latter disorder.

More recently, studies made headlines when they demonstrated that lycopene, a carotenoid found in the highest concentrations in tomato paste, also was associated with a lower risk of several types of cancer. Researchers found that lycopene inhibited the growth of prostate cancer cells, and that men who regularly eat ten servings of tomato products per week have a 35 percent lower risk of prostate cancer compared with men who eat only 1.5 servings. The most compelling evidence remains for prostate cancer, but lycopene also appears to inhibit breast cancer cells and large-scale studies in several countries show that women who consume high levels of carotenes in their diet have a significantly lower risk of breast cancer compared with women whose intake is low. Lycopene inhibits the cell growth of a particular type of leukemia. People who consume a lot of lycopene also have a lowered risk of cancers of the mouth and esophagus, and this carotenoid is also associated with a lower risk of skin cancer. In 2001, a study showed that women whose intakes of carotene, especially alpha-carotene and lycopene from food and supplements had a significantly lower risk of ovarian cancer. The two foods that were most strongly related to this reduction were raw carrots and tomato sauce.

Numerous studies have also shown that vitamin A and beta-carotene are useful in the treatment of existing cancers or precancers. Human studies have shown that high doses of vitamin A and beta-carotene supplements can cause a regression of a precancerous condition of the mouth called leukoplakia. Preliminary studies using high-dose vitamin A and/or beta-carotene in the treatment of cervical cancer have also been encouraging. In another study, performed in Italy and published in 1993, 307 patients with lung cancer had the cancerous lesions removed surgically. One group of patients was then given daily doses of 300,000 international units of vitamin A for one year, while the other group received no supplements. After a forty-six-month follow-up, 37 percent of those who took the supplements had a recurrence of the cancer, while 48 percent of the unsupplemented group had a recurrence.

Vitamin A and beta-carotene therapy have also been valuable adjuncts in the treatment of breast cancer. In animal studies, vitamin A has been shown to slow the spread of breast cancer to other parts of the body. In a study of women with breast cancer undergoing chemotherapy, women with higher blood levels of vitamin A responded twice as well to the therapy as did women with lower levels. There are two theories as to why these results were obtained. Vitamin A may have helped protect the women from the toxicity of the drugs, or it may have interacted with the drugs in a way that increased their effectiveness. In another study, Vitamin E and A levels were measured in women with breast cancer who were to undergo chemotherapy. These levels were then compared with those of healthy control subjects. Among the patients with vitamin A levels equal to or higher than those of the control subjects, 83 percent responded favorably to chemotherapy, and none experienced a progression of the cancer. Among patients with vitamin A levels below those of the control subjects, only 36 percent responded favorably to chemotherapy and 40 percent experienced a progression of the cancer.

Other human studies have shown similar results with other cancers. Scottish researchers reported that patients with melanoma (skin cancer), breast cancer, and bowel cancer all responded better to chemotherapy when their vitamin A levels were higher. In Finland, researchers treated cancer patients with both chemotherapy and a wide variety of vitamin and mineral supplements, including 15,000 to 40,000 international units of vitamin A, and 10,000 to 20,000 international units of beta-carotene. These patients lived longer and suffered fewer side effects than did unsupplemented patients.

In yet another study, one group of patients receiving conventional chemotherapy for metastatic gastric cancer also received antioxidant supplements containing vitamins A and E, while another group received only the chemotherapy. The supplemented group was found to have a significantly better response rate to their treatment and a prolonged survival time when compared with the unsupplemented group. At Cancer Treatment Centers of America's 1995 symposium, Adjuvant Nutrition in Cancer Treatment, Dr. Jae Ho Kim, professor of Radiology at Case Western Reserve University, explained that vitamin A works synergistically with chemotherapy and radiation. It appears to make the treatment more selective and, at the same time, it offers some protection against the toxic effects of the therapy.

The coauthor of this book, Nancy Bruning, experienced similar results during her cancer treatment. Luckily, Nancy's doctor recommended that she take vitamin A and other supplements during chemotherapy for breast cancer. I find it interesting that her side effects were relatively minor, and that twenty-two years after her diagnosis, she has no evidence of cancer.

Since 1994, a debate has raged concerning the use of beta-carotene supplements as a cancer preventive. In that year, a study conducted in Finland obtained negative results when using beta-carotene supplements in long-term smokers. Toward the end of 1995, another study, CARET (Beta-carotene and Retinol Efficacy Trial), reported similar results—in fact, they found that beta-carotene supplements might actually increase the risk of lung cancer in long-term smokers, as well as in asbestos workers.

Why were the results of these studies so different from those of previous studies? Some of the issues raised by the scientific community include the fact that the dose of beta-carotene used may have been too low. The CARET study, for instance, used about 55,000 international units of beta-carotene, rather than the 300,000 to 500,000 international units that have met with favorable results in other cancer studies. In addition, most scientists agree that antioxidant nutrients are more effective when taken together, rather than individually. Most important, perhaps, is the finding of the Finnish and CARET studies that was not highly publicized—that those individuals who had high beta-carotene intakes prior to the start of the studies were protected against lung cancer. Presumably, their high beta-carotene intake was from the food they ate, and by definition it was natural beta-carotene. In addition, their diet was probably higher in other carotenes and other antioxidants as well. This study used synthetic beta-carotene supplements and did not include other carotenoids or antioxidants. As I mentioned earlier, synthetic beta-carotene has been found to have virtually no beta-carotene activity, and this form may actually prove harmful, as it already has in some studies.

Studies like the CARET and Finnish studies should not simply be dismissed, since they do raise questions that need to be answered. Nevertheless, there are numerous human studies demonstrating the beneficial effects of beta-carotene on the incidence of oral, lung, and cervical cancers. For example, in a study published in 2001, researchers gave rather modest amounts of beta-carotene to women who had biopsy-proven cervical dysplasia, a precursor of cervical cancer, to see if this would cause the lesions to regress. The response rate to this treatment, compared with placebo, was most significant in women without human papilloma virus (a risk factor for cervical cancer) and who had a low to moderate form of cervical dysplasia.

At this time, the research, on balance, seems to support the merits of beta-carotene not only as a cancer fighter but also as a powerful weapon against a variety of other disorders. But it should be in its natural form to be safest and most effective.

SKIN

Studies indicate that vitamin A is useful in promoting healthy cell growth and is vital for healthy skin. As such, it has been found to be an effective means of treating acne. The type of vitamin A prescribed to treat severe forms of acne medically is a synthetic form of vitamin A called cis-retinoic acid. This form is available only by prescription and was developed so that the vitamin could be administered in very high oral doses—200,000 to 300,000 international units—without the level of toxicity that might occur if other active forms of vitamin A were used. Although this treatment is quite successful, there are toxicity problems even with this form of the vitamin. Beta-carotene, however, is nontoxic. When using beta-carotene, I have had excellent results without ever exceeding 100,000 international units per day. I must point out that beta-carotene works even for patients with severe acne that has not improved significantly with medical treatment, including antibiotics. I have also found beta-carotene to be a useful nontoxic treatment for dry skin, eczema, and psoriasis.

In addition to its use in the treatment of a variety of existing skin disorders, beta-carotene appears to offer protection from skin cancer and age-associated damage. Studies show that oral and topical applications of the antioxidants—including beta-carotene—can diminish ultraviolet-light–induced free-radical tissue damage, which is implicated in both skin cancer and aging. Researchers working in this field recommend that the products be used daily throughout the year for best protection. When taken orally, 50,000 international units of beta-carotene were found to protect against suppression of immune function caused by exposure to ultraviolet (UV) light. This immune suppression is thought to be a culprit in the development of skin cancers.

HIV INFECTION AND AIDS

Beta-carotene may also offer hope to people infected with the human immunodeficiency virus (HIV). In a study by Dr. Greg Coodley, HIV-infected patients, many of whom were taking the drug AZT (azidothymidine), were given either 180 milligrams (300,000 international units) per day of beta-carotene or a placebo for four weeks. Then treatments were switched, so that the beta-carotene group received placebos, and vice versa. It was found that CD4 cells and white blood cells—both of which are important for immune function—increased only during beta-carotene supplementation. Considering the immune system–enhancing effect of beta-carotene supplementation, as well as its lack of side effects, there is a possibility that the supplemented patients would not be as susceptible to opportunistic infection as would patients not receiving supplements, and that progression to AIDS (acquired immune deficiency syndrome) would also be delayed.

VISION

Vitamin A is known to be essential for healthy eyes. High dietary and supplemental intake of this nutrient, as well as high plasma levels of beta-carotene, have been associated with a decreased risk of cataracts and age-related degeneration of the macula (AMD). There is no effective medical treatment for AMD, which is the leading cause of vision impairment in people over sixty-five. High intakes of both lycopene and zeaxanthin as well as alpha-carotene may protect against the development of cataracts and macular degeneration. A 2001 study called the Age-Related Eye Disease Study involved over three thousand individuals with AMD. The study found that subjects with early signs of this condition who took antioxidants including beta-carotene, vitamin C, E, and zinc significantly reduced the likelihood that this disease would progress. Because it is such a serious condition and has no medical cure, the authors of this study recommended that people diagnosed with AMD take supplements to delay its progression. In a study funded by the National Eye Institute, researchers followed five thousand people. They found that a combination of beta-carotene and vitamin C and E reduced the risk of vision loss by 10 percent.

Other carotenoids also have been shown to protect eyesight, primarily by protecting the macula, the portion of the retina that gives us the ability to see the details that we need to be able to read, sew, and recognize people's faces. Recently, numerous studies have shown that lutein and zeaxanthin protect the macula. Supplementation with spinach (the most potent food source of lutein) or lutein supplements can effectively treat early-stage macular degeneration as well as prevent it. Subjects who were given five ounces of sauteed spinach four to seven times per week or a lutein-based antioxidant supplement had improvements in visual function. Studies show that this portion of the eye also responds to high intakes of other green leafy vegetables as well. When people with retinosa pigmentosa and other forms of retinal degeneration were given 40 milligram of lycopene supplements daily for twenty-six weeks, their vision and visual field were improved.

It turns out that carrots, a source of carotene, really *are* good for your eyes! So is spinach. But how many of us eat therapeutic amounts (for example, five ounces of cooked spinach) of these vision-sparing foods every day?

RDIs and Classic Deficiency Symptoms

The traditionally recognized deficiency symptoms of vitamin A are night blindness and other eye problems, skin disorders, suboptimal growth, and reproductive failure. Low-level night blindness is becoming more common in the United States, and in some cases may represent a sub-clinical deficiency. To prevent these severe deficiencies, the RDI is recommending 5,000 international units for men and women, and 8,000 international units for pregnant and lactating women.

Food Sources

Active vitamin A is found only in animal sources. It is especially high in the fish liver oil from cod, halibut, salmon, and shark. It is also found in beef and chicken liver, and in eggs and dairy products. Beta-carotene, the vitamin A precursor, is found only in green and yellow-orange fruits and vegetables, such as carrots, kale, kohlrabi, parsley, spinach, turnip greens, dandelion greens, apricots, and cantaloupe. Tomato paste is the best food source of lycopene.

When relying on food sources, be aware that vitamin A and carotenoids can be destroyed by heat; by alkalis such as baking soda, which is sometimes added to cooking vegetables to keep them green; by light; and by air. Because beta-carotene is especially susceptible to oxidation, carrot juice is rich in this substance only if it is consumed directly after pressing.

Supplements

Studies of the effects of vitamin A and beta-carotene on cancer have correlated with a decreased risk of cancer more often with a high beta-carotene intake than with a high intake of the vitamin A in fish liver oil. Since active vitamin A (from fish liver oil) and beta-carotene may have slightly different functions in the body, I recommend that my patients take a combination of beta-carotene and active vitamin A. My clinical experience has shown this combination to be most effective. Palmitate, the synthetic form of vitamin A, is water miscible (water soluble) and is therefore preferable for people who have difficulty absorbing fats.

There are over four hundred carotenoids, and it now appears that many if not all are vital for optimum health. That's why I now recommend a natural beta-carotene supplement that also contains mixed carotenoids. When buying carotenoid supplement, look for other carotenoids on the label in addition to beta-carotene, such as lycopene, lutein, alpha-carotene, and zeaxanthin.

Optimum Daily Intake—ODI

For optimum general health, the basic Optimum Daily Intakes for vitamin A and beta-carotene are:

Vitamin A: 5,000–25,000 IU for men and women
Beta-carotene: 11,000–25,000 IU for men and women

Vitamin A is always measured in terms of international units (IU). Beta-carotene and other carotenoids may be measured in terms of milligrams (mg) or international units. For simplicity's sake, in this book we use only international units. Based on a thorough scientific review of vitamin A and carotenoids, and on my clinical experience, the following amounts of vitamin A and mixed carotenoids appear to be valuable for:

CONDITION	SUGGESTED DOSAGE* VITAMIN A	SUGGESTED DOSAGE* BETA-CAROTENE WITH MIXED CAROTENOIDS
Acne, eczema, psoriasis	10,000–50,000 IU	50,000–200,000 IU
Cancer prevention	10,000–50,000 IU	25,000–100,000 IU
Skin problems	10,000–25,000 IU	25,000–100,000 IU
Enhancing immunity	10,000–25,000 IU	25,000–50,000 IU
Gastrointestinal ulcers	10,000–50,000 IU	25,000–50,000 IU
HIV/AIDS	5,000–25,000 IU	300,000–500,000 IU
Polluted air	5,000–25,000 IU	25,000–50,000 IU
Respiratory problems: allergies, asthma, bronchitis, emphysema, sinusitis	15,000–50,000 IU	100,000–200,000 IU

*Note that for each condition, you can use the lowest listed amount of vitamin A and the highest listed amount of beta-carotene, as I generally do, with excellent results.

If you have eye problems you may also wish to take up to 40 milligrams of lutein; if you are at high risk for cancer, you may wish to also take 10–20 milligrams lycopene.

Remember: If you have a medical condition, please consult with your physician before taking supplements. If you are pregnant or lactating, do not exceed 8,000 international units of vitamin A per day, as vitamin A may cause birth defects or be toxic to the infant.

Toxicity and Adverse Effects

All forms of active vitamin A—both fat- and water-soluble—are stored in the liver. This supplement can, therefore, be toxic in large amounts. In general, a normal, healthy adult must take at least 100,000 IU of vitamin A daily for a period of months in order to display any signs of toxicity. Early signs of toxicity are fatigue, nausea, vomiting, headache, vertigo, blurred vision, muscular incoordination, and loss of body hair. Although all of these symptoms are reversible when vitamin A supplementation is stopped, I would not recommend this dose unless you are under professional guidance.

Natural beta-carotene, on the other hand, can be given for long periods of time virtually without risk of toxicity. Since beta-carotene is a naturally occurring pigment, the only adverse effect of taking too much beta-carotene is the possibility of carotenemia, a harmless condition in which the skin turns a slight orange color. This is a signal that the body has converted as much beta-carotene to active A as it can, leaving the excess as an orange-yellow pigment. I often tell my patients that if they get carotenemia, they can cut back on their beta-carotene intake. On the other hand, such pigments are often given to sun-sensitive individuals, since the tinting of the skin affords some additional protection against sunburn. Carotene preparations are also used by some people for a cosmetic effect. The slight tint looks like a suntan and allows them to tan more easily and keep the tan longer. And, as we have seen, high levels of carotenoids may also be protective against skin cancer.

7 | Vitamin D

VITAMIN D is not truly a vitamin for two reasons. First, our bodies can make it upon exposure to sunlight. Second, in its active form, it is considered to be a hormone. Specifically, it has hormonelike effects on mineral absorption, bone mineralization, and some secretions.

Functions and Uses

Because of vitamin D's role in mineral absorption and bone mineralization, it is an extremely important vitamin in maintaining bone density. Studies show that calcium plus vitamin D supplements can prevent bone loss and improve bone density in the elderly. These two supplements together have also been shown to reduce the rate of hip fracture—a feat that hormone replacement therapy has not been proven to achieve.

While bone health is vitamin D's best-known function, studies have revealed other possible roles that vitamin D might play as well. For example, vitamin D combined with calcium has been found to possess anticancer properties. Studies have shown that the farther people live from the equator, the greater risk they have of dying from breast, colon, ovarian, and prostate cancer—probably because they are exposed to less sunlight and do not manufacture much vitamin D.

In some people, low levels of vitamin D may increase blood pressure, suggesting that therapeutic levels may help regulate it. When women who took vitamin supplements were followed for eleven years, researchers found that the risk of heart disease was 31 percent lower than women who did not take the supplement.

Vitamin D has also been found to play a role in the treatment of some immunological disorders such as multiple sclerosis and psoriasis. Children receiving vitamin D supplements from age one year on have an 80 percent decreased risk of developing type I diabetes. In addition, vitamin D has been found to improve psoriasis, as well as to affect biological rhythms, mood, and behavior. It may also improve muscle strength.

RDIs and Classic Deficiency Symptoms

In children, rickets is the classic deficiency disease of this vitamin. The symptoms of rickets include stunted growth, delayed tooth development, weakness, softened skull (in infants), and irreversible bone deformities.

In adults, hypocalcemia (low level of calcium in the bloodstream), osteomalacia (reduction of the mineral content of the bone), and osteoporosis (reduction in total bone mass) are associated with vitamin D deficiencies. Thinning bones that fracture easily—a classic sign of osteoporosis—have recently been recognized as a growing problem in postmenopausal women whose hormone production has changed from its premenopausal state. (Men can suffer, too, but are usually protected against bone loss by their higher testosterone levels.)

Additionally, women with a history of vitamin D deficiency may have irregularities in the pelvic bones, making it difficult to give birth. Calcium and magnesium, as well as other minerals and vitamins, should be taken along with vitamin D for these conditions, as these nutrients all work hand in hand in the body to form and maintain bone mass. In fact, when calcium supplements are taken alone—without vitamin D or other minerals—by postmenopausal women, the rate of bone loss is only slowed. The same is true of estrogen-replacement therapy.

The RDI for vitamin D is 400 international units. Surprisingly, the amount generally agreed upon by most professionals is 400 international units per day. According to recent government surveys, vitamin D deficiency is a major unrecognized epidemic in adult women of childbearing age, meaning women are not getting even the RDI. This is particularly disturbing when you look at research on colon cancer and vitamin D—

there is evidence that the recommendations made by the Institute of Medicine (400 international units for middle-aged adults and 600 international units for older adults) are too low.

Food Sources

Foods are generally low in this vitamin. The richest sources of vitamin D are fish liver oils and fatty saltwater fish such as sea bass, halibut, swordfish, herring, tuna, cod, and sable. Because milk is usually fortified with vitamin D, milk and dairy products are also a good source of this vitamin.

Supplements

There are two forms of vitamin D: Vitamin D_2 (ergocalciferol) and D_3 (cholecalciferol). Vitamin D_3 is the preferred form, since it is the naturally occurring form. But both D_3 and D_2 become the active hormone vitamin D after passing through the liver and kidney. Special active forms are available by prescription for patients who have a chronic liver or kidney disease that may impair their ability to convert the vitamin to its active form.

Optimum Daily Intake—ODI

For optimum general health, the basic Optimum Daily Intake for vitamin D is:

400–800 IU for men and women

Based on a thorough scientific review of vitamin D, and on my clinical experience, the following amounts of vitamin D appear to be valuable for:

CONDITION	SUGGESTED DOSAGE
High blood pressure	400–800 IU
Osteoporosis	400–800 IU
Cancer prevention	400–800 IU

Lifestyle, skin color, degree of air pollution, and geographical latitude all affect the degree of exposure to the sun and therefore the amount of vitamin D that can be made by the body. It is also questionable whether any vitamin D is synthesized during the winter months and whether the body's stores of this vitamin are able to meet the daily requirements during this period. Therefore, if you rarely spend time in the sun, have dark skin, live in the northern latitudes, avoid fortified dairy products, or have liver or kidney disease, you may be marginally deficient in this vitamin.

Recent research indicates that elderly people also may be at high risk for vitamin D deficiency. Anyone with osteoporosis who has not responded to calcium supplementation may be advised to add moderate vitamin D and magnesium supplementation to his or her regimen and to increase sunlight exposure. One study suggested that elderly women may actually require 600 to 800 international units, rather than 400 international units, per day. Most patients with Crohn's disease have low levels of vitamin D and should supplement with this nutrient to prevent osteomalacia.

Remember: If you have a medical condition, please consult your physician before taking supplements.

Toxicity and Adverse Effects

According to several studies, amounts of up to 1,000 international units per day of vitamin D appear to be safe for adults. Both the beneficial and adverse effects of exceeding this amount are controversial. Symptoms of too much vitamin D are nausea, loss of appetite, headache, diarrhea, fatigue, and restlessness. Mild cases of hypervitaminosis—a condition caused by vitamin overdose—are treatable. However, doses of more than 1,000 international units a day can cause hypercalcemia (high levels of calcium in the blood). This can lead to calcium deposits in soft tissues, such as those of the kidneys, heart, lungs, and vascular system—deposits that may be irreversible.

There is evidence that the synthetic active forms of vitamin D, available by prescription, may be a better treatment in individuals with malabsorption since smaller doses can be used, thus decreasing the risk of toxicity. These forms also act much more quickly to reverse deficiency symptoms.

8 | Vitamin E

NEXT TO VITAMIN C, vitamin E is America's most popular vitamin supplement. And its popularity seems well deserved, as recent studies suggest that this powerful antioxidant nutrient plays a vital role in the prevention of aging-related degenerative diseases, such as cancer and cardiovascular disease. But as you will see, vitamin E plays other important roles in maintaining optimum health that are not related to its ability as an antioxidant. That's why, by some estimates, if we all took adequate vitamin E supplements, we could reduce our health-care costs by $8 billion.

Vitamin E is really several compounds, including alpha-, beta-, delta-, and gamma-tocopherol; and alpha-, beta-, delta-, and gamma-tocotrienol. Most of the research has been done on alpha-tocopherol. Therefore, most supplements contain this form and in this chapter, when we say "vitamin E" we mean alpha-tocopherol, unless otherwise indicated. However, scientists have begun to expand the research on vitamin E compounds and the emerging research on gamma-tocopherol and the tocotrienols in particular is very exciting. These compounds have their own unique effects and, as with alpha-tocopherol, some are related to antioxidant activity and some are not. Potential benefits include the ability to prevent cancer, reduce cholesterol, reduce inflammation, protect the nervous system and prevent dementia and Alzheimer's disease. This research is too preliminary for us to make any firm recommendations as to their supplementation at this point, but we will be carefully monitoring this on-going and promising research on the family of vitamin E compounds over the years. Another development in the vitamin E arena is the realiza-tion that synthetic vitamin E has as little as one-eighth the potency of nat-ural vitamin E. Since most studies have used the synthetic form, this makes us wonder what results we'll be getting now that more researchers are switching to natural vitamin E in their studies.

Functions and Uses

VITAMIN E's ANTIOXIDANT POWERS

Studies indicate that vitamin E may slow the aging process and prevent premature aging by prolonging the useful life of our cells, thus main-taining the function of our organs. For example, it has been shown that the red blood cells of healthy people who receive vitamin E supplements age far less than do the red blood cells of those who receive no supple-ments. Human cells grown in a medium enriched with extra amounts of vitamin E divided and lived much longer than did cells grown in ordi-nary culture mediums. Further studies are needed, but the results of such experiments do indicate exciting possibilities.

What holds true for the cells in these experiments may hold true for other cells of the body, since vitamin E is utilized by practically all of our tissues. The bulk of it is stored in the muscles and fat tissue, but the high-est concentrations are found in the pituitary gland, adrenal gland, and testes. In animal studies, vitamin E deficiency has been implicated in widely diverse conditions, including cataracts, muscular and neuromus-cular disease, and the weakening of the cells of the lungs, liver, heart, and blood. In some studies, a deficiency of this nutrient also caused testicular degeneration and sterility in animals—a fact that resulted in vitamin E's reputed powers to improve your sex life.

Much of vitamin E's usefulness seems to stem from its role as a pow-erful antioxidant and anticarcinogen (for more information on antioxi-dants, see Chapter 3). There is a large body of evidence to support both this role and the synergy of vitamin E with selenium, another antioxi-dant. Part of vitamin E's benefits may be due to its ability to protect vita-mins A and C from oxidation, thus keeping them potent. In addition, vitamin E helps to increase the body's level of superoxide dismutase, an enzyme that, like vitamin E itself, is a powerful free radical scavenger. Vitamin E is also able to prevent the rancidity caused by the oxidation of polyunsaturated fats (PUFA), and thus prevent the free-radical damage that can result from ingesting these fats.

Because of its antioxidant capabilities, vitamin E helps protect the body from mercury, lead, carbon tetrachloride, benzene, the ozone, nitrous oxide, and a variety of other carcinogens and toxins that bring about harm through their ability to act as free radicals. Similarly, vitamin E has been shown to prevent the formation of nitrosamines from nitrites and nitrates found in cured meats, cigarette smoke, and polluted air. Interestingly, gamma-tocopherol seems to be able to protect us against a different class of free radicals than does alpha-tocopherol, and this type of free radical plays a central role in diseases that stem from chronic inflammation—in particular cancer, heart disease, and age-related brain disorders. In fact, high blood levels of gamma-tocopherol have been associated with lower risk of prostate cancer and preliminary evidence suggests it may also lower the risk of breast cancer, and perhaps colon cancer.

CANCER

Hundreds of human studies have been conducted on the role of vitamins in the prevention of cancer. These studies showed that vitamin E appears to protect us from lung, esophageal, and colorectal cancer, and possibly from cancer of the cervix and breast, as well. Animal studies indicate that the vitamin may protect against additional cancers, too. When vitamin E was given to animals who were exposed to potent carcinogens, it was found that the supplement reduced the incidence of cancer of the skin, mouth, colon, and breast. Additionally, topical vitamin E has been shown to protect the skin of animals against free radical damage caused by ultraviolet (UV) light.

Evidence indicates that vitamin E is also useful in the treatment of existing cancers. In animal studies, vitamin E has enhanced the ability of radiation treatments to shrink implanted cancerous tumors. In human studies, when vitamin E was given to cancer patients, the supplement appeared to protect normal cells from the damaging effects of chemotherapy drugs without protecting the cancer cells. Thus, it reduced some of the drugs' side effects without reducing their effectiveness.

Vitamin E's protective effect against cancer and cancer treatment may be due to its antioxidant powers, or to an ability to suppress the growth of the blood supply that feeds a tumor.

CARDIOVASCULAR DISEASE

Although studies examining the effects of vitamin E on circulation remain inconclusive and conflicting, this research has nevertheless yielded
tantalizing results. These studies aside, practitioners, myself included,
have found that vitamin E does improve blood flow to the extremities.
Some practitioners have reported positive results in treating circulatory
problems such as angina, arteriosclerosis, and thrombophlebitis. Others
have reported that supplementation helps relieve intermittent claudication—leg weakness and pain caused by poor circulation. This condition
is often found in the elderly and is usually treated with drugs that thin the
blood and widen the blood vessels to encourage normal blood flow. Vitamin E appears to relieve the condition through the same mechanisms,
without the accompanying side effects, while also reducing the inflammation that could damage arteries. Interestingly, a 2002 study found that men
whose blood had decreased levels of vitamin E (and beta-carotene) were
2.5 times as likely to have significant narrowing of the arteries (stenosis).

Some data indicates that vitamin E has the ability to increase the level
of high-density lipoproteins (HDLs, the good cholesterol) in men and
women with initially low levels of this substance. HDL is a substance recently discovered to be very protective against heart disease. Some studies have also shown that vitamin E lowers cholesterol levels in the blood.
In several studies, it was suggested that vitamin E plays an important role
in the metabolism of fats in the arterial wall.

Early studies linking vitamin E with possible heart disease prevention
were often conflicting or inconclusive. Then, in 1993, two large-scale
Harvard studies hit the scientific community like a bombshell. The Nurses'
Health Study followed 87,000 female nurses for eight years, during which
time subjects regularly filled out questionnaires about their lifestyles and
diets. After adjusting for factors such as age and the use of other antioxidant vitamins, researchers found that women who had the highest intake
of vitamin E—most of which was attributable to supplements—had a
36-percent lower risk of major coronary disease than did those with the
lowest intake. Only women who took the supplements for at least two
years showed any benefit.

The similarly designed Physicians' Health Study followed 22,000 male
physicians for four years. Researchers found that men who consumed at
least 100 international units of vitamin E for at least two years enjoyed a

40-percent reduction in risk of heart disease. These benefits occurred even when blood cholesterol levels did not change. It is interesting to note that the greatest protective effects were found in people who consumed between 100 and 249 international units of vitamin E per day, an amount impossible to get from food alone.

Another landmark study, from the Center of Human Nutrition of the University of Texas Southwestern Medical Center, gave subjects either 60, 200, 400, 800, or 12,000 international units of vitamin E over the course of eight weeks. Researchers found that only those groups of subjects who received at least 400 international units of vitamin E per day experienced a decrease in the susceptibility of LDL cholesterol to oxidation from free radicals. The less oxidation, the less chance of damage to the arteries.

These studies have strengthened the conviction of physicians who believe that there is ample evidence supporting the use of vitamin E supplements in the prevention of heart disease. However, many physicians are still reluctant to recommend supplementation to the general public, even though a growing number of practitioners are supplementing their own diets with vitamin E. There have been numerous editorials concerning this dichotomy.

Yet another study concerning coronary disease also showed the benefits of vitamin E supplementation. In this 1987 study, vitamin E supplementation was found to minimize the tendency of blood platelets to stick together (aggregate) in women taking oral contraceptives. This was an important finding, since stroke, which can result from platelet aggregation, is a disturbing side effect of taking birth control pills.

WOUND HEALING

Vitamin E may also play a role in the healing of wounds and the reduction of scar formation. Several studies have been performed to date, and many practitioners, myself included, recommend the topical application of vitamin E for these purposes. Some physicians prescribe oral vitamin E to lessen the risk of internal scar formation in women who have had breast implants following surgery for breast cancer. This is significant, as scar formation may lead to the hardening of the implants. Other practitioners recommend puncturing vitamin E capsules and applying the oil topically to any injury after a scab has formed to promote healing and reduce scarring.

THE IMMUNE SYSTEM

Animal studies have clearly shown that excesses of vitamin E enhance resistance to disease, and many human studies support these findings. Two studies of people with the autoimmune disease discoid lupus erythematosus showed that large doses of vitamin E had a beneficial effect, and some subjects experienced a complete clearing of symptoms. Patients suffering from rheumatoid arthritis, another autoimmune disease, have also benefited from vitamin E supplementation. In a study of seven patients who were given vitamin E and selenium along with their usual treatment, which was no longer effective, joint pain either diminished or disappeared completely.

In a study of people with osteoarthritis, 600 milligrams of vitamin E per day reduced pain as well as arthritis medication; and in another study, half the patients taking vitamin E experienced relief from pain and inflammation, compared with only 4 percent of those taking a placebo.

THE NERVOUS SYSTEM

Vitamin E may also be important for normal functioning of the nervous system. Certain children with progressive neuromuscular disease were shown to have a vitamin E deficiency. Their symptoms—which included difficulty walking, frequent falling, and abnormal reflexes—improved after vitamin E supplementation. Studies have also shown promising results in slowing neurological problems in older patients, in preventing these problems in children, and in treating Parkinson's disease.

In 2001, researchers discovered that vitamin E from food and supplements may help slow mental decline and reduce the risk of Alzheimer's disease. In one study, those with the highest intake of vitamin E had nearly a 40 percent reduction in the rate of mental decline. What's more, high intake of vitamin E was associated with a 70 percent reduction in risk of Alzheimer's disease over a four-year period.

WOMEN'S HEALTH

Some studies have shown that vitamin E helps lessen fibrocystic breast disease—benign lumps in the breast. In one study, 85 percent of the supplemented group responded to treatment, with a total disappearance of cysts and tenderness in 38 percent of the patients. My patients with fibrocystic disease have responded beautifully when vitamin E supplements were included in their health program.

Vitamin E also helps alleviate the pain and other symptoms associated with premenstrual syndrome (PMS). In one study, 76 percent of the women treated with vitamin E supplements improved, versus 29 percent of a control group that took a placebo. Many of my female patients have enjoyed marked improvement in their PMS symptoms in as short a period of time as two months. Many practitioners, myself included, have also had excellent results using vitamin E supplementation to reduce the incidence of hot flashes in menopausal women. Vitamin E may be the safest alternative to hormone replacement therapy in women who are at risk for breast cancer. Although some recommend soy products as a natural alternative to manage menopause symptoms, there is some debate about their safety in high-risk women. Vitamin E also appears to improve the type of vaginitis that affects older women whose vaginal tissues have atrophied.

Studies also indicate that vitamin E supplementation may be useful for treating excess bleeding due to insertion of an intrauterine device. Women who use the contraceptive device Norplant may also benefit from vitamin E supplements. In a study published in 2000, women who experienced breakthrough bleeding while on Norplant had higher levels of substances that indicated free-radical damage in the blood than normal menstrual blood. They also had lower than normal blood levels of vitamin E. Experiments with vitamin E suggest that this combination may cause the cells of the endometrium lining the uterus to be damaged, and that might lead to cancer. Vitamin E supplements may reduce this risk of increased free-radical damage.

OTHER USES

New functions and uses of vitamin E are being discovered all the time. In two studies, vitamin E has been shown to reduce the need for insulin in diabetes by improving insulin function. It may also reduce the oxidative stress that leads to many of the side effects of diabetes, including vascular disease and atherosclerosis. In diabetics, vitamin E also reduces the biochemical that indicates excess blood clotting, reduces cholesterol significantly, and increases HDL.

Vitamin E, along with vitamin C and beta-carotene, may also protect against cataracts. A 1991 study of 350 men and women found that people who took daily supplements of more than 400 international units of vitamin E per day had less than half the risk of developing cataracts as did people who took no supplements. Another study showed that taking a combination of antioxidants, including vitamin E, C, and beta-carotene, reduced vision loss by 10 percent.

There is also some evidence that vitamin E is good for the skin. It may be helpful in the treatment of lipofuscin—"age" or liver spots. A study using natural vitamin E supplements suggests this nutrient can help people with atopic dermatitis, with about one-fourth experiencing great improvement (compared to 1 percent of the control group) and 14 percent experiencing almost complete remission (compared to none in the control group). Topical vitamin E has also been found to improve scarring.

RDIs and Classic Deficiency Symptoms

Classic vitamin E deficiency symptoms include anemia caused by the premature aging and death of red blood cells, neurological disturbances such as difficulty in walking, and fragile capillaries. These symptoms generally appear only when there is the severe fat malabsorption that occurs in premature infants, or in people with disorders of the pancreas, tropical sprue, celiac disease, and cystic fibrosis. Vitamin E–deficient premature infants may also suffer from disorders of the retina, which can lead to blindness. The RDI to prevent these overt deficiencies is approximately 30 international units for men and women.

New data suggests that many people without severe fat malabsorption problems are at risk for prolonged marginal vitamin E intake, which may influence aging, cancer, and heart disease. In recent years, we've all been told to reduce our consumption of saturated fats, such as butter, and to increase our consumption of polyunsaturated fats, such as vegetable oil and margarine. This increase in PUFA is supposed to reduce the risk of coronary disease, but it also increases our need for protective vitamin E. Since the vegetable oils that are high in PUFA are also naturally high in protective vitamin E, this would seem to pose no problem. However, most of the commercial polyunsaturated oils are so highly processed, there is very little vitamin E left. So while we are increasing our PUFA consumption, we are not correspondingly increasing our intake of vitamin E, a situation that has many implications. For example, some studies have suggested that people who ingest high amounts of processed polyunsaturated vegetable oils with inadequate amounts of vitamin E may have a higher risk of cancer in general, and of breast cancer in particular.

Food Sources

Vitamin E generally occurs in the fats of vegetable foods. Natural (unprocessed) vegetable oils are a particularly rich source of vitamin E, with cottonseed, corn, soybean, safflower, and wheat germ oil having the highest concentrations. Smaller amounts of vitamin E are found in whole grains, dark green leafy vegetables, nuts, and legumes. Animal foods, such as meat and dairy products, have some vitamin E, but generally are low in this nutrient. Nuts—walnuts and pecans in particular—are high in gamma-tocopherol.

Cooking and processing cause foods to lose their vitamin E, since it is destroyed by heat, alkalis, light, air, and freezing. The milling of grains, for example, causes a loss of about 80 percent of the grain's vitamin E. As mentioned earlier, commercially processed vegetable oils are also low in vitamin E. In fact, the by-products of processed oils have become important sources for the production of vitamin E supplements! If you depend on vegetable oils for your vitamin E, choose cold-pressed or unrefined oils.

Supplements

Vitamin E actually consists of eight substances, of which alpha-, beta-, delta-, and gamma-tocopherol are the most active. There are natural and synthetic forms of all the tocopherols. The naturally occurring form of vitamin E is the D form, as in D-alpha-tocopherol. The synthetic form is the DL form, as in D,L-alpha-tocopherol, which contains only a small proportion of natural vitamin E. The natural form appears to be the most absorbable, and recent studies indicate that it is also the most potent (bioavailable). A supplement containing D,L-alpha tocopherol supplies only an eighth to half of the bioavailable vitamin E found in a comparable natural supplement.

Vitamin E supplements often contain alpha-tocopherols alone, because that has been shown to be the most active form. However, as mentioned earlier, other tocopherols appear to be important as well, which makes sense because this is how they occur in food. Also, there is evidence that taking large amounts of alpha-tocopherol alone depletes the body of gamma-tocopherol. In one study, researchers looked at the antioxidant effect of alpha-tocopherol versus mixed tocopherols. The mixed tocopherol was much more potent in inhibiting lipid peroxidation (a measure of free radical activity) than alpha-tocopherol alone. Now there are many more supplements that contain D-alpha-tocopherol and mixed tocopherols, and this is the type of supplement I now recommend. Because there is emerging research on the benefits of tocotrienols as well, some nutritionists are recommending that their patients take a tocotrienol supplement, too. In my opinion, adding a tocotrienol supplement to your program is fine, but since we have many unanswered questions about its bioavailablity and benefits in humans, I would not recommend taking it instead of the tocopherols.

Vitamin E succinate is a form of vitamin E that comes in a dry, oil-free powder. Since it is the water miscible (water-soluble) form of vitamin E, it can be tolerated by people who have a problem with fat malabsorption. The majority of the research on this form has focused on cancer treatment and prevention, rather than on cardiovascular disorders. Vitamin E succinate has been shown to be effective for prostate, breast, gastric, melanoma and other cancers in experimental animal models. It protects normal healthy cells against the negative effects of chemotherapy and radiation and makes cancer cells more susceptible to their effects. With the wealth of scientific research, it is a mystery as to why it is not routinely used as adjuvant cancer therapy. In addition, recent studies have demonstrated that it is also anti-atherogenic. However, for the best possible protection, I still recommend taking both vitamin E succinate (alpha-tocopherol succinate) and D-alpha tocopherol with mixed tocopherols. Vitamin E is measured in either international units (IU) or milligrams (mg). One milligram is equal to approximately 1.5 international units.

Optimum Daily Intake—ODI

For optimum general health, the basic Optimum Daily Intake for vitamin E is:

400–1,200 IU for men and women

Based on a thorough scientific review of vitamin E, and on my clinical experience, the following amounts of vitamin E appear to be valuable for:

CONDITION	SUGGESTED DOSAGE
Aging	400–800 IU
Cancer prevention	400–800 IU

Cardiovascular disease prevention	400–800 IU
Diabetes	800–1,200 IU
Fibrocystic breast disease	400–1,200 IU
Menopausal hot flashes	400–1,200 IU
Poor circulation	600–1,200 IU
Premenstrual syndrome	400–1,200 IU
Prevention of excessive bleeding with IUDs	100–400 IU
Wound healing	400–800 IU

Remember: If you have a medical condition, please consult your physician before taking supplements.

If you have high blood pressure and wish to take higher doses of vitamin E, start with 400 IU and increase it gradually and monitor your blood pressure. Over the course of time, vitamin E may actually lower blood pressure.

Toxicity and Adverse Effects

There is no well-documented toxicity of vitamin E in doses of 800 to 1,200 international units per day. However, with very high doses—over 1,200 international units per day—some adverse effects, such as nausea, flatulence, diarrhea, headache, heart palpitations, and fainting, have been reported. These are completely reversible upon reduction of the dose. For greatest safety, begin with a lower dose of vitamin E and increase the dose gradually to minimize the possibility of adverse effects.

9 | Vitamin K

VITAMIN K is found in food, but is also created by the bacteria in our intestines. For this reason, vitamin K is not strictly considered a vitamin.

Functions and Uses

BLOOD CLOTTING

Vitamin K's most important function is the role it plays in the production of coagulation (blood-clotting) factors in the body. It is required to make a substance called prothrombin, which is then converted to thrombin. Thrombin, in turn, converts fibrinogen to fibrin, which then creates the blood clot. (By the way, many rodent poisons work by counteracting vitamin K and thus causing the rodents to bleed to death.)

OTHER USES

Recent studies have revealed other possible roles for vitamin K. For example, low levels of vitamin K may be related to the development of osteoporosis (loss of bone density) and may also adversely affect behavior. Subclinical deficiency of vitamin K is also suspected to be related to atherosclerosis because it might increase the calcification of the blood vessels. What's disturbing is that people who are on the blood-thinning drug warfarin are told to reduce their intake of foods high in vitamin K. This would possibly *increase* their risk of atherosclerosis and at the very least negate whatever benefits might occur from the drug.

Anticoagulant drugs have been shown to reduce the metastasis (spread) of cancer, improving the survival of cancer patients. Since vitamin K is involved in coagulation, one would think it might be contraindicated in cancer patients. However, vitamin K not only has unique antineoplastic (antitumor growth) properties when used alone, but also augments patient survival when used in conjunction with radiation therapy. Paradoxically, vitamin K also increases the antimetastatic capacity of anticoagulant therapy.

RDIs and Deficiencies

Since vitamin K is easily obtained from the diet and synthesized in the body, deficiencies are rare and usually occur only when there is malabsorption due to bowel obstruction, sprue, bowel shunts, regional ileitis, ulcerative colitis, or chronic liver disease. Vitamin K is given prophylactically to infants at birth to prevent hemorrhage and presurgically to people who have bleeding and clotting disorders. The RDI for vitamin K is 80 micrograms for men and women.

Food Sources

Vitamin K is found in a wide range of foods, with the highest amounts found in spinach, turnip greens, broccoli, green cabbage, tomatoes, and liver. Smaller amounts are found in egg yolks, whole wheat, fruits, cheese, ham, and beef.

Supplements

Vitamin K is a general term used to describe a group of similar compounds, including K_1, which is found in foods; K_2, which is made by our intestinal bacteria; and K_3, a synthetic form that is available only by prescription. Since vitamin K is widely available in foods and made in our bodies, supplements are necessary only in cases of malabsorption or medical disorders, or at birth to prevent hemorrhaging in newborns.

Optimum Daily Intake—ODI

The ODI for vitamin K is the same as the RDI:

80 mcg for men and women

Remember: If you have a medical condition, please consult with your physician before taking supplements, especially if you are on anticoagulant therapy.

Toxicity and Adverse Effects

Only the K_3 form of vitamin K—the synthetic form—is known to have any degree of toxicity. The major symptom of vitamin K overdose is hemolytic anemia, in which the red blood cells die more quickly than the body can replace them.

10 | Vitamin B Complex

THE VITAMINS that belong in the B-complex group are B_1 (thiamin), B_2 (riboflavin), B_3 (niacin and niacinamide), B_6 (pyridoxine), B_{12} (cobalamin), folic acid, pantothenic acid, biotin, choline, inositol, and PABA (para-aminobenzoic acid). Although each B vitamin has its own unique biological role to play and its own individual properties, as a group, these nutrients have so much in common that they are often thought of as a single entity. In addition, the B vitamins work together in the body, and many of them are found in the same foods.

In this chapter I give you an overview of the group of vitamins known as B complex. I provide you with a general understanding of their uses, sources, RDIs, and ODIs. Then, in the following chapters I discuss each B vitamin individually.

Functions and Uses

The B vitamins are utilized as coenzymes (key components of enzymes) in almost all parts of the body. They are essential for maintaining healthy nerves, skin, hair, eyes, liver, and mouth; and for preserving good muscle tone in the gastrointestinal tract. The B vitamins also give us energy, as they are necessary for the metabolism of carbohydrates, fats, and proteins.

Research is always finding new functions of the B vitamins, as well as more clinical uses for B-vitamin supplementation. For example, the B complex's well-documented role in nervous system function has led many practitioners to use high doses to alleviate psychiatric symptoms such as mild depression, anxiety, nervousness, and poor memory. Additionally, specific vitamin B deficiencies have been found to be associated with psychiatric disorders such as schizophrenia, depression, delirium, and anxiety. In many cases, when B vitamin doses moderately above the RDAs were used to correct these deficiencies, the symptoms disappeared. In some instances, practitioners of orthomolecular medicine, such as Dr. Abram Hoffer, have treated schizophrenia and other psychiatric disorders with B vitamins in ranges far above the RDA. This, too, resulted in many positive case reports. Considering the low toxicity of B complex even in high doses, supplementation certainly seems worth a try.

Although the B vitamins are not antiaging nutrients per se, they are involved in preventing a variety of aging-related problems. B vitamins have also been linked with stress of many kinds. When you are under emotional stress; when you undergo surgery; and when you are sick, pregnant, or breast-feeding, your requirements for the B vitamins automatically increase. And yet it is a far from common practice to give hospital patients even RDI-level doses of the B vitamins—or of any other vitamins, for that matter. Nor is it common practice to give such supplements to elderly nursing-home patients, who are known to be at risk for nutrient deficiencies.

The B vitamins may also play a role in supporting your immune system. According to animal studies, all of the B vitamins enhance the immune system in some way when given in excess of the RDI. This is not because B vitamins themselves make white blood cells or antibodies, but because they are part of the enzymes that make these components of our immune system.

Considerable recent research has focused on the use of vitamins B_6, B_{12}, and folic acid in the treatment of homocysteinemia, a condition in which there are elevated amounts of the amino acid homocysteine in the blood. This disorder, which is sometimes found in the elderly due to deficiencies of these vitamins, is a risk factor for cardiovascular disease and has been implicated in many other disorders (see page 36). A similar condition, homocystinuria, is a hereditary disorder of metabolism that, if untreated, can cause death in late childhood or early adolescence. Again, high-dose therapy with vitamins B_6, B_{12}, and folic acid is being used to treat this condition.

RDIs and Deficiency Symptoms

The classically recognized deficiency diseases of the individual B vitamins include beriberi (thiamin) and pellagra (niacin). However, deficiency in a single B vitamin is rare; rather, people tend to have multiple deficiencies, making subtle deficiency symptoms more difficult to diagnose, yet more likely to be present. Researchers have found that activity originally attributed to individual B vitamins actually seems to depend on several vitamins acting in concert. The RDIs for the B vitamins vary (see the following chapters), but in general are quite low—around 2 milligrams each, or less.

Food Sources

The B vitamins are most plentiful in whole grains such as wheat, rice, oats, and rye; and in liver. They are also found in green leafy vegetables, meats, poultry, fish, eggs, nuts, and beans. Most of the B vitamins—and many other nutrients, as well—are removed when grains are highly refined. Although such products may have gone through the so-called enrichment process, this replaces only a few nutrients, leaving what was a nicely balanced source of B-complex vitamins sadly lacking.

Supplements

B complex is widely available as a supplement. Individual supplements of each B vitamin are also available. Brewer's yeast is a low-potency food supplement for a variety of B vitamins.

Optimum Daily Intake—ODI

As you will see from the chapters on the individual B vitamins, the approximate basic Optimum Daily Intake for B complex is:

25–300 mg in men and women (and 25–300 mcg for B_{12}, folic acid, and biotin)

The entire B complex is generally available in B-complex supplements and multivitamin formulas. If you buy a B complex 50, for example, it usually contains 50 milligrams of all the B vitamins measured in milligrams (B_1, B_2, B_3, B_6, choline, inositol, and PABA), and 50 micrograms of all those measured in micrograms (B_{12}, folic acid, and biotin). There are many physicians and other practitioners who prescribe as much as 2,000 milligrams (or micrograms) of a B vitamin. However, it is not recommended that you take this amount without professional supervision. And if you have a medical condition, it is not recommended that you take any amount without consulting your physician. The ratio of one B vitamin to another in supplements is generally 1:1. Never take high doses of a single B vitamin without increasing the amount you take of all the others. This is an important rule not just because the B vitamins tend to work together, but also because B vitamins compete in the intestines for absorption by the body. Thus, if you take an enormous amount of B_1, for instance, you might decrease the amount of B_3 being absorbed, and, ironically, wind up with a B-vitamin imbalance. Many well-meaning but insufficiently educated professionals mistakenly prescribe supplements of a single member of the B-vitamin complex. For example, professionals have often prescribed B_6 for carpal tunnel syndrome. In my opinion, some of the side effects ascribed to B_6 supplementation (see Chapter 14) may be due to the fact that other B vitamins were not given along with the B_6. This seems especially likely when massive doses of B_6—2,000 milligrams or more—have been taken.

To simplify matters, many people buy a B-complex or multivitamin supplement that contains all the B vitamins. Once you have established your basic ODI of the B vitamins, you can then add additional amounts of one or two individual B vitamins to suit your particular needs. In general, it is safe to take up to about two to three times the amount of the other Bs you are taking. For instance, if you take 100 milligrams of the entire B complex, you can then safely take a total of up to 200 to 300 milligrams of vitamin B_6.

Toxicity and Adverse Effects

In general, no toxicity of the B vitamins has been reported.

11 | Vitamin B₁ (Thiamin)

VITAMIN B$_1$, also known as thiamin, was the first B vitamin to be discovered, having been first isolated in the 1920s. Today we know that this nutrient has several important functions that contribute to good health.

Functions and Uses

Vitamin B$_1$ plays an essential role in the metabolism of carbohydrates, a major source of energy in our cells. This probably explains why the cells of the brain and the nervous system—which are extremely sensitive to carbohydrate metabolism—are the first to show signs of thiamin deficiency. Thiamin is also involved in converting fatty acids into steroid hormones such as cortisone and progesterone. This hormonal connection may explain why 100 milligrams of B$_1$ daily for ninety days cured 87 percent of adolescent women with moderate to severe menstrual pain and other problems. It is also necessary for proper growth and for the maintenance of healthy skin. Finally, there is some indication that thiamin, like all the B vitamins, plays a role in our resistance to disease.

Since thiamin is needed as a catalyst in the burning of carbohydrates, it should come as no surprise that if you increase your daily intake of either complex or simple carbohydrates, your need for thiamin increases, as the extra carbohydrates utilize more B$_1$. This affects both junk-food junkies and health-conscious people who have switched to high complex-carbohydrate diets. In fact, in one study, 28 percent of the subjects were deficient in thiamin, although they did not show classic symptoms of thiamin deficiency. The authors commented that this subclinical condition may be due to the placement of excess stress on the metabolism by a high-carbohydrate diet. In 2001, a study was published in which young men and women increased their carbohydrate intake from 55 percent to 75 percent of their total caloric intake. This reduced the levels of thiamin in their blood plasma and urine, suggesting that anyone who is on a high-carbohydrate diet may be at risk of a thiamin deficiency.

Thiamin requirements also rise during periods of increased metabolism, including times of fever, muscular activity, an overactive thyroid, pregnancy, and lactation, as well as during all forms of physical or emotional stress. In one study, surgical patients showed a significant fall in their thiamin levels forty-eight hours after surgery, indicating a higher rate of use. In another study, published in 2000, the researchers found that requirements for thiamin (as well as riboflavin and B_6) may be increased not only in athletes but also in individuals who are moderately active (2.5 to 5 hours a week). Oral contraceptives have been found to lower body levels of thiamin, too. Kidney patients undergoing long-term dialysis and patients being fed intravenously are also at risk of becoming thiamin deficient. Moreover, the consumption of large amounts of tea and coffee—whether decaffeinated or not—hinders thiamin absorption and therefore also increases the risk of deficiency. In fact, it is believed that many heavy tea and coffee drinkers have symptoms of nervous disorders associated with thiamin deficiency, but either have been misdiagnosed or have failed to seek medical help. Other foods with antithiamin activity are blueberries, red chicory, black currants, Brussels sprouts, red cabbage, and raw seafood. (Ascorbic acid, however, has been shown to protect against thiamin destruction in some of these foods.)

Schizophrenics are yet another group that tends to have low levels of thiamin. One survey of psychiatric patients showed 47 percent to be deficient in at least one of the three vitamins assessed. Thiamin deficiency was detected in 30 percent of the patients—although only one patient showed clinical symptoms of deficiency. In the mentally ill, the elderly, and people with poor diets, subclinical thiamin deficiency is common. Understandably, it has been found that an inadequate intake of vitamins, particularly of B_1, may result in mental illness. Some psychiatrists use B_1

in combination with other B vitamins to treat various emotional and psychiatric illnesses, often in conjunction with medication.

RDIs and Classic Deficiency Symptoms

The classic deficiency disease for B_1 is beriberi, a disease that affects the gastrointestinal, cardiovascular, and peripheral nervous systems. Advanced symptoms include indigestion, constipation, headaches, insomnia, a heaviness and weakness in the legs often followed by the cramping of leg muscles, and the burning and numbness of feet. In addition, the heart may become damaged or enlarged or beat rapidly and irregularly. Diuretics are commonly given to the elderly to prevent heart failure. Interestingly, two studies show that all diuretics increase the amount of B_1 excreted in the urine. This may lead to a subclinical deficiency of this vitamin and thus increase the severity and/or risk of heart failure! Severe vitamin B_1 deficiency also causes Korsakoff's syndrome, characterized by confusion, loss of memory, delusions, and amnesia; and Wernicke's disease, characterized by apathy, confusion, and delirium.

In this country, beriberi is usually confined to alcoholics. However, as we have seen, there are many other groups of people who are at risk of being deficient in this nutrient to a lesser extent and so may suffer more subtle effects on the nervous system, digestive system, and heart. As a result, many people may in fact be experiencing early subclinical symptoms of beriberi, including fatigue, apathy, mental confusion, the inability to concentrate, poor memory, insomnia, anorexia (loss of appetite), loss of weight and strength, emotional instability, irritability, depression, and irrational fears. To prevent these symptoms of thiamin deficiency, the RDI for vitamin B_1 is 1.5 milligrams for men and women, and 1.7 milligrams for pregnant and lactating women.

Food Sources

The richest sources of thiamin are organ meats (especially liver), pork, dried beans, peas, soybeans, peanuts, whole grains such as brown rice, wheat germ, rice bran, egg yolks, poultry, and fish. Sources of moderate amounts include plums, prunes, raisins, asparagus, beans, broccoli, oatmeal, Brussels sprouts, and a wide variety of nuts. In addition, many foods are fortified with this vitamin to prevent overt deficiency symptoms.

Foods lose their thiamin content if exposed to ultraviolet light, sulfites, nitrites, and live yeast. Cooking, too, destroys at least a portion of the nutrient. Baking, for instance, reduces the thiamin content of flour by 15 to 20 percent; broiling and roasting reduces the thiamin content of meat by 25 percent; and boiling reduces the thiamin in meat by 50 percent. Vitamin B_1 is also destroyed by thiaminase, an enzyme found in raw seafood, as well as by the tannins present in tea and coffee.

Supplements

B_1 (as thiamin hydrochloride or thiamin mononitrate) is available in individual supplements and in B-complex supplements in a wide range of potencies.

Optimum Daily Intake—ODI

For optimum general health, the basic Optimum Daily Intake for thiamin is:

25–300 mg for men and women

Based on a thorough scientific review of vitamin B_1, and on my clinical experience, the following amounts of thiamin appear to be valuable for:

CONDITION	SUGGESTED DOSAGE
Anxiety, depression	100–500 mg
Emotional or physical stress	100–500 mg
High complex-carbohydrate diet	50–100 mg

Remember: If you have a medical condition or psychiatric disorder, please consult with your physician before taking supplements.

Toxicity and Adverse Effects

Thiamin has no known toxicity.

12 | Vitamin B₂ (Riboflavin)

VITAMIN B₂—commonly known as riboflavin—was first isolated from milk in 1935. Although its function in the body was not at first understood, we now know that your body needs it to produce energy, and that it plays a role in many other processes as well.

Functions and Uses

ENERGY PRODUCTION AND TISSUE REPAIR

Riboflavin is important in the oxidation of amino acids, the synthesis and oxidation of fatty acids, and the oxidation of glucose—three processes involved in energy production. This vitamin also plays a role in thyroid hormone metabolism, which influences our metabolism and energy production.

In order for tissue repair to take place, the cells must be fueled by energy. Thus, an increased need for riboflavin is associated with many types of tissue damage, including that which occurs with burns, surgery, injuries, fever, and malignancies, as well as disorders such as tuberculosis, hypothyroidism, acute diabetes, and alcoholism.

THE BLOOD

The blood, too, requires riboflavin, a deficiency of which can lead to vitamin B₂ anemia. It is thought that this disorder occurs either because the deficiency inhibits red blood cell production, or because it causes the cells to die too early. There is also evidence that riboflavin may work in conjunction with iron to correct iron-deficiency anemia. Researchers have discovered that some sickle-cell anemia patients are deficient in B_2 and thus may have an increased need for this vitamin.

THE IMMUNE SYSTEM

Riboflavin may also play a role in the immune system, since animal studies have indicated that riboflavin deficiency reduces the body's ability to produce antibodies. Animal experimentation also suggests that riboflavin deficiency may increase the susceptibility of the tissues of the esophagus to cancer.

VISION

Riboflavin is essential for healthy eyes. Found in the pigment of the retina, this vitamin enables the eyes to adapt to light. Thus, B_2 deficiencies can manifest themselves as photophobia, an excessive sensitivity to light that causes the eyes to water and become inflamed and bloodshot. Vision may become blurred, and the eyes may easily become tired. Animal studies have shown that there is also a correlation between cataracts and a lack of B_2, leading many practitioners to treat the early stages of cataracts in humans with the vitamin. The encouraging results indicate that this vitamin may either prevent cataracts or delay their progress.

THE NERVOUS SYSTEM

Like B_1 and the other B vitamins, B_2 is often found to be deficient in patients with psychiatric disorders and is sometimes given to these patients along with their medication. Another indication that B_2 is useful for neurological problems is its beneficial effect on carpal tunnel syndrome. Practitioners, including myself, have had success with carpal tunnel patients using this nutrient and vitamin B_6, and even B_3 (niacin).

RDIs and Classic Deficiency Symptoms

The classic deficiency symptoms of vitamin B_2 involve the lips, tongue, eyes, skin, and nervous system. Early signs of deficiency include changes in the eyes, such as increased light sensitivity, tearing, burning and itching, eye fatigue, and decrease in the sharpness of vision. Cheilosis—tiny lesions in the mouth or cracks in the corner of the mouth—is another early warning sign, as are sore or burning lips, an inflamed or purple tongue, and discomfort in eating and swallowing. There may also be flaking of the skin around the nose, eyebrows, chin, cheeks, earlobes, or hairline. Additionally, dermatitis and sores may occur on the vulva and scrotum. Behavioral changes, too, are common, and include depression, moodiness, nervousness, and irritability.

To prevent these overt deficiencies, the RDI for vitamin B_2 is 1.7 milligrams per day for both men and women, and 2 milligrams for pregnant and lactating women. Many people may be marginally deficient in B_2 as the result of taking antibiotics, oral contraceptives, or other medications; or as the result of alcohol consumption. These substances deplete or interfere with the absorption or utilization of riboflavin. In addition, exercise may increase the need for B_2, as can a weight-loss diet. As we have learned, requirements also increase during any kinds of stress, including pregnancy and lactation.

Food Sources

Foods naturally high in B_2 are cheese, yogurt, and eggs; meat, especially kidney and liver, poultry, and fish; beans; and spinach. Other good sources are avocados, currants, asparagus, broccoli, Brussels sprouts, and nuts. Unless they are made with whole grains, cereals and grains are ordinarily low in riboflavin; however, they are often enriched with B_2. Milk, which begins as a good source of B_2, loses 10 to 12 percent of this nutrient when it is pasteurized, irradiated, evaporated, or dried. Storing it in clear glass bottles leads to losses of up to 75 percent in three-and-a-half hours. Cooking causes meat to lose about 25 percent of its B_2. Adding sodium bicarbonate to preserve the green color of vegetables during cooking also destroys riboflavin.

Supplements

Riboflavin is available in many potencies, both individually and in B-complex supplements.

Optimum Daily Intake—ODI

To maintain and achieve optimum general health, the basic Optimum Daily Intake for B_2 is:

25–300 mg for men and women

Based on a thorough scientific review of vitamin B_2, and on my clinical experience, the following amounts of riboflavin appear to be valuable for:

CONDITION	SUGGESTED DOSAGE
Anxiety, depression	100–500 mg
Carpal tunnel syndrome	100–500 mg (with an equal amount of B_6)
Cataract prevention	100–500 mg
Emotional or physical stress	25–200 mg
Oral contraceptive use	100–300 mg
Strenuous exercise	50–100 mg

Remember: If you have a medical condition or psychiatric disorder, please consult with your physician before taking supplements.

Toxicity and Adverse Effects

Riboflavin has no known toxicity.

13 | Vitamin B₃ (Niacin and Niacinamide)

V ITAMIN B₃ comes in two forms: niacin (or nicotinic acid) and niacinamide. Our bodies can make niacinamide from tryptophan, an amino acid found in animal foods, but this accounts for only a small fraction of our needs. We also convert niacin into niacinamide.

Vitamin B₃ is a coenzyme in several important biochemical functions, particularly those needed to maintain healthy skin and a properly functioning gastrointestinal tract and nervous system. This nutrient is involved in other important processes, as well, including the metabolism of lipids (fats).

Functions and Uses

CARDIOVASCULAR DISEASE

Because of niacin's role in metabolizing fats, much of the therapeutic use of niacin (not niacinamide) involves the treatment of high levels of cholesterol. An overwhelming number of studies have shown that niacin is effective in reducing both "bad" cholesterol and triglyceride levels in the blood. Other studies show it can raise the "good" cholesterol. For example, in one study, extended-release niacin was compared with gemfibrozil, and the niacin was more effective at raising HDL cholesterol and apolipoprotein A-1 levels than was the drug. In another study, researchers gave patients simvastatin along with niacin, and the results were remarkable—nearly 70 percent less deaths, heart attacks, strokes, and hospitalizations for cardiovascular disease during the three-year follow-up. When niacin was given with lovastatin, it was shown to be safe and effective, especially for raising HDL. Another study compared the efficacy of niacin with that of clofibrate, a widely prescribed cholesterol-lowering drug. Niacin was much more effective than the drug in lowering serum cholesterol, very-low-density lipoproteins (VLDLs), and triglycerides. It also significantly increased high-density lipoproteins (HDL, or the good cholesterol). Still other studies show that extended release niacin, even in high doses, is safe for treating Type II diabetics, who often have low HDL levels. The authors of these studies and others concluded that because of these effects, as well as niacin's low cost and low toxicity, niacin should be considered the treatment of choice for many patients with elevated cholesterol levels. Others suggest combining niacin with cholesterol-lowering drugs because of its efficacy and also because it works by mechanisms different from the drugs being used. The option of using niacin seems particularly attractive when one considers that many of the medications used to treat this condition can have serious side effects, including a higher incidence of gastrointestinal cancer and an increased risk of gallbladder disease.

In my clinical practice, I have found niacin to be extremely effective in lowering cholesterol and triglycerides. When patients using niacin returned to their physicians for follow-up exams, the doctors were delighted with the results. When I gave one particular patient niacin supplements as part of his overall health program, he was able to reduce his cholesterol from 350 to 225 and his triglycerides from 225 to 90.

Niacin is especially useful for people who, like me, have a stubborn hereditary predisposition to high cholesterol. By following a strict diet and exercise regimen, I was able to lower my cholesterol from 270 to 245. This reflected an improvement, but not an adequate improvement. Now that I have added extra niacin to my plan, my cholesterol stays around or below 200, and my HDLs at 90 or above.

Vitamin B_3 has other cardiovascular functions, as well. In the form of niacin, it is a vasodilator—an agent that relaxes and widens the blood vessels. Thus, niacin is also used in the treatment of various circulatory problems.

THE NERVOUS SYSTEM

Some of the early symptoms of niacin deficiency include apprehension, irritability, depression, weakness, and loss of memory—all nervous system-related disorders. These symptoms may be followed by disorientation, confusion, and hysteria. Because of the importance of niacin to the nervous system, many practitioners use niacin and/or niacinamide alone or in conjunction with other medications in the treatment of mental disorders such as anxiety, nervousness, depression, and even schizophrenia. Perhaps this treatment would be more effective if we also considered other nutrients as well. For example, we need a sufficient amount of omega-3 fatty acids (see Chapter 34) in order for B vitamins to work properly. One researcher suggests that a major cause of mental illness in today's society may be due not only to a deficiency in B vitamins and particularly niacin, but in omega-3 fatty acids as well. Studies have suggested that niacinamide—as well as vitamins E and B_6, and calcium pantothenate—may also be useful in the treatment of epilepsy, when used with anticonvulsants.

MENSTRUAL PROBLEMS

Two studies using niacin relieved menstrual cramps in about 90 percent of the subjects. In both studies the subjects, who ranged in age from about fourteen to forty-four, took 100 milligrams of niacin twice a day and increased this to every two to three hours while they were experiencing cramps. In one study, they added 60 milligrams of rutin and 300 milligrams of vitamin C, and this enhanced the effect of the niacin. The effectiveness of the therapy lasted for several months, even after it was discontinued. The women who best responded to the treatment experienced flushing, and those who did not respond did not flush. The researcher suggests that this may indicate that the nonresponders needed a higher dose.

CANCER

It appears from several studies that niacinamide is effective against more than one type of carcinogen. Thus, this nutrient may be useful in preventing several forms of cancer.

RDIs and Classic Deficiency Symptoms

Severe niacin deficiency is a major factor in the development of pellagra, a disease characterized by the three Ds: dermatitis, diarrhea, and dementia. To prevent these deficiency symptoms, the Reference Daily Intake for vitamin B_3 is 20 milligrams for men and women.

Easily observable deficiencies of vitamin B_3 generally occur only in alcoholics and other severely malnourished people. Niacin deficiency is also quite common in people who eat corn-based diets, because the niacin contained in the corn is unabsorbable. (An exception is corn that has been soaked in lime water, as is done in Mexico. This process releases the niacin.) Vitamin B_3 requirements may be higher in people who have cancer; people who are taking the drug isoniazid, used to treat tuberculosis; women who are taking oral contraceptives; and people who have protein deficiencies.

Food Sources

Vitamin B_3 is found in beef, pork, fish, milk and cheese, whole wheat, potatoes, corn and corn products, eggs, broccoli, tomatoes, and carrots. However, some B_3 is often present in a form that is not absorbable. Since B_3 may be lost in cooking water, it is advisable to steam, bake, or stir-fry vegetables to spare as much of this vitamin as possible.

Supplements

Both niacin and niacinamide are widely available as supplements. If you are treating circulatory problems or trying to lower your cholesterol and triglycerides, I recommend niacin as the choice rather than niacinamide.

Several types of niacin supplements are now on the market. They include immediate-release (IM) niacin; sustained- or time-release (SR) niacin; and inositol hexaniacinate (IHN), which contains niacin plus inositol. When using higher levels of IM niacin, individuals generally experience a flushing sensation, which often limits its use. Although SR niacin was designed to eliminate this sensation, it still produces flushing and gastrointestinal upset in some individuals. SR niacin is generally better tolerated, but at levels above 1,500 milligrams a day, elevated liver enzymes and liver toxicity have been reported. On the other hand, IHN, or flush-free, niacin appears to be completely safe and without any flushing effect. Human studies using as much as 4,000 milligrams daily have shown IHN niacin to be free of side effects and adverse reactions. IHN has been shown to be beneficial for circulatory disorders, including Raynaud's disease and intermittent claudication. However, it appears that in some individuals, IM or SR niacin may be more effective than IHN in lowering serum cholesterol and LDL levels. So if IHN doesn't work for you, consider trying one of the other forms.

Optimum Daily Intake—ODI

For optimum general health, the basic Optimum Daily Intake for vitamin B₃ (10 to 25 percent of which should be niacin) is:

25–300 mg for men and women

Based on a thorough scientific review of vitamin B₃, and on my clinical experience, the following amounts of B₃ appear to be valuable for:

CONDITION	SUGGESTED DOSAGE
Anxiety, depression	100–500 mg niacin or niacinamide (under professional advice)
Circulatory problems	50–500 mg niacin
Emotional or physical stress	100–500 mg niacin or niacinamide
High triglycerides and/or cholesterol	250–1000 mg niacin (up to 2,000 mg under professional advice)

Remember: If you have a medical condition or psychiatric disorder, please consult with your physician before taking supplements.

Toxicity and Adverse Effects

There is no known toxicity of this vitamin in doses of 2 grams (2,000 milligrams) or less. In individuals with liver disorders, though, high-dose niacin therapy needs to be closely monitored by a physician, since it can cause elevations in liver function tests. Also consult with a professional if you have a history of ulcers, as high doses may exacerbate a pre-existing gastric or duodenal ulcer.

In healthy people, the only adverse effect of niacin supplementation is a temporary flush, which makes you turn red and you perhaps feel slightly itchy. However, by taking niacin after a meal, or by taking an aspirin an hour before you take the niacin, you can lessen or prevent the flush without losing the beneficial effects. Caution must be exercised when using time- or sustained-release (SR) niacin, since taking higher doses of sustained-release niacin, even under professional advice, yielded reports of liver toxicity. The newer flush-free form, inositol hexaniacinate (IHN), appears to be much safer.

14 | Vitamin B$_6$ (Pyridoxine)

VITAMIN B$_6$, also known as pyridoxine, is one of the most essential, widely utilized vitamins in the body. As a coenzyme, B$_6$ participates in over sixty enzymatic reactions involved in the metabolism of amino acids (the building blocks of protein) and essential fatty acids. It is, therefore, needed for the proper growth and maintenance of almost all our body structures, and for almost all our body functions.

Functions and Uses

THE NERVOUS SYSTEM

One of the many systems dependent on vitamin B$_6$ is the nervous system. For instance, vitamin B$_6$ is necessary for the production of serotonin and other neurotransmitters in the brain—substances that, when deficient, appear to be associated with depression. Although megavitamin therapy for psychiatric symptoms is controversial, many studies indicate an association between B$_6$ deficiency and emotional illness, including depression and schizophrenia. Many practitioners, including myself, feel that there is enough evidence to warrant its use as an alternative treatment when psychotropic drugs fail or result in toxicity. Others suggest that it be used along with psychotropic drugs to enhance the effectiveness of the treatment. In one study, of schizophrenic men and women, adding B$_6$ to their previous drug regimen eventually replaced their lack of drive and motivation with feelings of well-being; they also reported feeling more energetic, alert, and responsive.

Research shows that B_6 may have a much greater effect on the nervous system than previously thought. For example, a number of studies report that patients with carpal tunnel syndrome—a neurological condition that leads to weakness and pain of the wrist and hand—respond positively to B_6 supplementation, especially when combined with vitamin B_2. In addition, infants fed formulas low in vitamin B_6 have suffered epileptic-like convulsions, weight loss, nervous irritability, and stomach disorders. These problems, as well as other forms of childhood epilepsy, have been found to respond to B_6 supplementation. Autistic children also have been shown to improve when given B_6 along with magnesium.

CARDIOVASCULAR HEALTH

Vitamin B_6 is needed for healthy blood and blood vessels. It is required by the body to turn iron into hemoglobin and to produce red blood cells and antibodies. A deficiency can therefore cause anemia and a depression of immune system responses.

Studies also indicate that vitamin B_6 may help prevent arteriosclerosis (hardening of the arteries), and that low levels may increase the risk of heart attack. Vitamin B_6 is one of the B vitamins that are receiving increasing attention because of their ability to lower homocysteine, a risk factor for cardiovascular disease. In one study, healthy volunteers without high homocysteine levels were given one of three different regimens. In regimen #3, which contained B_6 at 100 milligrams along with high-dose B_{12} and folic acid, only by adding a high level of B_6 were total homocysteine levels significantly reduced. Another finding was that therapeutic levels of vitamin B_6 interact with folic acid and deplete it, supporting the view that you should not give high levels of one B vitamin alone.

Reducing homocysteine alone would likely reduce your risk of heart attack or stroke. B_6 has another role to play, when given along with a cholesterol-lowering drug, fenofibrate. When given alone, fenofibrate was shown to raise homocysteine levels 44 percent, which may counteract the cardioprotective effect of the drug. However, when you add B_6, B_{12}, and folic acid to the regimen, homocysteine levels rose only 13 percent. This remarkable result prompted the authors of this study to recommend that these three vitamins routinely be given along with fenofibrate. My question is: Why settle for 13 percent? Why not give higher doses of the B vitamins to completely prevent the rise in homocysteine levels?

These three B vitamins also have been given after coronary angioplasty and have decreased the rate at which the treated blood vessel closed again (restenosis). Therefore, supplementation should be considered in anyone who has had this procedure.

WOMEN'S HEALTH

B$_6$ is also important for women who suffer from menstrual problems, including premenstrual syndrome (PMS). Symptoms of PMS can include depression, irritability, fatigue, painful and swollen breasts, bloated abdomen, swollen fingers and ankles, headache, stomachache, and backache. In some women these symptoms are relieved when menstruation begins. In other women, menstruation can bring on increased appetite, sweet cravings, weight gain, cramping, sleep disturbances, increased susceptibility to stress, and decreased energy. Many studies have shown that B$_6$ reduces or eliminates these symptoms for most women. The reason for this is unclear, but it may be that high estrogen levels after ovulation result in an increased need for B$_6$ or a decreased ability to absorb it. In addition, B$_6$ tends to act as a natural diuretic, promoting the formation and release of urine. This would also help reduce PMS symptoms. Certainly, I have seen remarkable results in my own patients with B$_6$ supplementation, and many researchers suggest that B$_6$ be tried before progesterone is considered.

A number of studies have shown that women who take oral contraceptives tend to have lower blood levels of this vitamin. This may be responsible for the lethargy, fatigue, and mental depression experienced by some women on oral contraceptives, since B$_6$ supplementation improves these symptoms.

B$_6$ is of special concern for both pregnant and lactating women, as studies have shown that the requirement for this nutrient increases at these times. Moreover, studies have found that pregnant women consume only 50 percent of the RDA during the last month of pregnancy, and that breast-feeding women consume only 60 percent of the RDA after delivery. These figures are of importance not only for the expectant mother, but for her infant, too. For instance, according to one study, B$_6$ supplementation can reduce or cure the nausea and vomiting of pregnancy. Another study found that Apgar scores—a measure of a newborn's health—were significantly better for infants of mothers who took an amount several times the RDA of B_6 than for those who took an amount close to the RDA. Adequate levels of B_6 are also vital in lactating women because of the previously mentioned association of B_6 deficiency with convulsions and irritability in some infants.

OTHER USES

Asthmatics may benefit from B_6 supplementation, as may those with sickle cell anemia; diabetes; and Chinese restaurant syndrome, an adverse reaction to monosodium glutamate (MSG), the symptoms of which include facial pressure, tingling and burning of the skin, chest pain, headache, and heartburn. This nutrient has also been shown to be of use in the treatment of recurring kidney stones in adults, and in kidney failure in some infants. In addition, experiments with animals suggest that a diet deficient in B_6 may be involved in premature aging. Another experiment suggests that B_6 holds promise as a treatment for melanoma, a deadly form of cancer.

RDIs and Classic Deficiency Symptoms

The most frequently diagnosed and well-recognized deficiency symptoms of vitamin B_6 occur in the skin and nervous system. The changes in the skin and mucous membranes are similar to those caused by other members of the B-complex group and include seborrheic dermatitis, particularly around the nose, eyes, eyebrows, the skin behind the ears, and the mouth; acne; cheilosis and stomatitis, which are characterized by tiny sores and cracks in and around the mouth; and glossitis (inflamed tongue). B_6 deficiency is also associated with nervous system problems such as depression, confusion, dizziness, insomnia, irritability, nervousness, a pins-and-needles feeling in the hands and feet, and even brain wave abnormalities and convulsions.

While the list of benefits and uses of B_6 is a long one, it is difficult for men and women to obtain even their RDIs of 2 milligrams, and pregnant and lactating women to obtain their RDI of 2.5 milligrams, from food. Certain members of the population, such as women, dieters, adolescent girls, alcoholics, and the elderly, have consistently been found to take in less than the RDA. For instance, one study of seventy-four female college students (excluding those taking oral contraceptives) determined that only one of them was getting the full RDA of B$_6$. In addition, many people may require more than the RDI. Among the situations that raise B$_6$ requirements are exposure to radiation; the use of certain medications, including oral contraceptives, the antituberculosis drug isoniazid, the antiparkinsonain drugs benzerazide and carbidopa, penicillamine, and cycloserine; tobacco use; air pollutants; cardiac failure; and, of course, stress.

Food Sources

All foods contain small amounts of B$_6$. Those foods thought to contain the highest amounts of this nutrient include eggs, spinach, carrots, peas, meat, chicken, fish (especially herring and salmon), brewer's yeast, walnuts, sunflower seeds, and wheat germ. Sources of moderate amounts of B$_6$ include brown rice and other whole grains, blackstrap molasses, avocados, cantaloupes, bananas, cabbage, and beans.

However, it has recently been discovered that data on the vitamin B$_6$ content of foods is unreliable, since the amount of B$_6$ in foods does not necessarily represent the amount that is bioavailable—active in the tissues after ingestion. This is true to some degree of all nutrients, but studies have shown that the bioavailability of the B$_6$ content of foods may in fact be quite limited. In addition, this content is affected by heat, oxygen, and light. In fact, up to 70 percent of the B$_6$ in foods may be lost during cooking, processing, and refining.

Supplements

The most commonly available form of vitamin B$_6$ is pyridoxine hydrochloride. However, a form called pyridoxine 5 phosphate(P5P) may be better absorbed and utilized in some people. People who are not responding to B$_6$ therapy might consider switching to P5P, which is the more active form of this vitamin. Also, some individuals lack the optimal amount of enzyme activity to metabolize B$_6$ to its active form, P5P.

Optimum Daily Intake—ODI

For optimum general health, the basic Optimum Daily Intake for vitamin B$_6$ is:

25-300 mg for men and women

Based on a thorough scientific review of vitamin B_6, and on my clinical experience, the following amounts of B_6 appear to be valuable for:

CONDITION	SUGGESTED DOSAGE
Anxiety, depression	100–500 mg
Asthma	50–300 mg
Carpal tunnel syndrome	50–500 mg
Emotional or physical stress	100–500 mg
Kidney stones (oxalate)	100–300 mg
Oral contraceptive use	50–300 mg
Premenstrual syndrome	50–300 mg
Water retention	100–300 mg
Cardiovascular disease	100–300 mg
High levels of homocysteine	100–500 mg (consider P5P)

Remember: If you have a medical condition or psychiatric symptoms, please consult with your physician before taking supplements. High doses of B_6 should not be used in people who are taking levodopa, a drug used in the treatment of Parkinson's disease.

Toxicity and Adverse Effects

B_6 is relatively nontoxic, but some problems with the nervous system have been reported. This occurs only with huge doses of 2,000 to 6,000 milligrams of B_6 daily, although there are isolated cases of toxicity with smaller doses. These side effects appear to be reversible when the dosage is discontinued. In addition, dependency has been induced in healthy adults who were given 200 milligrams daily for thirty-three days. This dependency results in a deficiency when supplementation is stopped abruptly.

15 | Vitamin B$_{12}$ (Cobalamin)

I N 1926, scientists determined that a certain form of anemia could be reversed or controlled by eating a half pound of raw or lightly cooked liver daily. By 1948, B$_{12}$, the nutrient that was responsible for eliminating the anemia, had been isolated. We now know that this B vitamin, also known as cobalamin, is a coenzyme needed by the body to form healthy blood and perform a variety of other functions, as well.

Functions and Uses

THE BLOOD AND BLOOD VESSELS

As already mentioned, the best-known function of vitamin B$_{12}$ is the role it plays in blood formation. Specifically, this nutrient is needed to form red blood cells in the marrow. Without an adequate amount of B$_{12}$, pernicious anemia results, with symptoms that include pallor and fatigue.

Recent research also demonstrates another blood-related function for this vitamin. B$_{12}$, along with B$_6$ and folic acid, helps keep homocysteine in check (see page 124 for information about homocysteine and cardiovascular disease). Therapeutic amounts of B vitamin supplements would therefore lower the risk of cardiovascular disease.

Supplementation with these three B vitamins also counteracts the increase in homocysteine caused by cholesterol-lowering drugs. In an amazing study, even conservative amounts of these nutrients reduced the 44-percent increase in homocysteine from the drug fenofibrate down to 13 percent. This study not only may demonstrate why therapy with cholesterol-lowering drugs does not reduce the death rate; it also suggests that we include therapeutic amounts of B vitamin supplements in cholesterol-lowering therapy so that the therapy actually helps people.

Another study using B_{12}, B_6 and folic acid decreased the rate at which blocked arteries closed up again after angioplasty, as well as reduced homocysteine.

THE NERVOUS SYSTEM

Vitamin B_{12} is involved in the production of myelin, a fatty substance found in the sheath that covers our nerves. Therefore the association between B_{12} deficiency and impaired nervous system function is well established. B_{12} deficiency may play a part in many mild to severe physical and emotional symptoms such as confusion, moodiness, memory loss, peripheral neuritis, leg and finger incoordination, depression, and psychosis. These can occur even when there are no signs of changes in the blood to indicate either low levels of B_{12} or anemia.

Recent studies have also uncovered a possible link between Alzheimer's-like dementia and low vitamin B_{12} levels in the blood. Although it is not known whether there is a direct causal relationship between the two, it may be that prolonged low blood levels of B_{12} produce the irreversible neurological changes seen in this disease. One theory is that uncontrolled homocysteine is contributing to the destruction of the myelin sheaths that encase the nerves and that may be related to the dementia or other changes. In a 2001 paper, the author found that the method used to measure B_{12} in the blood is inadequate to determine whether homocysteine is responsible for the symptoms of Alzheimer's-like dementia. He recommends directly testing homocysteine levels because this indicates low levels of the other homocysteine-lowering B vitamins.

CANCER

Vitamin B_{12} may also play a role in cancer prevention. When combined with ascorbic acid, this nutrient has been shown to inhibit the formation of cancer in laboratory mice. In addition, a study of smokers found low levels of both B$_{12}$ and folate, especially in those with precancerous changes. Vitamin supplementation decreased these abnormal cells.

RDIs and Classic Deficiency Symptoms

The classic deficiency disease of B$_{12}$ is pernicious anemia, whose symptoms can include weight loss, weakness, pale skin, and psychological disturbances. This type of anemia is rather common and appears most frequently in alcoholics, the elderly, and strict vegetarians (non–lacto-ovo). It is imperative to use diagnostic tests to distinguish B$_{12}$ anemia from folic acid anemia. If folic acid is given to someone already deficient in B$_{12}$, severe B$_{12}$ deficiency will develop, as the body needs vitamin B$_{12}$ to utilize folic acid. If B$_{12}$ is given to someone already deficient in folic acid, severe folic acid deficiency will develop. To prevent overt deficiencies, the RDI for vitamin B$_{12}$ is 6 micrograms for men and women, and 8 micrograms for pregnant and lactating women.

Certain conditions can cause B$_{12}$ deficiency even when there is adequate dietary intake of the nutrient. When an inherited defect prevents the body from manufacturing sufficient quantities of a substance called intrinsic factor, normal absorption of the vitamin cannot take place. In addition, prolonged excess exposure to nitrous oxide (laughing gas) may result in lowered blood levels of this vitamin. Although early studies suggested that vitamin C supplementation may also destroy B$_{12}$, subsequent studies using improved technology have shown that large doses of vitamin C do not have this effect. On the contrary, the absorption of the cyanocobalamin form of B$_{12}$ is slightly increased in the presence of vitamin C. Some medications, though, do interfere with absorption of this nutrient. (See the Drug-Nutrient Interaction Table on page 270.)

Although we have the ability to produce B$_{12}$ in the intestines, we are not sure how much of this can be absorbed by the body.

Food Sources

Generally, the amount of B$_{12}$ in foods is small. All sources are animal in origin: lamb and beef kidneys; and lamb, beef, calf, and pork livers are among the foods highest in B$_{12}$. Good sources include beef, herring, and mackerel. Egg yolk, milk, cheese, clams, sardines, salmon, crabmeat, and oysters also have reasonable amounts.

Vitamin B_{12} is not stable in the presence of heat, acid, or light, and is susceptible to oxidation, so care is required during the storage and cooking of foods.

Supplements

Cyanocobalamin is the form of B_{12} that is most widely used in oral supplements. Hydroxycobalamin is the form of B_{12} used in injections, which are recommended in cases of B_{12} malabsorption.

Optimum Daily Intake—ODI

For optimum general health, the basic Optimum Daily Intake for vitamin B_{12} is:

25–500 mcg for men and women

Based on a thorough scientific review of vitamin B_{12} and on my clinical experience, the following amounts of B_{12} appear to be valuable for:

CONDITION	SUGGESTED DOSAGE
Anxiety, depression	100–500 mcg
B_{12} anemia	250–500 mcg (injections by your physician may be necessary if you have malabsorption)
Emotional or physical stress	100–500 mcg
Cardiovascular disease	500–1000 mcg
Elevated homocysteine levels	500–1000 mcg

Remember: If you have a medical condition or psychiatric symptoms, please consult with your physician before taking supplements.

Toxicity and Adverse Effects

Vitamin B_{12} has no known toxicity.

16 | Folic Acid

FOLIC ACID, also known as folate or folacin, was identified and named in the 1940s. This nutrient takes part in a variety of body processes, ranging from the synthesis of genetic material to the transmission of nerve signals. In one of its most important roles, folic acid works closely with vitamin B_{12} in the metabolism of amino acids and the synthesis of proteins, including the production of genetic material (RNA and DNA). Thus, it is vital to healthy cell division and replication and to tissue growth. As you will see, a number of its therapeutic uses are related to this function.

Functions and Uses

THE BLOOD AND BLOOD VESSELS

Like vitamin B_{12}, discussed in the previous chapter, folic acid is needed for the proper formation of red blood cells. Without adequate amounts of folic acid, a specific type of anemia results, characterized by oversized red blood cells. Folic acid shares other blood-related functions with B_{12} and B_6 as well, in particular the ability to lower homocysteine. As mentioned in the chapters on these other two B vitamins, homocysteine is a naturally occurring body chemical that is part of your daily metabolism. However, when it accumulates, it increases your risk of cardiovascular disease. Many studies show that folic acid, B_6, and B_{12} work together to lower this deadly chemical. In one study, subjects were given one of three different regimens. In regimen #3, which contained the highest doses of B_6, B_{12}, and folic acid, total homocysteine levels were significantly reduced. Although the subjects were healthy volunteers without high homocysteine levels, it is likely the same effects would occur in people with high homocysteine. Another finding was that therapeutic levels of vitamin B_6 interact with folic acid and deplete it—a reminder that we should not take high levels of only one B vitamin alone.

Reducing homocysteine would likely reduce your risk of heart attack or stroke, but most conventional therapy aims to lower cholesterol. In one study, when the cholesterol-lowering drug fenofibrate was given alone, fenofibrate was shown to raise homocysteine levels 44 percent, which may counteract the cardioprotective effect of the drug. However, when the researchers added modest amounts of B_6, B_{12}, and folic acid to the regimen, homocysteine levels rose only 13 percent. As my friend and colleague Kirk Hamilton commented about this study in his Clinical Pearls Abstract Service: "This type of truly integrative medicine is what I get most excited about. If we are going to include nutraceuticals and less toxic therapies in mainstream medicine, we are going to have to start by comingling traditional and nontraditional treatments, as in this case. Key points in this article are that the authors encouraged the B-complex vitamins to be used routinely with lipid-lowering fenofibrate therapy to help prevent the adverse consequences of elevated homocysteine. Secondly, these nutrients are given at such a minimal dose that these results could easily be achieved with one extra supplemental pill." I couldn't have said it better myself! But I would add: why settle for a 13 percent rise in homocysteine? Why not give higher doses of the B vitamins to keep the rise down to 0 percent, since they are harmless?

Similarly, folic acid has been given along with B_6 and B_{12} after coronary angioplasty and has decreased the rate at which the treated blood vessel closed again (restenosis). Therefore, supplementation should be considered in anyone who has had this procedure—another example of integrative medicine at its best.

Further evidence that folic acid supplements may reduce your risk of stroke and cardiovascular disease (CVD) comes from a study done at Tulane University. Researchers looked at nearly 10,000 men and women who did not have CVD at the start of the study. After following them for an average of nineteen years, they found that those who got the most folic acid from their diet experienced fewer strokes and less CVD than those who consumed the least folic acid.

DYSPLASIA

Because of folic acid's role in cell division, a deficiency of this nutrient is associated with dysplasia, an abnormal growth of tissues. Researchers have had some success in using folic acid to treat various types of dysplasia, including the very common cervical dysplasia. Evidence suggests that in some women, the use of oral contraceptives causes a localized folate deficiency in the cells of the cervix, somehow making them more susceptible to cancer-causing viruses or chemicals. Because dysplasia is considered precancerous, when the condition is severe, surgical removal of the suspicious cells is generally recommended. Fortunately, folate has helped stop or reverse cervical dysplasia in a number of women taking oral contraceptives. I have recommended folic acid to many patients whom physicians have referred to my office for this problem. When their physicians gave them follow-up exams, they were delighted to find a reversal of the dysplasia.

Researchers are always trying to find particular groups that are at risk so they can design treatments geared toward that group. For example, they have found that some women have a particular genetic defect that, when paired with a folic acid deficiency, increases their risk of cervical cancer. These women should obviously be getting folic acid supplements. But since women are never tested for this defect unless they are part of a study, and so many women are deficient in folic acid, why not just recommend that all women take folic acid supplements, which would easily counteract the risk of having this defect as well as confer all the other benefits discussed in this chapter?

BIRTH DEFECTS

Because of the rapid cell multiplication that takes place during pregnancy, the mother's need for folate is great. Pregnancy may deplete the mother's supply of folic acid as the rapidly growing fetus makes increased demands on her body's nutrient stores. This may cause anemia in the mother and birth defects in the child. In one study, one group of mothers whose children were born with harelips—one or more splits in the upper lip—were given folic acid prior to and during the first trimester of their next pregnancy, while another group remained unsupplemented.

Only one of the supplemented mothers gave birth to another child with harelip; in the unsupplemented group, there were fifteen recurrences. Since oral contraceptives may also affect the level of folate in the blood throughout the body, any woman who discontinues use of the pill to become pregnant should make sure she has adequate folate stored in her body before she conceives.

The greatest attention received by folic acid is due to its ability to prevent defects of the neural tube, the structure in the embryo that gives rise to the brain, the spinal cord, and other parts of the central nervous system. In 1992, the U.S. Public Health Service released an advisory stating that "in order to reduce the frequency of neural tube defects and their resulting disability, all women of childbearing age in the United States who are capable of becoming pregnant should consume .4 milligrams (400 micrograms) of folic acid per day for the purpose of reducing their risk of having a pregnancy affected with spina bifida or other neural tube defects. However, the current RDI for pregnant and lactating women is twice that amount—800 micrograms. Recent data from Britain suggests that to maximize the reduction of homocysteine it appears that you also need a daily dose of 800 micrograms. In 1998, the United States made it mandatory to fortify cereal products with folic acid, but fortification adds only about 100 micrograms of folic acid a day to the diet. How are we supposed to protect ourselves from heart disease and our babies from birth defects without taking folic acid supplements?

And, interestingly, the studies showing the most remarkable results did not use supplementation of folic acid only. In one study, for example, B_{12} supplementation along with folic acid actually demonstrated superior results in preventing neural tube defects. In another study, multivitamins containing 800 micrograms of folic acid along with a multimineral supplement also demonstrated excellent results. So, although food fortification with folic acid is a step in the right direction, it does not supply enough folic acid to get optimum results, and folic acid–fortified foods are not necessarily also fortified with optimum amounts of the other B vitamins with which folic acid works so well.

THE NERVOUS SYSTEM

Folic acid supports healthy nervous system function in several ways. Folic acid derivatives are coenzymes for neurotransmitters—the chemicals that permit the sending of signals from nerve fiber to nerve fiber. Because of this important function, folic acid may cause certain nervous system—related disorders. Some studies have suggested that a folic acid deficiency can produce minor and major mental problems and mood changes, including depression, schizophrenia, and dementia. A study from Boston University and Tufts University found that people with high levels of homocysteine in their blood had double the risk of Alzheimer's disease than those with low or normal levels. And an animal study conducted at the National Institute of Aging found that mice fed folic acid could repair Alzheimer's-like brain damage but those who did not get folic acid could not.

Studies suggest that up to one-third of people with severe depression may have a folate deficiency. However, it is difficult to detect this particular group of people because blood tests are not sensitive enough. Some researchers suggest we measure blood levels of homocysteine as a marker for folate deficiency so we can treat this group with folic acid supplements. But this type of testing is not routine; nor, in my opinion, is it really necessary. Folic acid supplements have been shown to improve mood, arousal, and cognitive and social function, so why don't we treat all people with mood disorders such as depression with folic acid? Interestingly, when people taking the antidepressant drug fluoxetine also took supplemental folic acid, they experienced significantly greater improvement than those taking only the drug. The author of the study suggests that folic acid supplementation would probably improve the effect of other antidepressants as well.

Finally, since large doses of this vitamin have been reported as improving the condition of a certain congenital form of mental retardation, folate may also be connected with other forms of mental retardation and low IQ (intelligence quotient).

THE IMMUNE SYSTEM

Many aspects of the immune system are affected by a deficiency in folic acid, including the ability to recognize invading microbes and the number and strength of our white blood cells. Thus, folic acid, when deficient, may render us less resistant to disease.

RDIs and Classic Deficiency Symptoms

The classic deficiency disease of folic acid is a type of anemia in which the red blood cells are improperly formed. The symptoms of this condition include irritability, weakness, sleeping difficulties, and pallor. Diagnostic tests must be used to distinguish folic acid anemia from B_{12} anemia. If B_{12} is given to someone already deficient in folic acid, severe folic acid deficiency will develop. If folic acid is given to someone already deficient in B_{12}, severe B_{12} deficiency will develop. Classic folic acid deficiency symptoms most often occur in alcoholics and people with intestinal malabsorption usually due to the aging process, gastrointestinal surgery, or some other disease or condition of the digestive system. To prevent such overt deficiency, the RDI is 400 micrograms for men and women, and 800 micrograms for pregnant and lactating women.

Studies have shown that aspirin; nitrous oxide, an anesthetic gas; anticonvulsants; sulfasalazine, used for inflammatory bowel disease; and methotrexate, an anticancer drug, may interfere with folate absorption or utilization. In addition, there may be an increased need for this nutrient during illness, injury, and surgery, during which times the body repairs itself. It logically follows that folic acid requirements increase during any time of stress.

A word should be said about folinic acid, a synthetic derivative of folic acid that is used in very high doses to rescue cancer patients from methotrexate toxicity. It should not be confused with the vitamin folic acid. Folic acid does not interfere with the efficacy of methotrexate. Unfortunately, many patients are still advised not to take folic acid with this chemotherapy drug, thus putting them at risk for folic acid deficiency.

Food Sources

Folic acid is found in many types of foods. The best natural sources of folic acid are beef liver, lamb liver, pork liver, and chicken liver; deep-green leafy vegetables, such as spinach, kale, and beet greens; and asparagus, broccoli, whole wheat, and brewer's yeast. However, it has been estimated that only 25 to 50 percent of the folic acid in food is biologically available. In addition, cooking and other types of processing can reduce folic content by 50 to 90 percent. For instance, 68 percent of the folic acid in whole wheat is removed when the grain is processed into white flour.

Supplements

Folic acid is available without a prescription in amounts up to 800 micrograms, either as an individual supplement or as part of a multivitamin formula. Stronger supplements are available only with a doctor's prescription.

Optimum Daily Intake—ODI

For optimum general health, the basic Optimum Daily Intake of folic acid is:

400–1,200 mcg for men and women

Based on thorough scientific review of folic acid, and on my clinical experience, the following amounts of folic acid appear to be valuable for:

CONDITION	SUGGESTED DOSAGE
Anxiety, depression	400–800 mcg
Cervical dysplasia	800–5,000 mcg (5 mg)
Emotional or physical stress	400–800 mcg
Folic acid anemia	800–2,000 mcg (2 mg)
Cardiovascular disease	1–5 mg
Elevated homocysteine levels	1–5 mg

Remember: If you have a medical condition, or any psychiatric symptoms, please consult with your physician before taking supplements.

Toxicity and Adverse Effects

There is no known toxicity of folic acid. However, women who are taking folic acid supplements, especially if they are current or former users of oral contraceptives, are at risk for lower plasma zinc concentrations. I recommend that these women take additional zinc to prevent lowered zinc levels. Also, make sure you are taking B_{12} supplements along with your folic acid supplements. Before prescribing high therapeutic doses, I recommend a screening for both folic acid and B_{12} anemia.

17 | Pantothenic Acid

I n 1933, pantothenic acid was recognized as a substance that stimulates growth. We now know that this nutrient is needed for a wide range of processes throughout the body.

Functions and Uses

Our bodies convert pantothenic acid to coenzyme A, which is used in a variety of biological processes involving the metabolism of fats, carbohydrates, and proteins, and the synthesis of hormones, bile, and hemoglobin. It is also needed for the production of sphingosine and acetylcholine, two very important substances involved in nerve transmission. Some of the ways in which this nutrient specifically affects function are discussed below.

EMOTIONAL AND PHYSICAL STRESS

There are no documented cases of naturally occurring pantothenic acid deficiency. However, when deficiencies were artificially created in humans, headache, fatigue, insomnia, and nervous system–related symptoms such as anxiety and depression did occur. Some of these symptoms are no doubt due to the fact that pantothenic acid is used in nerve transmissions and in the production of hormones that control our reactions to emotional and physical stress and the fight-or-flight response. This is why this vitamin has long been considered an antistress vitamin. Interestingly, laboratory animals fed a pantothenic-rich diet show significant improvement in exercise tolerance. This may hold true for humans, too. Some studies actually show that pantothenic acid helps delay the onset of fatigue, especially when combined with other members of the B complex. One study in particular showed that human subjects given 10 milligrams of pantothenic acid daily were significantly better able to withstand cold-water stress. This may be connected with the nutrient's role in helping us resist stress in general.

There is some indication that pantothenic acid helps improve our ability to heal and withstand the stress of physical injury. For example, the surgical scars of supplemented laboratory animals healed better than did the scars of unsupplemented animals. In another study, a preparation that included pantothenic acid reduced the effects of ultraviolet radiation on animals. Another preparation containing a pantotheniclike substance was applied to human subjects with sports-related injuries. As a result, there was significant decrease in swelling and increase in joint mobility.

THE IMMUNE SYSTEM

Deficiencies in pantothenic acid have been shown to adversely affect the immune system in both humans and animals, indicating that the nutrient also has a role in our system of defense. It has been found that some people with rheumatoid arthritis—an autoimmune disorder—have significantly lower blood levels of pantothenic acid than do people without this disorder. The lower the levels of this nutrient, the more severe the symptoms appear to be. Studies have shown that when rheumatoid arthritis patients are given pantothenic acid, their symptoms of stiffness, disability, and pain are often alleviated. When the treatment is withdrawn, symptoms reappear. Similar results were achieved in patients with osteoarthritis.

Pantothenic acid has also proved effective in the treatment of chronic discoid lupus, another autoimmune disorder. In one study, the condition of thirty out of thirty-seven patients improved with massive doses of 6 to 10 grams per day, followed by lower maintenance levels of 2 to 4 grams.

CARDIOVASCULAR DISEASE

Because of pantothenic acid's role in metabolizing fats, this nutrient has been used to lower blood cholesterol levels and treat related problems. In one study, supplementation of pantethine—a more active form of pantothenic acid—in amounts of 900 milligrams per day—brought about a statistically significant lowering of serum cholesterol levels and improved lipid metabolism in 1,045 hyperlipidemic patients, some of whom were diabetic (Types I and II). The authors concluded that pantethine should be considered for the treatment of high cholesterol and lipid abnormalities in patients with diabetes mellitus, and in other patients at high risk for such cardiovascular disorders.

RDIs and Deficiency Symptoms

The RDI for pantothenic acid has been established at 10 milligrams per day.

Food Sources

Pantothenic acid appears in a wide variety of foods. The best sources are eggs, potatoes, saltwater fish, pork, beef, milk, whole wheat, peas, beans, and fresh vegetables. Significant amounts of pantothenic acid are lost in foods when they are canned, cooked, frozen, or otherwise processed. For example, 50 percent of the pantothenic acid in grains is lost during the milling process.

Supplements

Pantothenic acid is available in two forms: as calcium pantothenate, which is 92 percent pantothenic acid and 8 percent calcium; and as a more active metabolite known as pantethine, which is very unstable and extremely expensive.

Optimum Daily Intake—ODI

For optimum general health, the basic Optimum Daily Intake for pantothenic acid is:

25–500 mg for men and women

Based on a thorough scientific review of pantothenic acid, and on my clinical experience, the following amounts of pantothenic acid appear to be valuable for:

CONDITION	SUGGESTED DOSAGE
Anxiety, depression	100–500 mg
Emotional or physical stress	100–500 mg
High cholesterol	900 mg pantethine
Joint inflammation	100–2,000 mg
Lupus	6–10 g, gradually tapering to 2–4 g as maintenance
Osteo- and rheumatoid arthritis	50–2,000 mg
Cardiovascular	900 mg pantethine

Remember: If you have a medical condition or psychiatric symptoms, please consult with your physician before taking supplements.

Toxicity and Adverse Effects

Pantothenic acid has no known toxicity. Nevertheless, doses of over 2,000 milligrams per day should be taken only with professional advice.

18 | Biotin

BIOTIN IS an important coenzyme that is involved in a number of processes. It is not considered to be a true vitamin since it is made in our bodies by intestinal bacteria.

Functions, Uses, and Deficiencies

Like several of the other B vitamins, biotin is necessary for the metabolism of carbohydrates, fats, and protein. Biotin deficiency symptoms include seborrheic dermatitis, which is most commonly seen in infants; and hair loss. When due to a deficiency, these conditions do respond to supplementation. While there has been no research to support the widely touted use of biotin as a cure for hair loss, there are anecdotal reports that do.

Just as biotin deficiency can cause hair loss, it has also been known to result in appetite loss, nausea, numbness, depression, and high blood cholesterol. There is some evidence that biotin supplementation helps to prevent and treat nervous system disorders seen in patients undergoing long-term hemodialysis. These patients' symptoms are similar to those of Alzheimer's patients and include disorientation, speech disorders, memory loss, restless legs, tremors, and difficulty in walking.

Because biotin is both manufactured by the body and found in many foods, only a few small groups of people have been found to be overtly biotin deficient. These groups include infants who are born with a genetic defect; bodybuilders and other people who eat large quantities of raw eggs, which contain a substance that inhibits biotin absorption; and people who are undergoing long-term therapy with antibiotics or sulfa drugs—substances that may reduce the synthesis of biotin by intestinal bacteria. (For more information about drug interactions, see the Drug-Nutrient Interaction Table on page 270.)

New research suggests that biotin deficiency may be more prevalent than previously thought. No one ever quantified how much biotin our intestines actually produce. If our intestines and intestinal flora are not 100 percent healthy—if we have bacterial overgrowth, or "leaky-gut syndrome" that prevents adequate nutrient absorption, if we have an autoimmune disease, skin disease, ulcerative colitis, cancer, or irritable bowel syndrome—are we still making sufficient biotin? This new thinking is why when a patient comes in to see me, if she has chronic fatigue and is also suffering from hair loss, I think "biotin."

RDIs

The RDI for biotin has been established at 300 micrograms per day.

Food Sources

Foods high in biotin are chicken, lamb, pork, beef, veal, liver, brewer's yeast and other nutritional yeasts, soybeans, milk, cheese, saltwater fish, whole wheat flour, and rice bran. Biotin is stable during normal cooking and processing. Eggs, another excellent source of biotin, contain a substance that inhibits biotin absorption in the body. However, cooking destroys this substance.

Supplements

Biotin is available as d-biotin and is included in most B-complex and multivitamin supplements. Although it is also available as an individual supplement, I have never felt the need to supplement biotin individually.

Optimum Daily Intake—ODI

For optimum general health, the Optimum Daily Intake for biotin is:

100–300 mcg for men and women

Remember: If you have a medical condition or psychiatric symptoms, please consult with your physician before taking supplements.

Toxicity and Adverse Effects

Biotin is considered to be nontoxic.

19 | Choline, Inositol, and PABA

ELATIVELY LITTLE is known about these three nutrients. These members of the B-complex group are synthesized in the body and therefore are not considered essential vitamins. However, they are involved in many important body processes.

Functions and Uses

Both choline and inositol seem to be involved in the body's use of fats and cholesterol and have been shown to alleviate or prevent the accumulation of abnormal quantities of fat in the liver. Choline is used in the transport and metabolism of fats. Inositol is involved in the synthesis of phospholipids, which are essential to the digestion and absorption of fats, facilitate the uptake of fatty acids by the cells, and regulate the transport of material in and out of the cells.

Choline is also used by the body to make acetylcholine, a neurotransmitter that permits the sending of messages from nerve fiber to nerve fiber. Thus, an adequate supply of choline is critical for optimum nerve function. It has been demonstrated, for example, that a deficit of this nutrient may play a role in the development of certain neurologic disorders, such as Huntington's chorea, Parkinson's disease, and Alzheimer's disease. In doses of 500 to 3,000 milligrams per day, choline has resulted in a significant improvement in children who were seriously developmentally delayed.

Recently, inositol has been found to be effective for treating depression, panic disorder, and obsessive-compulsive disorder (OCD). In 2001, a study was published that compared inositol directly against fluvoxamine, a drug used to treat panic disorder. The results showed that inositol was as effective as the drug, and that it caused milder side effects. The authors point out that only 70 percent of patients respond to treatments for panic disorder, and that inositol is a natural compound that has few known adverse effects. Therefore, it is attractive to people who may not want to take psychiatric medication. Although the human studies of inositol as a treatment for these psychiatric disorders are small, animal studies support the results.

Lecithin (phosphatidyl choline), a natural source of choline, is a structural component of cell membranes. It is used successfully to treat some cases of tardive dyskinesia, another neurological disorder. This condition, which results in facial twitches, is a common side effect of the heavy use of tranquilizers such as Thorazine. Lecithin has also been widely advocated in the treatment of high serum cholesterol. However, studies have generally failed to prove its effectiveness except at extremely high intakes of 12 to 35 grams per day.

PABA (para-aminobenzoic acid) appears necessary for the body's formation of folic acid and for the metabolism of protein. Although it has proved to be effective in combating gray hair in animals, there is only anecdotal evidence that this nutrient has the same effect in human beings. Because of its ability to protect against sunburn when applied to the skin, PABA is a common ingredient in some sunscreens. There is no evidence that oral doses of PABA have a similar effect.

RDIs and Deficiencies

There have been no known cases of naturally occurring choline, inositol, or PABA deficiency, and RDIs for these nutrients have not been established.

Food Sources

Choline is found in legumes, organ and muscle meats, milk, and whole grain cereals, and is particularly high in egg yolk. Inositol is distributed in fruits, vegetables, whole grains, meats, and milk. PABA is found in brewer's yeast, liver, kidney, whole grains, and molasses.

Supplements

Choline, inositol, and PABA are generally included in B-complex and multivitamin formulas, in amounts similar to those of the other B vitamins. They are also available as individual supplements.

Choline comes in three forms: choline bitartrate, choline dihydrogen citrate, and phosphatidyl choline (lecithin). I usually recommend lecithin, a natural substance high in this nutrient, since it is more absorbable and less irritating at higher levels than are the other two forms. Lecithin comes in several forms: capsules that contain oil, liquid, and granules.

Inositol is available in tablet and powder form. The tablets are preferable, as they are easier to take and cheaper than the powder. (It has been said that the price of the powder is high because it is allegedly purchased by those who intend to use it to cut cocaine. There is no evidence that inhalation of inositol confers any additional effects, or is of any therapeutic benefit.) PABA is included in nutritional supplements as para-aminobenzoic acid.

Optimum Daily Intake—ODI

For optimum general health, the Optimum Daily Intake is:

Choline: 25–500 mg for men and women
Inositol: 25–500 mg for men and women; anxiety and panic attacks: 15–18 g
Lecithin: 12–35 g for men and women (therapeutic dose for lipid, neuro-
     logic, and psychiatric disorders)
PABA: 25-500 mg for men and women

There is not enough evidence at this time to warrant a high intake of these nutrients for most people, since large doses may cause some adverse effects if taken over an extended period of time. However, if you are suffering from a neurologic, psychiatric, or lipid disorder, you may want to try taking large amounts of lecithin under the advice of a professional. Other practitioners and I have had good results recommending lecithin to patients with mild cases of shingles—up to two capsules of 1,200 milligrams each three times a day.

Toxicity and Adverse Effects

There may be adverse effects if these nutrients are taken in high doses. Patients who have been treated with high oral doses of lecithin (choline) have complained of dizziness, nausea, diarrhea, depression, and a fishy odor on their breath and skin. Recent studies show that high doses of PABA (8 to 48 grams daily) are associated with side effects such as malaise, fever, liver disease, and lowered white blood cell counts.

20 | Vitamin C (Ascorbic Acid)

ASCORBIC ACID—or vitamin C, as it is commonly known—has spent a good deal of time in the limelight over the years. The nutrient first came to the public's attention through the work of Linus Pauling, who researched the vitamin's ability to help the body combat the common cold and other disorders. Later, vitamin C's role as an antioxidant began to receive a lot of attention. While these are, of course, important functions, they are only part of the picture of this key nutrient. Despite decades of media hype, most people don't realize just how widespread is the role of vitamin C in maintaining and restoring optimum health.

Functions and Uses

VITAMIN C'S ANTIOXIDANT POWERS

A good deal of vitamin C's usefulness seems to stem from its role as an antioxidant. In this role, vitamin C prevents the free-radical damage that contributes to aging and an entire spectrum of degenerative and aging-related diseases, including cancer and cardiovascular disorders. In addition, ascorbic acid prevents other antioxidant vitamins, including A and E, from being oxidized, thus keeping them potent.

THE IMMUNE SYSTEM

Perhaps foremost among vitamin's C's many functions is the major role it plays in the immune system, where, according to growing evidence, it helps increase resistance to a range of diseases, including infections and cancer. Studies of both animals and humans have shown that excesses of vitamin C stimulate the production of lymphocytes, an important component of our immune system. Ascorbic acid also appears to be required by the thymus gland (one of the major glands involved in immunity), and increases the mobility of the phagocytes, the type of cell that eats bacteria, viral cells, and cancer cells, as well as other harmful foreign invaders.

Since vitamin C levels in the blood and body tissues decrease with age, it is not surprising that some elderly subjects who receive vitamin C supplements show enhanced immunity. Many laboratory studies have indicated that vitamin C inactivates a variety of viruses and bacteria in test-tube conditions. Combined with the ability of vitamin C to boost our immune system's ability to combat bacteria and viruses, this has implications also for heart disease and gastric cancer, the risk for both of which appears to be increased by bacterial infection.

Although the research regarding vitamin C and the prevention of colds is inconsistent, what is consistent is that vitamin C supplementation can shorten the duration and lessen the intensity of the symptoms of upper respiratory infections and results in fewer sick days in all types of acute illness. So while taking vitamin C may not lessen the number of colds you get, it may make them milder. Vitamin C has also been used to reduce the symptoms of asthma and allergies, particularly in cases of seasonal allergic rhinitis. Like many other practitioners, I have used vitamin C with my own patients with superb results.

EMOTIONAL AND PHYSICAL STRESS

Another important role of vitamin C is the one it plays in our ability to handle all types of physical and mental stress. Vitamin C is needed by the adrenal glands to synthesize hormones, and the normally high levels of ascorbic acid in these glands are especially depleted during high-stress occurrences, such as surgery; any kind of illness, including infections and injuries; cigarette smoking; and the use of birth control pills. Research reveals that recovery from injury or surgery can be dramatically accelerated through the use of vitamin C supplementation. In a study in which subjects were given eight to fifty times the RDA (460 to 3,000 milligrams), recovery time was reduced by 50 to 70 percent. The higher the dosage, the shorter the recovery time.

Although physical exercise has many physical benefits, it also is a stress on the body. Fortunately, vitamin C supplementation has been shown to attenuate the physical stresses of exercise and allowed marathon athletes to run faster. A similar effect occurs with other types of stress, which is good news for us nonmarathoner runners. A study from Germany, for example, further supports the role of vitamin C and stress. This research showed that people who took 1,000 milligrams of vitamin C per day dealt better with psychological stress than those who did not take the supplement. On both subjective and objective tests, such as blood pressure and cortisol levels, subjects exhibited fewer physical and mental signs of stress and they recovered faster.

CANCER

The studies of vitamin C as a means of cancer treatment are, unfortunately, conflicting at this point. However, some research has indicated that the vitamin may be an effective form of cancer therapy.

In 1976, pioneering research conducted by Drs. Edwin Cameron and Linus Pauling studied one hundred terminally ill cancer patients and concluded that the patients who received supplemental ascorbic acid lived an average of 4.2 times longer than did those who did not receive the supplement. Some supplemented patients lived 20 times longer.

A 1990 follow-up study conducted by Drs. Abram Hoffer and Linus Pauling looked at the effects of high-dose vitamin C therapy (12 grams a day) on cancer patients whose disease was progressing despite treatment with surgery, chemotherapy, and radiation. Patients were also given large daily doses of other nutrients, including 1.5 to 3 grams of niacin, 250 milligrams of vitamin B_6, other B vitamins, 800 international units of vitamin E, 30,000 international units of beta-carotene, and 200 to 500 milligrams of selenium. Included in the study were forty patients with cancer of the breast, ovary, uterus, or cervix, and sixty-one with other types of cancer; all of these patients received the nutritional regimen. A control group of thirty-one cancer patients did not receive the regimen. For those patients not receiving the supplements, the mean survival time was 5.7 months. Of those patients who did receive the supplements, 80 percent were considered to be good responders, with a mean survival time of 122 months for patients with cancer of the breast, ovary, uterus, and cervix; and 72 months for patients with other types of cancer. Even the 20 percent considered poor responders lived twice as long, on average, as did the unsupplemented cancer patients.

Another remarkable study, of people with colon polyps, showed that vitamin C supplementation could reduce the polyp area as well as the actual number of polyps. This is a very exciting finding, because it involves not just prevention of a condition—but actual reversal. What's more it's a reversal of a potentially lethal condition—polyps of the colon are quite common as we age and are associated with a greater risk of colon cancer. That's why physicians remove any polyps they find during a colonoscopy. Interestingly, this study used 3,000 milligrams of vitamin C per day, which is significantly higher than the amounts used in other studies, and which did not have this result. This suggests to me that we see significant results only when higher levels of supplements are used.

Laboratory research has borne out the results of these human studies. Such research has shown that ascorbic acid can inhibit the growth of leukemia cells and increase the cell-killing ability of various drugs and hormones. Since vitamin C appears to enhance chemotherapy in addition to boosting immunity, many practitioners, including myself, recommend vitamin C supplements to their patients who have cancer, usually in addition to conventional cancer therapy. Hospital protocol is supposed to recommend that 500 milligrams of vitamin C be given to cancer patients. Unfortunately, not all hospitals follow this protocol.

Even traditionalists such as the National Cancer Institute and the American Cancer Society feel that the evidence is strong enough to warrant a diet high in vitamin C as a possible preventive measure. Vitamin C's ability to enhance the immune system, discussed earlier, is just one way in which the nutrient contributes to cancer prevention, as is the vitamin's antioxidant function. Another protective mechanism involves nitrosamines and similar substances. Nitrosamines are proven carcinogens in animals and humans. Our bodies are exposed to nitrosamines in food and cigarette smoke. In addition, we ingest nitrites and nitrates, the precursors of nitrosamines, in food (vegetables and cured packaged meats such as bacon, sausage, hot dogs, and ham), water, polluted air, and cigarette smoke. Studies have shown that vitamin C blocks the process by which the body uses these substances to make nitrosamines and should therefore also block the formation of the tumors that nitrosamines could generate. Studies have correlated a high intake of dietary vitamin C with a reduced risk of cancer of the stomach, colon, bladder, lung, esophagus, and cervix.

It is especially important that cigarette smokers take in adequate amounts of vitamin C. One study showed vitamin C to be anticarcinogenic in laboratory rodents who were exposed to benzopyrene, a very potent carcinogen found in cigarette smoke, including secondhand smoke. Another study found that smokers need a daily intake of nearly two and a half times the RDA to maintain the concentration of ascorbic acid found in nonsmokers.

In addition to the protective properties of orally administered vitamin C, various studies have shown that topical application of vitamin C may protect the skin from the free-radical damage associated with ultraviolet (UV) light. Many companies are now adding vitamin C and other antioxidants to their sunscreens and skin-care products. Animal studies have demonstrated a protective effect of vitamin C administration during radiation treatment for cancer. Both topical and oral vitamin C may prove to be protective during this treatment in humans, as well.

CARDIOVASCULAR DISEASE

A recent study demonstrated that men who consume 300 milligrams of vitamin C daily, through food and supplements, have a 40-percent lower death rate from heart disease and other causes than do those whose intake is less than 50 milligrams. Vitamin C also acts in many ways to help prevent high blood pressure and atherosclerosis—the hardening of the arteries that can lead to heart attack and stroke. Both human and animal studies have linked increased levels of vitamin C with a reduction of serum cholesterol. It is thought that vitamin C may play a role in moving cholesterol from the arteries to the liver, where it is converted into bile acids and then, eventually, eliminated from the body along with fiber. Vitamin C may also help repair damaged arterial walls and so prevent cholesterol deposits from forming. In addition, as an antioxidant, it reduces the oxidation of LDLs (low-density lipoproteins, the bad cholesterol), and thus helps prevent any damage from occurring in the cell wall in the first place. Some studies have shown that an increase in vitamin C is associated with higher levels of high-density lipoproteins (HDLs). Often called good cholesterol, HDLs appear to protect the body from heart disease.

It has been discovered that elevated levels of lipoprotein(a), another fatty substance that can be measured in the blood, is a risk factor for stroke. Drs. Linus Pauling and Matt Rath have found that optimal vitamin

C also prevents the deposition of lipoprotein(a) in the vascular wall. In a wonderful study of older men and women, men with high blood levels of vitamin C had less narrowing of the arteries. This effect did not show up in women—perhaps because women need higher levels than do men.

But do any of these effects translate into better quality of life or a longer lifespan? Some studies suggest that they do. For example, researchers demonstrated that men who consume 300 milligrams of vitamin C daily, through food and supplements, have a 40 percent lower death rate from heart disease and other causes than do those whose intake is less than 50 milligrams.

In another clinical trial, patients with atherosclerosis who were given 1,000 milligrams of vitamin C daily could walk farther without feeling pain or breathlessness than could unsupplemented patients. In another study, surgical patients given 1,000 milligrams of vitamin C daily, when contrasted with unsupplemented patients, had a 50 percent lower incidence of deep vein thrombosis—a blood clot that can cut off the blood supply to a major organ such as the heart, lung, or brain.

VISION

As we age, we face many possible serious vision problems that reading glasses can't fix. Fortunately, there are very exciting studies using vitamin C and other antioxidants that provide hope for the aging eye. Take for example, a study funded by the National Eye Institute. This huge study involved 5,000 people and found that a combination of vitamin C, E, and beta-carotene reduced risk of vision loss by 10 percent.

Another study of older people, conducted in Spain, found that those with the highest blood levels of vitamin C had a 64 percent reduced risk of cataract. And a 2001 study called the Age-Related Eye Disease Study involved over 3,000 individuals and a condition called age-related degeneration of the macula (AMD). AMD is the leading cause of vision impairment in people over sixty-five. The study found that subjects with early signs of this condition who took antioxidants including vitamin C, E, beta-carotene, and zinc significantly reduced the likelihood that this disease would progress. There is no effective medical treatment for this condition, and the researchers recommend that people diagnosed with AMD take supplements to delay its progression. Interestingly, this same study did not find that the antioxidant supplements reduced incidence of cataracts, but perhaps this is because the dosage was too low to elicit this effect.

OTHER USES

Vitamin C has other functions, as well. It is essential for the growth and repair of tissues in all parts of the body. It is needed for the formation of collagen, present in connective tissue, and for the formation of bone and cartilage. It is needed for the repair of fractured bones. When given before and after dental extraction, vitamin C causes the gum tissues to heal more rapidly.

Vitamin C seems to be a valuable adjunct to medical treatment in general. Researchers in the Netherlands have done a study suggesting that patients who have recently undergone an operation experience less breathing problems after they have been given a "cocktail" of vitamins C and E. Breathing problems, which are a side effect of the sedatives and painkillers given to surgery patients, can increase the heart rate and blood pressure and eventually lead to an unexpected heart attack. In another study, people with Graves' disease (a hyperactive thyroid) were given vitamin C and other antioxidants along with their medication. This group experienced a reduction in symptoms and did better than those who got the medication without the supplements.

A study published in 2002 found that a high intake of vitamins C and E was associated with a decreased risk of Alzheimer's disease. The theory is that free radicals are involved in this disease and those at risk should be protecting themselves by increasing their intake of these antioxidants.

Finally, vitamin C helps other nutrients do their job. It is needed to convert folic acid, a B vitamin, into its active form. It increases our ability to absorb iron from nonanimal foods, such as raisins and spinach. It also plays a role in the storage of iron in the bone marrow, spleen, and liver, and improves the bioavailability of selenium.

RDIs and Classic Deficiency Symptoms

The classic deficiency disease for vitamin C is scurvy. Early symptoms of scurvy are subtle and difficult to diagnose: listlessness, weakness, irritability, vague muscle and joint pains, and weight loss. Symptoms of advanced scurvy are bleeding gums, gingivitis, loosening of the teeth, and extreme weakness and fatigue. The RDI established to prevent these overt symptoms of scurvy is 60 milligrams for men and women.

Yet, many experts feel that the RDI is far too low, and that we are at high risk of not getting the amount of ascorbic acid we need. Unlike most other animals on this planet, we are incapable of producing vitamin C in our bodies. Neither can we store it for very long. Therefore, we must depend upon our food to supply us with what we need every day. Many researchers argue that optimum intake of vitamin C is the amount that would be synthesized by humans if we had the enzyme necessary to make vitamin C. Animals that produce their own vitamin C have high levels of ascorbic acid in their tissues. It has been shown that mammals synthesize the equivalent of 3,000 to 19,000 milligrams per day, when calculated for a human weighing 154 pounds. In humans, maximum body pools—the highest level of a substance that the tissues can absorb until they are saturated—have been estimated at 1,500 milligrams per day, but have been reevaluated by others at 5,000 milligrams of vitamin C for a 154-pound person. It is estimated that a daily dose of about 200 milligrams of vitamin C would maintain a body pool of this size in a healthy individual if he or she were totally devoid of stress of any kind. Even the government has begun to question the adequacy of the RDI for vitamin C. A 1996 study completed by Dr. Mark Levine and colleagues of the National Institutes of Health examined vitamin C requirements in healthy volunteers. The researchers concluded that the current recommendation of 60 milligrams should be increased to 200 milligrams per day.

As another means of calculating optimum daily intake, scientists have studied the handful of other animals that do not produce vitamin C: guinea pigs, other primates, and certain fish. Their discovery has startling implications for human beings: Per body weight, primates and guinea pigs consume the equivalent of 2,000 milligrams of vitamin C per day. When under stress, they may ingest the equivalent of up to 7,000 to 10,000 milligrams of vitamin C per day. By law, animal chow for guinea pigs and monkeys must provide, respectively, the equivalent of 1,100 milligrams and 1,250 milligrams daily. This data suggests that an optimum intake for humans may be 1,000 milligrams or more daily—an amount far higher than the RDI of 60 milligrams!

Food Sources

The foods that are highest in vitamin C include broccoli, Brussels sprouts, black currants, collards, guava, horseradish, kale, turnip greens, parsley, and sweet peppers. Also high on the list are cabbage, cauliflower, chives, kohlrabi, orange pulp, lemon pulp, mustard greens, beet greens, papaya, spinach, strawberries, and watercress. Sources of moderate amounts of ascorbic acid are asparagus, lima beans, Swiss chard, gooseberries, red currants, grapefruit, limes, loganberries, melons, okra, tangerines, potatoes, and turnips. (Notice that citrus fruits such as oranges and grapefruits do not have the highest ascorbic acid content; however, their skin is high in bioflavonoids, substances that increase the amount of vitamin C that is absorbed.)

Ascorbic acid is easily destroyed when exposed to oxygen, and this process is accelerated by light and heat. Vegetables begin to lose vitamin C as soon as they are cut. Freshly squeezed orange juice, which is not likely to be that high in vitamin C in the first place, quickly begins to lose its supply of this nutrient, too. As a result, there is almost no vitamin C to speak of in the juice sold in bottles and cartons. When researchers analyzed orange juice, they found that, on average, the juices lost 2 percent of their vitamin C content every day once opened. Ready-to-drink juice had less vitamin C than juice made from concentrate to begin with and dipped as low as zero after one week of opening. Since vitamin C is sensitive to heat and is lost when large quantities of water are used in cooking, vegetables should be eaten raw, lightly steamed, or cooked in a small amount of water to retain the greatest amount of this nutrient.

Supplements

Vitamin C supplements are available both as ascorbic acid and as mineral ascorbates. You should be aware that the vitamin C in most supplements has been synthesized from natural, inexpensive substances such as starch, molasses, or sago palm. The natural vitamin C found in supplements is extracted from rose hips, which contain 1 percent ascorbic acid. Rosehips vitamin C supplements actually contain mostly synthetic vitamin C, as a vitamin C supplement made entirely from rose hips would be enormous in size and very expensive. However, rose hips probably contain complementary substances that enhance the absorption of the vitamin, so that there may be some advantage to taking supplements that contain them. I do recommend that you buy ascorbic acid supplements that contain bioflavonoids (see Chapter 35), as these substances have been shown to increase vitamin C absorption.

In some supplements, ascorbic acid has been mixed with minerals to form mineral ascorbates. The most readily available mineral ascorbate is calcium ascorbate, which is sometimes mixed with other mineral ascorbates, such as magnesium ascorbate and sodium ascorbate. The advantage of calcium and other mineral ascorbates is that these are buffered forms of vitamin C—a desirable trait for some individuals, because they are nonacidic and gentler to the stomach. People who have difficulty with oral doses of straight ascorbic acid can use these buffered products without getting acid stomach or diarrhea. Vitamin C is widely available in the form of chewable tablets. Although convenient, high intakes of these tablets are not recommended for two reasons. First, they are usually loaded with sugar. Second, they may cause the pH of the saliva to fall so low that calcium is leached from tooth enamel.

Ascorbic acid is also available in the form of a powder that is to be dissolved in liquids. Although cheaper than tablets and capsules, the powder is less convenient to take. In addition, it, too, can damage tooth enamel, and so should be sipped through a straw if high dosages are taken frequently during the day.

Optimum Daily Intake—ODI

For optimum general health, the basic Optimum Daily Intake for vitamin C is:

500–5,000 mg for men and women (along with 500–5,000 mg
   bioflavonoids)

Based on a thorough scientific review of vitamin C, and on my clinical experience, the following amounts of vitamin C appear to be valuable for:

CONDITION	SUGGESTED DOSAGE
Allergies or asthma	3,000–7,000 mg
Bleeding gums	1,000–3,000 mg
Cancer prevention	5,000–10,000 mg
Coronary heart disease prevention	500–4,000 mg
Enhanced immunity	1,000–5,000 mg
Exposure to cigarette smoke and polluted air	1,000–5,000 mg
High levels of stress	1,000–5,000 mg
Surgery, wounds, injuries	5,000–10,000 mg

Your Optimum Daily Intake may vary from day to day, depending on various factors. For example, you may want to raise your intake temporarily during times of stress, or when you have a cold or another type of infection. After such a period of time, remember to decrease your supplementation gradually until it is back to your normal ODI.

It is best to spread your total intake of vitamin C over the course of the day. For example, if you take 3,000 milligrams total, take 1,000 milligrams at each meal. There are two advantages to this. First, because vitamin C is rapidly excreted from the body, divided doses ensure a more constant level of blood and tissue saturation. Second, divided doses reduce the likelihood of any adverse effects, such as acid stomach or diarrhea.

Absorption varies widely from person to person. Studies have shown that one person may be able to absorb 3 grams of this vitamin without any excess spilling over into the urine. Other subjects are able to absorb only 100 milligrams at a time and will excrete anything over that.

Remember: If you have a medical condition, please consult with your physician before taking supplements.

Toxicity and Adverse Effects

There is no proven toxicity for vitamin C. You may have heard that vitamin C causes kidney stones, but no studies show any relationship between vitamin C and the formation of kidney stones (calcium oxalate) in healthy people. Keep in mind, though, that vitamin C may actually interfere with the accuracy of certain commercial kits used by physicians to determine oxalate in the urine. A 1993 study suggests that kits using decarboxylase may be preferable. However, if you have a history of kidney problems of any kind, you should take vitamin C only under the guidance of a qualified professional. With alterations in kidney function, the mechanism that handles vitamin C excretion may not be working properly, so that caution may be warranted.

Early studies suggested that large doses of vitamin C destroy vitamin B_{12} in the body. Subsequent studies using improved techniques have shown that vitamin C does not have this effect.

One common adverse effect of very high levels of vitamin C—5,000 milligrams a day and up—is intestinal gas and loose stools. This effect is benign and completely reversible. In fact, many practitioners, including myself, advise using this effect as a guide to finding your personal Optimum Daily Intake, particularly if you suffer from chronic fatigue, HIV infection, or AIDS. Many practitioners recommend that you start with lower daily doses of vitamin C (2 to 6 grams) and add 1 to 2 grams each week until bowel intolerance symptoms—gas, bloating, and/or diarrhea—appear. Then cut back on the dosage just until the symptoms are eliminated. Interestingly, it often appears that as someone gets better, their bowel tolerance decreases, and they need less vitamin C. I have noticed this occurring in myself. When I have a cold or the flu, I can take as much as 10 grams of vitamin C a day, with no bowel intolerance symptoms. But when I'm well, this amount does cause symptoms.

Some practitioners believe that if you take very high doses of vitamin C, and then suddenly stop supplementation, you may experience rebound scurvy. A recent review study found that there is no basis for this belief. However, if you are concerned, you can easily prevent this by reducing your dosage slowly over a period of a few weeks.

Vitamin C is used by the liver to detoxify drugs and other chemicals and appears to protect the body from the side effects that accompany many drugs. For instance, it has been shown to prevent acetaminophen (e.g., Tylenol) toxicity to the liver without hindering the drug's effectiveness. However, when taking other long-acting drugs, you may want to consult with a professional about taking high doses of ascorbic acid.

Part 3

The Minerals

21 | Calcium

OUR BODIES contain approximately 1,200 grams—about 2.5 pounds—of calcium, 99 percent of which is stored in our bones and teeth. The remaining 1 percent of calcium—10 to 12 grams, or about a third of an ounce—is distributed throughout the body in the bloodstream and the fluids surrounding our cells. Most people are aware by now that calcium is needed for strong bones—but few realize that sufficient calcium is also needed for healthy blood pressure, cancer prevention, and even cardiovascular health.

Functions and Uses

THE BONES

Most of the attention paid to calcium is due to its role in maintaining strong, healthy bones. As I just mentioned, although most of the calcium in the body is found in the bones, calcium performs various vital functions throughout the body. Thus, our bones are designed to provide more than a rigid framework for our bodies. They also function as a kind of bank from which the body can draw the calcium it needs for other purposes. This is an ongoing dynamic process during which bone—which, despite its seeming permanence, is a live tissue—is constantly being broken down and re-formed. In the process, about 600 to 700 milligrams of calcium are exchanged in the bone of normal adults every day. Normally, if there is sufficient calcium being absorbed from the diet, the blood and bone calcium levels stay in balance and fluctuate only slightly. However, from the body's point of view, it is more important to maintain enough calcium in the blood to keep the heart beating regularly than it is to keep the bones strong and hard. So if the diet is deficient in calcium, the body will always choose to maintain a certain level of calcium in the blood by drawing it out of the bone. This is accomplished through a complex system involving hormones, especially the parathyroid hormone, and vitamin D. Even if there is adequate calcium in the diet, a lack of vitamin D will seriously impair the body's ability to make use of the mineral.

The survival mechanism just discussed can cause some problems if a calcium-deficient diet is consumed over a long period of time. Eventually, there is so much calcium lost from the bone that osteoporosis—loss of bone mass, or thinning of the bone—occurs. The bones become porous, brittle, and so weak that a person may easily suffer a fracture from such normal activities as sneezing, bending over, or receiving a hug. The vertebrae of the spinal column may compress or fracture, causing pain, disability, loss of height, and a hunched-over appearance. If calcium is lost from the bones of the jaw, periodontal disease may result. Hip fracture is also a common sign of osteoporosis and is a major source of disability among the older population. Indeed, osteoporosis is occurring in epidemic proportions in an estimated 15 to 20 million Americans. Women over the age of fifty (postmenopausal) are especially at risk, but many younger people and older men are affected as well. Osteomalacia, or softening of the bone, is another common problem that is caused by inadequate calcium intake.

The growing consensus is that osteoporosis is not a disease that comes on suddenly in middle or old age. Many studies have correlated a long-term low-calcium diet, perhaps beginning at the age of thirty or earlier, with the development of osteoporosis and periodontal disease. In children, the deficiency symptom of poor calcium intake is rickets, a condition in which the bones grow too weak to support the weight of the child, with deformity being the highly visible result. There is some recent evidence that a suboptimum calcium intake in childhood may help set the stage for bone loss in later life, even when there are no obvious problems during childhood.

Because the body gives top priority to the maintenance of normal calcium levels in the blood, blood tests are an ineffective means of determining calcium levels in either the bone or the diet. The blood may be perfectly normal, while the bone level is poor. The clinical signs of calcium depletion from the bone are insidious and so are not usually apparent until the symptoms of osteoporosis begin to appear. Even X rays are incapable of picking up bone loss until 30 to 40 percent of the bone has disappeared! Once osteoporosis is diagnosed, it can usually be slowed or halted with appropriate therapy, but it can be difficult to reverse. For this reason, I feel that the best course of action is prevention. That is why I recommend that calcium supplementation be started as early as possible, preferably by age twenty. Studies show that when we supplement our diets with 500 to 1,500 milligrams of calcium daily, it improves bone mass in people at any age—including adolescents, young adults, older men, and postmenopausal women. When we add trace minerals and vitamin D as well, studies show a reduction in risk of fracture.

HYPERTENSION

Recent studies indicate that the high incidence of hypertension (high blood pressure) in the United States may be a result of low calcium intake combined with high sodium intake. In one study, forty-eight hypertensive men were treated with 1,000 milligrams of calcium for eight weeks. Twenty-one of them (44 percent) achieved a therapeutically meaningful reduction in their blood pressure. In many cases, the result was similar or superior to that achieved with blood pressure medication.

In another study, women with high blood pressure were given either 1,500 milligrams of calcium or hypertensive medication for four years. The calcium-supplemented group achieved a significant drop in their systolic blood pressure. The unsupplemented group experienced a rise in their blood pressure, even though they were taking hypertensive medication.

Studies have also revealed a worldwide correlation between pregnancy-related hypertension and low calcium intake. In countries characterized by an average calcium intake of 1,000 milligrams per day or more, pregnancy-related hypertension occurs in fewer than 1 out of 200 pregnancies. In societies in which calcium intake is under 500 milligrams per day, the incidence is ten to twenty times higher.

Calcium supplementation is free of the unpleasant side effects so frequently encountered with antihypertensive drug treatment, including impotence, fatigue, exercise intolerance, weight gain, dizziness, and impaired concentration. As the studies indicate, calcium therapy can be an effective, medication-free means of treating high blood pressure. Hypertensives who are salt-sensitive seem to benefit most.

COLON CANCER

There is also some evidence that calcium helps prevent colon cancer. Epidemiological studies have shown that colon cancer incidence is lower in people who receive more sunlight exposure and consume more dairy foods. Several studies suggest that people who eat a typical high-fat diet may be protected from colon cancer by consuming 1,200 to 1,500 milligrams of calcium daily. The authors found that within two to three months after supplementation was begun, tests of the subjects' colon linings showed that the number of fast-growing cells associated with cancer had significantly decreased. In a Dutch study of over 2,500 people, those with a low intake of calcium had a higher risk of being diagnosed with colorectal cancer and a higher death rate from this form of cancer, as well. It should be noted that one source of dietary calcium—yogurt—provides the body with two forms of protection. In addition to the calcium, yogurt contains friendly bacteria (acidophilus) that inhibit the effects of known colonic carcinogens.

OTHER FUNCTIONS

In addition to the functions just discussed, recent evidence demonstrates that calcium supplementation plays a significant role in cardiovascular health. In 2002, for example, researchers studied hundreds of women who were fifty-five years of age or older and who were at least five years postmenopausal. Half the women were given calcium supplements of 1,000 mg per day—in addition to the estimated 900 milligrams they were getting from food. After one year, the supplemented women experienced a 7 percent increase in their HDL cholesterol. This translates into a 20 to 30 percent drop in cardiovascular events and is similar to the result you get with statin drugs, but without the side effects of those drugs. The women also experienced a 6 percent decrease in their LDL cholesterol. The women who did not get the supplement experienced none of these beneficial effects. Can someone please explain to me why we are giving women statin drugs, when calcium accomplishes the same thing and with the extra added benefits discussed in this chapter? (As we saw in Chapter 13, niacin also significantly elevates HDL, when given alone or with statins.)

Calcium's functions do not stop there. This mineral is used to activate the enzymes involved in fat and protein digestion and in the production of energy. It is involved in blood clotting and the transmission of nerve impulses. Calcium also regulates the contraction and relaxation of the muscles, including the heart. And it aids in the absorption of many nutrients, especially vitamin B_{12}.

RDIs, Deficiencies, and Factors that Influence Absorption

Although calcium intake is clearly a major factor in the development of the diseases of calcium deficiency—osteoporosis, osteomalacia, and rickets—it is not the only factor. There are many other circumstances that influence the absorption and utilization of the calcium you consume. These include other elements of the diet, exercise, and any medication taken.

Some studies have linked diets high in protein and fat—especially when the fat and protein come from foods of animal origin—with the loss of calcium from the bone. However, it is difficult to isolate other factors such as vitamin D, calcium, and phosphorus intake in these studies. Therefore, the results have been conflicting.

One important dietary element is phosphorus intake. Most researchers advise that the ratio of calcium to phosphorus should be at least 1 to 1. In other words, you should take in at least as much calcium as you do phosphorus. If phosphorus intake is much higher, it may impair the absorption of calcium, as well as increase the amount drawn out of the bone. So if your diet contains many phosphorus-rich foods such as meats, soft drinks, and food additives, your phosphorus intake may be too high to maintain a good calcium balance.

There's good evidence that an adequate amount of all the micronutrients can make a significant difference in the body's proper and efficient metabolism of calcium. One group of women was given a calcium and vitamin D supplement and experienced an improvement in bone density. The other group received a balanced supplement of calcium, vitamin D, and 100 percent of the RDA for over fifteen other vitamins and minerals. This group experienced a two to three times greater increase in bone density. A growing body of evidence seems to indicate that several trace minerals, including zinc, manganese, copper, and boron, and essential fatty acids, as well as vitamin D and the B vitamins, all play a role in preventing, halting, and reversing osteoporosis.

The RDI for calcium has been established at 1,000 milligrams for everyone over the age of four, except for pregnant or lactating women, for whom the RDI is 1,300 milligrams. However, research has shown that a large percentage of people develop osteoporosis even when their intake is at this level. This suggests that 1,000 milligrams may not be enough, especially during the early time in your life when you are developing peak bone mass and, for women, after menopause. In fact, the American Medical Association and many research scientists recommend at least 1,500 milligrams for postmenopausal women.

Interestingly enough, recent research has discovered that our ancient human ancestors who lived during the Paleolithic Age ingested approximately 1,600 milligrams of calcium per day, and some estimates go as high as 2,000 milligrams. Evolutionary theory suggests that we are genetically programmed to require a similar amount, yet today we get only a quarter to a third that amount, on average. The richest food source is milk and dairy products. Over three glasses of milk or the equivalent is needed to attain the RDI of 1,000 milligrams, but many people do not drink anywhere near this amount of milk every day. While the lactose in milk may increase calcium absorption, we are not sure whether lactose-intolerant people—who have trouble digesting milk—experience an impairment in calcium absorption. They are likely, however, to avoid milk products and so are at particularly high risk of calcium deficiency.

Twelve thousand years ago human bones were 17 percent denser than they are today. This in spite of the fact that they were not milk drinkers. By and large, they got their calcium from wild plants, not milk or animals. The wild plants gathered and eaten then were approximately four times higher in calcium than the cultivated cereal plants that now dominate our diet.

One study found that two-thirds of the women in America between the ages of eighteen and thirty—the period during which peak bone mass is developing—ingest less than the RDI. After the age of thirty-six, three-fourths have calcium intakes less than the RDI. Fully one-fourth of all American women ingest less than 300 milligrams on any given day. Further exacerbating the situation is that absorption of whatever calcium is in the diet begins to decrease during the ages of forty to fifty, and in some cases, perhaps as early as thirty. After menopause, estrogen levels decrease, an event that has also been implicated in bone loss. Estrogen therapy, which may have some disturbing side effects, is often prescribed in an attempt to prevent bone loss in postmenopausal women. In fact, estrogen therapy slows bone loss, at best. Many practitioners prefer calcium therapy over estrogen therapy, as calcium, when taken with other nutrients, appears to increase bone density.

I also advise my patients to get regular physical exercise, because studies have shown that physical exercise may improve calcium absorption and utilization and may therefore play a crucial role in the prevention and treatment of osteoporosis. Aerobic exercise and weight training have been shown to increase bone mass in athletes, in the elderly, and in people recovering from a decrease in bone mass that occurs during a decrease in physical activity. Loss of bone mass is most pronounced in people undergoing full bed rest, who lose 200 to 300 milligrams of calcium per day. A diet that is adequate for a healthy adult may not provide enough calcium to offset prior illness-related losses. Increasing the calcium intake alone during the illness will not offset these losses, either. However, resumed physical activity combined with adequate calcium intake will restore normal bone mass.

As mentioned earlier, another factor that can affect calcium absorption is any medication being taken. Among the many medications that can affect the absorption and utilization of calcium are antibiotics, oral contraceptives, anticonvulsants, and laxatives (for details, see the Drug-Nutrient Interaction Table on page 270.) When such medications are taken, calcium intake should be increased. While calcium should be taken when on tetracycline, it must be taken several hours before or after taking the medication. The same holds true for dairy products. Unfortunately, calcium can interfere with the effectiveness of tetracycline when taken at the same time.

Food Sources

Dairy foods such as milk, cheese, and yogurt are outstanding sources of calcium. If you do not consume such foods, it is extremely difficult to achieve a satisfactory intake of dietary calcium. In addition to its being a superb source of calcium, milk contains lactose, a substance that may increase the absorption of calcium in our bodies. Other foods that can make a substantial contribution include canned salmon and sardines (including the bones), and green leafy vegetables such as collard greens, turnip greens, and mustard greens. Clams, oysters, and shrimp are also good sources of calcium, followed by kale, broccoli, soybeans, and soybean products such as tofu.

It has been estimated that we actually absorb as little as 20 to 40 percent of the calcium in our food. Part of the problem may be oxalic acid, a substance found in spinach, Swiss chard, beet greens, cocoa, and rhubarb. This substance may bind with calcium to prevent its absorption in the colon. Phytic acid, or phytates—substances found in the outer layers of cereal grains—may also interfere with calcium absorption. However, the evidence is inconclusive, and many scientists discount it. In addition, the inhibitory effect of such substances appears to occur only when calcium intake is low and oxalic acid or phytate intake is quite high. In addition, the fermentation of yeast, as found in leavened bread, destroys much of the phytate in the flour. In fact, when vegetarians were studied, it was found that they have less incidence of osteoporosis than nonvegetarians. Since vegetarians as a group eat a diet high in phytates, it seems unlikely that calcium absorption is significantly affected by this substance.

Supplements

Calcium supplements are available as tablets, flavored chewable squares, and in liquid form. The supplements generally combine pure, or elemental, calcium with other chemicals or salts. The forms most commonly available are calcium aspartate, calcium carbonate, calcium citrate, calcium gluconate, and calcium lactate. When buying calcium supplements, remember to consider the amount of elemental calcium, not the amount of calcium salts. Of the three forms, calcium carbonate contains the greatest amount of elemental calcium: 40 percent. Many people prefer this form because the higher calcium content allows them to take fewer pills to obtain their Optimum Daily Intake. However, the other forms may have specific therapeutic value. Another factor to consider is absorbability. I generally recommend calcium carbonate and calcium lactate, since they appear to be generally absorbable. Calcium citrate or citrate-malate are the most absorbable, particularly in the elderly. Often, elderly individuals have low levels of hydrochloric acid in their stomachs, which is necessary for calcium absorption. Calcium citrate or citrate-malate requires little hydrochloric acid for absorption.

I advise you to take your calcium supplements along with magnesium and vitamin D, as these three nutrients work together to enhance one another's absorption and utilization in the body. Also, if calcium supplements are taken without magnesium, it may result in a magnesium deficiency—a deficiency that has been implicated in osteoporosis. The calcium-to-magnesium ratio should be approximately 2 to 1. Fortunately, there are now many supplements that contain calcium carbonate or calcium lactate and magnesium in the proper proportions. There are also supplements that combine calcium with vitamin D.

Dolomite is a supplement that contains both calcium and magnesium. However, because this product contains these minerals in their least absorbable form, I do not recommend its use. Bone meal, another source of calcium, is highly absorbable. However, this form contains substantial amounts of phosphorus, and most people get quite enough—and often too much—phosphorus from their diets.

Many antacids are being promoted as calcium supplements since these products contain calcium carbonate. However, some of these also contain aluminum, a toxic mineral that can interfere with calcium absorption and have many deleterious effects on the body. One study showed that these adverse effects include high levels of calcium excreted in the urine, bone resorption (loss of minerals from the bone), impaired fluoride absorption, and phosphorus depletion, all of which may ironically contribute to bone disease. If you choose to use antacids as your source of calcium, be sure to read the label to check that aluminum is not an ingredient.

Optimum Daily Intake—ODI

For optimum general health, the basic Optimum Daily Intake for calcium is:

1,000–1,500 mg for men and women

Based on a thorough scientific review of calcium, and on my clinical experience, the following amounts of calcium appear to be valuable for:

CONDITION	SUGGESTED DOSAGE
Broken bones and fractures	1,000–2,000 mg
High blood pressure	1,000–1,500 mg
Osteoporosis	1,200–2,000 mg
High LDL and/or low HDL	1,200–2000 mg

As mentioned, calcium should be taken with magnesium in a ratio of at least 2 to 1, and with vitamin D to aid in absorption. Since the body is unable to absorb 1,000 milligrams all at once, divide your total ODI into halves or thirds and take them two or three times a day. Bear in mind that the above doses include food sources.

Remember: If you have a medical condition, please consult with your physician before taking supplements.

Toxicity and Adverse Effects

Calcium has no known toxic effects. A panel of the Food and Drug Administration (FDA) concluded that calcium intakes of 1,000 to 2,500 milligrams daily do not result in hypercalcemia—high levels of calcium in the blood. Although hypercalcemia may be seen in certain medical conditions and in cases of vitamin D overdose, a high intake of calcium is not in itself a causative factor. The development of kidney stones in connection with high calcium intake is rare. One study demonstrated that calcium citrate does not cause kidney stones.

Some people report a feeling of relaxation and drowsiness after taking calcium supplements. This has never been documented in a scientific study. However, if you experience this particular effect, you can do what I suggest to my patients: Take advantage of the drowsiness by scheduling your calcium supplements in the evening before retiring.

22 | Phosphorus

PHOSPHORUS is the second most abundant mineral in the body, after calcium. There are approximately 600 to 700 grams of this mineral—1.25 to 1.5 pounds—in the average-size person, which represents about 1 percent of total body weight. As is the case with calcium, most of the body's phosphorus (80 to 90 percent) is found in the bones and teeth. The rest is distributed throughout the body in the cells and in the blood and other fluids. The ratio of calcium to phosphorus in the bone is about 2 to 1. However, in the soft tissues, the proportion of phosphorus is much higher.

Functions and Uses

First and foremost, phosphorus strengthens bones and teeth. But this mineral also plays a part in almost every important chemical reaction in the body. Most of its actions have to do with the utilization of fats, protein, and carbohydrates. One function is to combine with fats in the blood to make phospholipids, which, in turn, become the part of the cell that regulates the transport of materials in and out of the cell walls. Phosphorus is also involved in the transport of fats in the circulatory system.

Phosphorus is involved in energy metabolism, storage, and regulation. It also plays a role in such cellular processes as muscle contraction, the transfer of nerve impulses, hormone secretion, and protein synthesis. Additionally, it is a component of the nucleic acids—RNA and DNA—that control heredity and the replication of cells. Moreover, many of the B vitamins are effective only when combined with this mineral in the body. Finally, phosphorus plays an important part in our buffer system, which maintains the proper acid-base balance (pH) within the body.

RDIs and Deficiency Symptoms

Considering the many ways in which phosphorus is used within the body, it is fortunate that most people have no trouble getting more than the Reference Daily Intake of 1,000 milligrams for men and women, and 1,300 milligrams for pregnant and lactating women. Although there is some evidence that phytates—substances found in whole grains—interfere with the absorption of essential minerals, there is doubt as to whether this occurs on a large enough scale to be of practical importance. Although long-term phytate consumption has not been specifically investigated, vegetarians, who consume a high-fiber diet rich in phytates, have not been found to be deficient in phosphorus. The long-term use of aluminum-containing antacids, however, may deplete the body of phosphorus to such a degree that deficiency is a real possibility. Symptoms of phosphorus deficiency include weakness, loss of appetite, loss of bone mass, and loss of calcium.

The actual absorption, storage, and excretion of phosphorus is dependent on mechanisms involving vitamin D and parathyroid hormone. Like calcium, phosphorus exists in a complex give-and-take relationship between the bones, blood, and soft tissues of the body. It is continuously being deposited and released from the bone bank as blood levels fluctuate in response to dietary intake and excretion. In addition, phosphorus levels and calcium levels influence each other. It has been suggested that phosphorus and calcium intake should be approximately equal—in a ratio of 1 to 1—even though the ratio in bone is 2 to 1. However, excess phosphorus consumption is common, with an average daily intake of 1,500 to 1,600 milligrams. This means that in most diets, phosphorus intake exceeds calcium intake. A convincing body of evidence suggests that this overly high phosphorus intake, coupled with long-term low calcium intake and high protein intake, is a major dietary factor in the demineralization that leads to osteoporosis. For instance, in a study of female athletes, those who drank carbonated beverages—which are rich in phosphorus—

had more than twice as many fractures as did those who did not include high-phosphorus beverages in their diet (see Chapter 21 for more information on calcium and osteoporosis).

Food Sources

Phosphorus is found in nearly all foods, but is especially high in carbonated soft drinks, milk and other dairy products, meat, and fish. Nuts, beans, and grains are also high in phosphorus.

Supplements

Rather than adding phosphorus supplements to their diet, most people appear to require a reduction of phosphorus. Foods that are particularly high in phosphorus include meat and carbonated beverages. Traditionally, a calcium-to-phosphorus ratio of 1 to 1 is recommended. However, as a general rule, a higher percentage of phosphorus (70 percent) than calcium (40 percent) is absorbed from the diet. In addition, the calcium-to-phosphorus ratio in the bone is 2 to 1. Bearing this in mind, you may want to manipulate the ratio slightly in favor of calcium to maintain a more favorable balance in the body.

Optimum Daily Intake—ODI

For optimum general health, the Optimum Daily Intake for most people can usually be met through dietary sources. Possible exceptions may include the elderly, menopausal women, and individuals on restricted diets. For this population, the ODIs are:

200–400 mg for men and women

Remember: If you have a medical condition, please consult with your physician before taking supplements.

Toxicity and Adverse Effects

Too much phosphorus may lead to an increase in the excretion of calcium, and, consequently, to osteoporosis.

23 | Magnesium

Your body contains between 20 and 28 grams of magnesium. Half of this amount is found in the bones. The remainder activates hundreds of enzymes throughout the body and is critical for proper cell function.

Functions and Uses

BONES AND TEETH

Like calcium and phosphorus, magnesium is required for strong, healthy bones and teeth. This mineral plays an important part in bone growth and helps prevent tooth decay by holding calcium in tooth enamel. Understandably, poor magnesium intake has been implicated in bone disorders such as osteoporosis.

MUSCLES

One of magnesium's most important roles is that of helping the muscles to relax. When calcium flows into muscle tissue cells, the muscle contracts. When calcium leaves and magnesium replaces it, the muscle relaxes. These functions are no doubt related to the association of magnesium deficiency with the occurrence of muscle spasms, tremors, and convulsions. Many professionals now successfully use magnesium malate supplements—a combination of magnesium and malic acid—in the treatment of fibromyalgia, a disorder characterized by many tender points in the muscles; and in the treatment of chronic fatigue, which may also involve muscle aches and pains.

PSYCHIATRIC DISORDERS

Low magnesium appears to be associated with psychiatric problems. In a study of 165 boys, it was found that those with symptoms of depression, schizophrenia, and sleep disturbances had lower levels of magnesium in the blood than did boys without these disorders. In another study, it was found that the average magnesium levels of autistic children were also well below average. In fact, there is some evidence that autistic children may improve when given large doses of magnesium along with vitamin B_6.

In adults, insufficient magnesium may be accompanied by a loss of sensation in the extremities and, if severe, tremors, convulsions, muscle contractions, confusion, delirium, and behavioral disturbances. One study found that psychiatric patients who had attempted suicide had lower magnesium levels than did nonsuicidal psychiatric patients and healthy individuals.

CARDIOVASCULAR DISEASE

Magnesium—along with sodium, potassium, and calcium—appears to affect the muscle tone of the blood vessels, which may explain why magnesium supplementation has been shown to help control cardiovascular disease. For example, research indicates that magnesium supplementation is effective in lowering some types of high blood pressure in individuals with low magnesium levels. In addition, research has shown that people suffering from angina, which can be caused by a spasm of the blood vessel leading to the heart, are benefited by magnesium supplementation. People with high blood pressure often experience spasms in the blood vessels of the retina, which can eventually affect vision. In studies, these people, who tend to have low levels of magnesium, have experienced a regression of this disease when taking magnesium supplements. Diabetes is another disease that can damage the blood vessels of the retina, possibly leading to severe vision problems and even blindness. Again, there is evidence that low levels of magnesium may be an additional risk factor in the development and progression of this complication.

In several studies, magnesium supplementation has improved the balance of lipids (fats) in the blood. Yet, treatment with two lipid-lowering drugs (gemfibrozil and simvastatin) decreased blood levels of magnesium in diabetics. This in turn affected their glucose levels and, one could theorize, compromised the beneficial lipid-lowering effects of the drugs.

MENSTRUAL PROBLEMS

Several studies suggest that magnesium supplements may be useful in treating menstrual problems. In one study, magnesium supplementation decreased lower back pain, lower abdominal pain, and lost days from work. In another, magnesium and vitamin B_6 together reduced the intensity and duration of menstrual cramps, and symptoms continued to improve over a four to six month period. In another study twenty-one out of twenty-five women given magnesium experienced reduced menstrual symptoms, compared with twenty-five women who did not get the supplement. The authors of this study suggest these improvements may be due to the dramatic drop in the blood levels of a certain prostaglandin as a result of the magnesium therapy, as well as magnesium's well-known ability to relax muscle spasms and dilate blood vessels.

OTHER FUNCTIONS

Magnesium has many functions other than those just discussed. For instance, magnesium plays an important role in maintaining the function of the nerves. It also stabilizes the enzymes that produce cellular energy and thus is involved in energy regulation and metabolism. It also plays a role in proper insulin production. Finally, this nutrient may prove useful in preventing certain complications of pregnancy, such as prematurity and intrauterine growth retardation.

RDIs and Deficiencies

Since magnesium is widely distributed in foods, severe deficiencies are most often found in those whose food intake is low or imbalanced, such as alcoholics and diabetics. However, many other groups of people may be at risk. It has been estimated that as much as 60 percent of the United States population is at risk for magnesium deficiency. For instance, people using a number of drugs, including antibiotics and diuretics, may have depleted magnesium. Oral contraceptives, too, have been found to lower blood magnesium. Since low magnesium levels result in blood clots, this may help explain why there is a higher incidence of thrombosis among women on the pill. (For more information on the effect of drugs on magnesium levels, see the Drug-Nutrient Interaction Table on page 270.) In addition, magnesium may be too low in people with malabsorption syndromes or gastrointestinal disorders such as Crohn's disease. We are also beginning to recognize that bulimics are at risk because of their prolonged diarrhea and/or vomiting. Stress has also been implicated in depleted magnesium levels, which may account for the typical Type A personality's increased risk for cardiovascular disease. One study suggested that stress may also be in part responsible for the lowered magnesium levels in women with premenstrual tension.

The RDI for magnesium is 400 milligrams for men and women, and 450 milligrams for pregnant and lactating women.

Food Sources

Magnesium is widely distributed in foods. Those foods with the highest magnesium content include milk and other dairy products, meat, seafood, nuts, blackstrap molasses, soybeans, seeds, and wheat germ. Whole grains such as oatmeal, cornmeal, and rice are also good sources.

Bear in mind, however, that the magnesium content of food varies considerably with the magnesium content of the soil in which the food is grown. In addition, much of the magnesium in food is lost during processing. For example, milling removes 59 percent of the magnesium from whole wheat. Cooking foods in water also causes this mineral to leach out.

Supplements

The potency of magnesium supplements is determined by the amount of elemental magnesium. I recommend taking magnesium supplements as either magnesium carbonate or magnesium oxide, as these forms have the greatest potency. Magnesium oxide contains the greatest percentage of magnesium—60 percent—while magnesium carbonate is 40 percent magnesium. Other forms of magnesium, such as chelated magnesium, which is bound to amino acids; magnesium citrate; magnesium malate; and magnesium aspartate, are also available. Many practitioners prefer these forms in specific therapeutic regimens. Although they provide less magnesium per tablet or capsule than do magnesium oxide and magnesium carbonate, these forms do contain compounds that appear to have their own beneficial effects. Citrate, for example, is important for energy production. In addition, the magnesium in these supplements may be more bioavailable than that in the higher-magnesium products.

Magnesium works together with other nutrients, such as calcium and vitamin D. As explained in Chapter 21, calcium and magnesium supplements should be taken together. The consensus is that the calcium-to-magnesium ratio should be about 2 to 1, which is what I usually recommend. There are supplements that contain both calcium and magnesium in this ratio. While practitioners have reported success using a ratio that is closer to 1 to 1, studies supporting this ratio are lacking at this time. Many people compromise by taking calcium and magnesium in a ratio of 2 to 1.5

Optimum Daily Intake—ODI

For optimum health, the basic Optimum Daily Intake for magnesium is:

500–750 mg for men and women

Based on a thorough scientific review of magnesium, and on my clinical experience, the following amounts of magnesium appear to be valuable for:

CONDITION	SUGGESTED DOSAGE
Angina	500–1,000 mg
Fibromyalgia and chronic fatigue	6–12 tablets of magnesium malate*
High blood pressure	500–750 mg
Oral contraceptive use	500–750 mg
Osteoporosis	500–1,000 mg
Menstrual problems	500–750 mg

*Six tablets supply approximately 300 milligrams of magnesium and 1,200 milligrams of malic acid.

Remember: If you have a medical condition, please consult your physician before taking supplements.

Toxicity and Adverse Effects

Magnesium toxicity is rare, except in individuals with kidney failure. In healthy individuals, large amounts of magnesium salts—3,000 to 5,000 milligrams daily—have a cathartic effect, and magnesium-containing products are often used as over-the-counter laxatives. These products, which include Epsom salts (magnesium sulfate), milk of magnesia (magnesium hydroxide), and magnesium citrate, work by drawing fluid into the intestines and thereby stimulating contractions. Toxicity symptoms have been noted in subjects treated with 9,000 milligrams of this mineral.

24 | Zinc

OUR BODIES contain approximately 2 to 3 grams of zinc, which is distributed throughout the body. Zinc is an essential component of over twenty enzymes associated with many different metabolic processes. The highest concentrations of zinc are found in the eyes, liver, bones, prostate, semen, and hair.

Functions and Uses

GROWTH AND REPRODUCTION

Perhaps the most critical role zinc plays is in the synthesis of the nucleic acids RNA and DNA, which are essential for cell division, cell repair, and cell growth. Thus, zinc is needed for reproduction and for growth and development. Several studies have linked low zinc levels with complications during pregnancy, including miscarriage and birth defects.

Studies have also found large percentages of children to be deficient in zinc. These children showed symptoms of suboptimal growth, in addition to a loss of taste acuity and poor appetite. When their zinc intake was increased, the symptoms improved. Animal studies and human studies of children and adults suggest that lethargy, passivity, and apathy are symptoms of marginal zinc deficiency, since these behavioral problems improve with zinc supplementation.

VISION

One of the highest concentrations of zinc in the human body is found in the eye, especially the iris and retina. Although the exact mechanisms of its functions are largely unknown, zinc seems to be involved in the activation of vitamin A, and thus is a factor in night vision. It is also an antioxidant and may protect vision by reducing damage from free radicals. Zinc deficiency may be contributing to the development or progression of chronic eye diseases, such as macular degeneration, the major cause of vision loss among older people. In one study, the risk of vision loss was reduced by 10 percent in people taking supplements of 80 milligrams of zinc and 2 milligrams of copper. In addition, there is a growing body of evidence that indicates that poor zinc intake is related to such eye conditions as impaired color discrimination; cataract formation; and optic neuritis, the inflammation of the optic nerve.

PHYSICAL AND MENTAL STRESS

There is some evidence that zinc levels fall following physical and mental stress. For instance, strenuous exercise has been shown to lead to significant losses of zinc, probably due to the increase in glucose metabolism, which requires zinc. According to one estimate, up to 90 percent of athletes may not be getting enough zinc. It has also been discovered that zinc is depleted during upper respiratory infection accompanied by fever. In addition, severe burn victims have only two-thirds the normal amount of zinc in their blood. Studies have shown that zinc supplements may have therapeutic value in cases of physical stress. When hospital patients who were marginally deficient in zinc were given extra zinc, it helped restore the rate of healing to normal. Zinc may therefore be of benefit to people who have undergone surgery or have sustained broken bones or wounds. Some physicians prescribe zinc to stimulate the healing process.

TASTE AND SMELL

Zinc is especially important in body systems that undergo a rapid turnover of cells. This includes the gastrointestinal system, and particularly the taste buds—a fact that may explain why a change in the ability to taste foods is often an early sign of zinc deficiency. This symptom may be accompanied by similar changes in the ability to smell. Foods may either have no taste or smell at all, or taste or smell unpleasant. All these factors contribute to a loss of appetite, but may be so insidious that they go unnoticed. Many of my elderly patients report a heightened sense of taste after a few weeks of zinc supplementation. They often find this development quite remarkable, since prior to supplementation, they may not have recognized the loss of taste sensitivity. The elderly may benefit from zinc supplementation in another way, too, as zinc appears to play a role in increasing bone density in postmenopausal women.

THE IMMUNE SYSTEM

Zinc may exert a protective influence by boosting the immune system. Many studies have shown that a zinc deficiency can impair a large variety of immune functions and defense mechanisms in animals, and some studies have shown similar effects in humans. These effects—which include abnormalities and eventual shrinking of the spleen, thymus, and lymph nodes; and impaired production of antibodies—have been found to be correctable with zinc supplementation.

Low zinc levels, often accompanied by high copper levels, have been reported in people with many types of cancer. We've known since 1981 that people with a certain type of lung cancer survived for a significantly longer period of time when they had high levels of zinc in their blood. It's not surprising that low levels of zinc are also found in people with AIDS. Diabetics tend to have less zinc in their tissues and this may be related to many of their complications. Zinc deficiency may be related to the body's inability to produce the enzymes used in glucose metabolism, insulin resistance, immune problems, loss of ability to taste, and conditions related to oxidative stress.

Since the beneficial effects of zinc on immunity are so well documented, and the therapy is nontoxic and inexpensive, some researchers suggest further studies involving immune deficiency diseases. Many of my patients who get frequent colds and sore throats have shown a marked decrease in these outbreaks with zinc supplementation.

DIABETES

Diabetics tend to have less zinc in their tissues and this may be related to many of their complications. Zinc deficiency may be related to the body's inability to produce the enzymes used in glucose metabolism, insulin resistance, immune problems, loss of ability to taste, and conditions related to oxidative stress.

ANOREXIA NERVOSA

Many studies suggest that there is a relationship between zinc depletion and anorexia nervosa. Researchers theorize that inadequate levels of zinc might somehow help trigger the development of this disease, which further depletes zinc levels, which further worsens disease symptoms, and so on, in a vicious cycle. My anorexia patients, as well as those of other practitioners, have improved with zinc supplementation, indicating that zinc may be helpful both in the treatment and in the prevention of this serious disease.

HORMONE LEVELS

Zinc has been shown to inhibit the production of prolactin, a pituitary hormone, and so is used therapeutically in men and women with abnormally high prolactin levels. Elevated prolactin levels can lead to distressing effects such as secretion of breast milk, enlarged breasts, sexual dysfunction, and breast cancer.

THE PROSTATE GLAND

The prostate gland has one of the highest concentrations of zinc in the body. In general, low levels of zinc in the prostate appear to be associated with diseases of the gland. Zinc supplementation has been shown to reduce the size of the prostate and symptoms of benign prostatic hypertrophy (BPH) in the majority of patients. Zinc also inhibits the binding of androgens to receptors in the prostate gland, an action that may play a role in the prevention of prostate cancer and other diseases of the prostate gland.

OTHER PROTECTIVE FUNCTIONS

Aside from its support of the immune system, zinc may protect the body in a variety of other ways. For instance, zinc has been shown to protect the liver from damage due to poisoning from the common cleaning solvent carbon tetrachloride. Zinc is also known to prevent the absorption of lead and cadmium, which we may be exposed to through our drinking water, car and bus exhaust fumes, and many other environmental factors. Through its influence on cell membrane stability, zinc may even help protect us from substances known to contribute to cancer, heart disease, and a variety of other disorders. Zinc is an essential component of superoxide dismutase (SOD), an antioxidant made by the body to combat free radicals.

RDIs and Deficiency Symptoms

Despite the fact that zinc is so necessary, there are no true storage depots for this mineral. Although relatively large amounts are found in the bone, along with other minerals, it does not appear that this zinc is readily available to the body. Instead, the body is dependent upon a continual external supply, as the relatively small body pool of biologically available zinc appears to be used rather rapidly. Therefore, deficiency signs tend to appear quite soon after depletion. It is now recognized that subclinical zinc deficiency may manifest itself as impaired ability to heal, impaired acuity of taste and smell, loss of appetite, and impaired night vision. Prolonged zinc deficiency may result in failure to grow, mental disturbances, lethargy, skin changes, and susceptibility to frequent infections. Testicular function may also be adversely affected. This is probably the origin of the oyster's reputation as an aphrodisiac, as oysters have a high zinc content.

The RDI for zinc is 15 milligrams for all men and women. In spite of its importance and seemingly wide availability in food, evidence indicates that many people do not get enough zinc from their diets. Marginally low intakes are common in large areas of the country because the soil is deficient in this mineral. (In fact, at one time, many farm animals were found to be deficient in this mineral, and they now receive zinc-enriched feed.) A 1979 study detected an average intake of 8.6 milligrams per day for humans, or just over half the RDI. In another survey, the zinc intake of elderly people was on the average less than half the RDI, indicating that this group is particularly at risk. It is worthwhile noting that the people in this survey suffered from the loss of taste sensitivity so common in this age group. In another study of the elderly, it was found that senile purpura—purple spots under the skin caused by bleeding—may also be due to a zinc deficiency. Indeed, zinc is used, both orally and topically, in the treatment of many skin conditions, including folliculitis (inflammation of the hair follicles); acrodermatitis enteropathica (a severe genetic skin disorder); acne vulgaris (common adolescent acne); alopecia areata (a usually temporary form of hair loss); and leg ulcers.

Certain individuals are unable to absorb zinc, or absorb the mineral only poorly, and thus are at risk for zinc deficiency. These include babies with the hereditary disease acrodermatitis enteropathica, mentioned above; as well as people with malabsorption syndromes such as Crohn's disease, celiac disease, and short bowel syndrome. Also at risk are people with chronic kidney disease, sickle cell anemia, cystic fibrosis, pancreatic insufficiency, and other chronically debilitating disorders. These individuals may have subtle signs of zinc deficiency, including loss of appetite, impaired night vision, and depressed immune and mental functions. In one study, patients with highly active Crohn's disease had only 60 percent of the normal blood level of zinc.

Several drugs have been found to interfere with zinc absorption and metabolism. These include such commonly used substances as alcohol, diuretics, and oral contraceptives.

The dip of zinc levels associated with the use of oral contraceptives is probably the result of the drugs' hormone content, as zinc levels are also lower during pregnancy. In addition, the use of oral contraceptives has been found to reduce folic acid levels in some women, and so often leads to folic acid supplementation. Unfortunately, in large doses, folic acid has been found to lower zinc concentrations in the blood, which may make these women particularly prone to zinc deficiency.

Research on the use of diuretics for hypertension suggests that some unexplained side effects of the drugs may be the result of zinc depletion, rather than the drugs themselves. Impotency, for example, appears to be connected to low zinc levels. The association of diuretic therapy with zinc deficiency may have important implications for patients who suffer heart attacks, as the deficiency may retard the healing of the injured heart.

The water you drink may also affect zinc levels. Excessive copper intake, commonly resulting from copper pipes, worsens an already existing zinc deficiency. In addition, there is some evidence that the calcium bicarbonate found in hard tap water may interfere with zinc absorption and utilization.

Food Sources

Although some zinc is found in nearly all foods, the mineral is especially plentiful in meats, poultry (particularly dark meat), fish and other seafood (oysters are notably high), liver, eggs, legumes such as peanuts, and whole grains. Approximately 73 percent of the zinc is removed from whole grains during the milling process that produces white flour. The flour is then enriched, a process that replaces several vitamins and iron, but not zinc.

The biological availability of zinc in different foods varies. It is estimated that as little as 40 percent of dietary zinc is actually absorbed. Some studies have suggested that the zinc in meats and seafood is better absorbed than the zinc in grains. Zinc deficiency is known to occur in populations whose zinc intake is far in excess of the RDI, but is derived solely from grain sources. This has led to the concern that vegetarians may need a higher intake of zinc. However, when vegetarians were recently studied, it was found that they had adequate zinc levels. It may be that the soybean products popular in vegetarian cuisine help supply the extra zinc and enhance its absorption.

Supplements

Zinc is available as individual supplements and as part of many multivitamin and multimineral formulas. In supplements, pure or elemental zinc is combined with other compounds. Of these, I feel that zinc gluconate and zinc citrate, which are sometimes referred to as chelated zinc, are the best choices for most people, as they are relatively inexpensive and well tolerated. Zinc sulfate is the least expensive, but can be very irritating to the stomach. Many practitioners use other forms of zinc, such as zinc picolinate and zinc orotate, because they believe they are the most absorbable forms or have experienced better clinical outcomes. Unfortunately, there is still no scientific data comparing the absorbability of different forms of zinc.

Since zinc supplements combine elemental or pure zinc with another compound, when buying supplements you must consider the amount of elemental zinc, which is commonly listed on the product label. For example, 80 milligrams of zinc gluconate usually contain 10 milligrams of elemental zinc, and 220 milligrams of zinc sulfate supply 50 milligrams of elemental zinc.

Optimum Daily Intake—ODI

For optimum general health, the basic Optimum Daily Intake for zinc is:

22.5–50 mg for men and women

Based on a thorough scientific review of zinc, and on my clinical experience, the following amounts of zinc appear to be valuable for:

CONDITION	SUGGESTED DOSAGE
Decreased sense of taste and smell	30–50 mg
Enhanced immunity	30–50 mg
Enhanced wound healing	30–50 mg
Poor night vision	30–50 mg
Prostatitis	30–50 mg (up to 100 mg under professional advice)
Diabetes	25–50 mg
Skin problems	22.5–50 mg

Higher doses of zinc (above 50 mg per day) should be taken only under profesional advice.

Remember: If you have a medical condition, please consult with your physician before taking supplements.

Toxicity and Adverse Effects

The symptoms of zinc toxicity are gastrointestinal irritation and vomiting. Zinc is actually recognized as an emetic—a substance that induces vomiting. However, this form of toxicity occurs only when 2,000 milligrams or more have been ingested. Studies have shown that even when up to ten times the RDA of 15 milligrams is given for prolonged periods of time, there are no adverse reactions.

There is some evidence that an excessive intake of zinc—more than 50 milligrams per day taken for an extended period of time—may lower copper levels and aggravate a marginal copper deficiency. This may, in fact, be a beneficial, rather than adverse, effect for some people. Although copper is an essential nutrient, there are people with copper levels that are far too high for optimum health. In fact, high-level zinc supplementation has been used therapeutically to treat Wilson's disease, a potentially fatal disorder characterized by excessive copper accumulation in tissues. Nevertheless, researchers recommend that patients on long-term zinc supplementation of more than 50 milligrams a day have their copper levels, lipids, and immune function monitored.

Short-term experiments suggest that 150 milligrams of zinc twice a day decrease levels of high-density lipoproteins (HDLs, or good cholesterol) and raise levels of low-density lipoproteins (LDLs, or bad cholesterol) and/or serum cholesterol, causing a less desirable ratio. However, studies are needed to assess long-term effects. The results of another study, using 50 milligrams of zinc per day, showed the opposite effect: HDL cholesterol increased and overall cholesterol decreased. In addition, diastolic blood pressure decreased.

25 | Iron

E VERY CELL in the body contains and requires iron, a mineral that is needed for all body functions. Thus, iron stores are carefully guarded by the body and, when depleted, cause diverse symptoms.

Functions and Uses

OXYGEN TRANSPORT AND STORAGE

Approximately 75 percent of the body's iron is found in our red blood cells in the form of hemoglobin, a protein-iron compound responsible for carrying oxygen from our lungs to all of the parts of our body. About 5 percent of our iron is found in a substance called myoglobin. This protein, a form of hemoglobin that is found in the muscles, carries and stores oxygen for the muscles. The iron helps hemoglobin and myoglobin to carry and hold the oxygen, and then release it for use by every cell in the body.

ENERGY PRODUCTION

Iron is present in a variety of enzymes—catalysts that help chemical changes take place throughout the body. Many of the iron-containing enzymes are involved in the production of energy.

THE IMMUNE SYSTEM

Iron is also of key importance in maintaining many of the functions of our immune system. While either too much or too little of the mineral may create problems, most problems are due to a deficiency.

HEART DISEASE

Studies have shown that high blood levels of iron along with other markers of iron nutriture that are elevated may be risk factors for heart disease. Everyone should have these levels monitored by a professional.

RDIs and Deficiency Symptoms

The major deficiency disease for iron is hypochromic microcytic anemia, often called iron deficiency anemia. In this form of anemia, the red blood cells are smaller than normal and pale in color due to low amounts of hemoglobin. Because of the low hemoglobin content of the blood, the tissues of the body become oxygen-starved, leading to symptoms such as listlessness, fatigue, irritability, difficulty swallowing, paleness, heart palpitations during exertion, and a general lack of well-being.

However, because the symptoms of anemia appear only after all the body's stores of iron have been depleted, the usual tests for anemia are an unsatisfactory means of detecting iron depletion. Moreover, numerous studies have shown that even in the absence of anemia, iron deficiency may have a detrimental effect on learning ability, endurance, and general well-being. For example, when chronically fatigued women were studied, the researchers concluded that some of these women might have been suffering from iron deficiency, even though their hemoglobin was in the accepted range. Apparently, their normal range for hemoglobin was higher than average. In other studies, women who were clearly iron deficient and women who had low to normal hemoglobin levels were found to have a low tolerance for cold, which improved when they received iron supplements. Runners who are iron deficient but nonanemic have been found to have less endurance. When college students were studied, it was found that low iron may play a part in faulty attention spans. Another study indicated that iron supplementation of iron-deficient children improves their ability to learn. Finally, both infants with anemia and infants with signs of iron deficiency but no anemia have shown significant improvement in mental development scores when supplemented with iron.

Because iron plays a role in immune system function, other deficiency symptoms include increased susceptibility to infection, reduced white blood cell counts, and impaired antibody production. Other widely diverse signs of possible iron deficiency are becoming increasingly recognized. Angular cheilosis, an inflammation of the corners of the mouth, has most frequently been seen in vitamin B deficiencies. However, according to one report, iron deficiency was present in a much higher percentage of sufferers. Animal experiments suggest that iron deficiency may contribute to high levels of fat in the blood and liver. In addition, new data indicates that a craving for salt may be a sign of iron deficiency.

Of all the nutrient allowances, the allowance for iron is the most difficult to obtain from dietary sources. This is why iron deficiency is the most common single nutrient deficiency in the world. Vast numbers of individuals become deficient in iron at some time in their lives, and large segments of the population are chronically deficient.

While iron deficiency is far from uncommon in men, children, and the elderly, the highest risk category is menstruating women. Healthy men have an iron reserve of 1,000 milligrams, and lose an average of 1 milligram of iron per day. In menstruating women, the iron reserve is not more than 200 to 400 milligrams. These women lose an average of 1.5 milligrams per day, and sometimes as much as 2.4 milligrams per day. In a study of female college students, only six of the seventy-four women studied—about 12 percent—were getting the RDA for iron. Other surveys have shown that 10 to 30 percent of women have iron deficits. In 2001, a national survey found that in 5,300 children six to sixteen years of age, iron deficiency was most common in girls (nearly 9 percent), and iron deficient children were more than twice as likely to have below average math scores than children with normal iron levels. The RDI for iron is 18 milligrams for all men and women. Yet women and girls have lower caloric requirements and consequently cannot meet their needs even when they follow a diet of carefully selected foods.

Pregnant women are at particularly high risk for low iron, with deficiencies as high as 60 percent. I usually recommend supplements for these women because their needs cannot be met by the average diet. Often, they had a marginal iron intake before becoming pregnant. Therefore, their iron stores are below optimum, putting them and their babies at risk.

Some researchers have expressed concern that vegetarian women may be at an even higher risk for low iron intake than nonvegetarians. Based on an actual analysis of their diet, the average intake is 11 to 14 milligrams per day for lacto-ovo vegetarian women. Although this is below the RDI, nonvegetarian women appear to have similarly low intakes.

Even when iron intake is sufficient, various factors can affect iron absorption. Low stomach acid, removal of part of the stomach, and malabsorption syndromes have all been shown to reduce iron absorption. In addition, calcium phosphate salts, tannic acid in tea, and antacids tend to interfere with absorption. Phytates, a substance found in whole grains, may interfere with iron absorption, too. However, the evidence for this is inconclusive.

Food Sources

Foods that are highest in iron are meat (especially liver), poultry, and fish. Other substantial sources are eggs, breads and cereals (either whole grain or iron-enriched), leafy vegetables, potatoes and other vegetables, fruit, and milk.

The absorbability of iron from foods varies widely. The organic iron found in red meats is the most absorbable (10 to 30 percent). Plants contain inorganic iron, only 2 to 10 percent of which is absorbed by our digestive tracts. In addition, large quantities of iron are lost from food that is cooked in water. However, when you cook acidic foods in cast-iron cookware, iron from the cookware leaches out into the foods, increasing its iron content considerably. Vitamin C also enhances the absorbability of iron in nonanimal foods and prevents it from being converted into its unstable form, which may cause oxidative stress and cell damage from free radicals.

Supplements

Iron is available as an individual supplement and as part of many vitamin-mineral formulas. The most common form is iron sulfate, which is very inexpensive and can be irritating to the digestive tract. I recommend iron glycinate, iron fumarate, and iron gluconate, since they are less irritating to the digestive tract and less likely to cause constipation. As when buying other minerals, look for the elemental content when choosing an iron supplement.

Optimum Daily Intake—ODI

For optimum general health, the basic Optimum Daily Intake for iron is:

15–25 mg for men
18–30 mg for women

Based on a thorough scientific review of iron, and on my clinical experience, the following amounts of iron appear to be valuable for:

CONDITION	SUGGESTED DOSAGE
Chronic fatigue	15–20 mg
Iron deficiency anemia	20–30 mg
Poor attention span	15–20 mg

Remember: If you have a medical condition, please consult your physician before taking supplements.

Anemia due to iron deficiency will respond fairly rapidly to supplementation. Nevertheless, supplements should be continued for several months to fully replenish the body's stores. You should be aware that anemia may also be due to a vitamin B_{12} or folic acid deficiency (see Chapters 15 and 16 for details). Other possible causes of anemia are internal bleeding, the adverse effects of certain drugs, and the presence of toxins in the body. There is also a condition called sports anemia. Not a true anemia, this problem is due to abnormal destruction of red blood cells through mechanical injury, rather than inadequate iron intake. Thus, routine iron supplementation is not justified. Be sure to consult with your doctor if you show signs of anemia.

Toxicity and Adverse Effects

The toxicity of iron is low, and harmful effects of daily intakes of up to 75 milligrams per day are unlikely in healthy individuals. The body has a highly effective mechanism that prevents an overload of iron from entering it and causing toxicity. The amount of iron the body absorbs is carefully regulated by the intestines according to the body's needs. The greater the need, the higher the rate of absorption. Growing children, pregnant women, and anemic individuals have higher rates of absorption. When a deficiency occurs, the rate of absorption increases to two to three times higher than normal. Unfortunately, this response does not appear to be sufficient to prevent anemia in iron-deficient subjects who are only mildly anemic and whose iron intake is marginal.

There have been conflicting scientific reports concerning iron and the risk of coronary heart disease. Some studies have shown that high iron levels and other markers of iron status in the blood appear to increase the risk of heart disease, while other studies have failed to confirm these findings. Some studies have demonstrated that high levels of serum ferritin (a complex in which iron is stored in the tissues) or of total iron-binding capacity (TIBC) appear to increase the risk of heart disease, while other studies have failed to confirm these findings, as well. Iron-related oxidative stress may also increase free radical damage to our DNA and hence increase the risk of cancer. The strongest evidence is for colorectal cancer, but again studies are conflicting. What does all this mean?

We know that antioxidants are our natural defense against free radical oxidative stress, and that iron is a very powerful pro-oxidant—an initiator of oxidative stress (for more information about oxidative stress, see Chapter 3). The discrepancies in the study findings may be the result of the balance of antioxidants and iron. Even though iron is essential to the functioning of our bodies, too much iron combined with poor antioxidant defense, due to poor intake of antioxidants, would put anyone at high risk for increased oxidative stress, which is believed to be a culprit in heart disease and cancer. Since we can easily measure iron, TIBC, and ferritin levels in our blood, these levels should routinely be screened during physical exams. If high levels are present, a reduction of iron intake should be discussed with your physician. Current research supports taking iron supplements above the RDI only if necessary. Patients with inflammatory bowel disorders such as Crohn's disease and ulcerative colitis should not take iron supplements unless under professional advice.

In some cases, a dangerous condition known as hemochromatosis can cause the excessive absorption of iron. This results in a build-up of excess iron in the tissues of many organs, possibly leading to damage to the liver, heart, pancreas, and other organs. In genetic hemochromatosis, there is inappropriately high absorption of dietary iron from birth. Acquired hemochromatosis may occur as a result of transfusions, medical conditions, or excessive long-term iron intake. This condition, too, can easily be detected through blood tests. If the tests confirm the condition, steps should be taken to avoid iron in food and supplements and to avoid foods cooked in cast iron cookware or stored in metal cans.

26 | Copper

T HE BODY CONTAINS about 100 to 150 milligrams of copper. It is stored in the liver, brain, heart, and kidneys and is found in the hair.

Functions and Uses

Copper helps your body absorb and use iron to synthesize hemoglobin. It also plays a role in maintaining the integrity of myelin, the fatty substance that is a constituent of the covering of some nerves. Copper is needed for taste sensitivity; the maturation of collagen, a component of connective tissue, bone, cartilage, and skin; the formation of elastin, a protein that forms certain tissues; and bone development. It is also an important part of a number of enzymes required for energy production; the oxidation of fatty acids; and the formation of melanin, a skin pigment. Copper is also involved in the metabolism of ascorbic acid. And copper plays a role in the immune system. It is, in fact, an essential component of superoxide dismutase (SOD), an antioxidant made by the body to combat free radicals. This function may explain the association between copper and blood levels of homocysteine, an excess of which is related to many conditions, including heart disease and cancer. Experimentally induced copper deficiencies or excesses have each been reported to increase the severity of a wide variety of infections in laboratory animals.

Drugs containing copper complexes have been shown to be effective in combating many inflammatory diseases, including rheumatoid arthritis, osteoarthritis, ankylosing spondylitis, rheumatic fever, and sciatica. Copper-containing drugs are also used in the treatment of ulcers, convulsions, chorea, cancer, and diabetes. It is thought that the drugs' positive effects are due to the copper complexes' ability to facilitate or promote tissue repair processes that use copper-dependent enzymes.

While human copper deficiency is not a common problem, abnormally high blood copper levels are often seen in people with viral infections, rheumatoid arthritis, rheumatic fever, lupus erythematosus, myocardial infarction, leukemia, and certain cancers, although the causes for the increased levels of copper are unexplained. It may be that excess copper plays a role in the development and progression of these diseases, or it may be that the body is circulating more copper in an attempt to deal with the diseases. When experimental animals were given oral contraceptives, their blood copper levels were significantly elevated. Copper is best measured in a blood component known as ceruloplasmin—the copper-protein compound in which 95 percent of the body's circulating copper is found. This measurement can be made as part of any routine blood test.

RDIs and Deficiency Symptoms

The RDI for copper is 2 milligrams for all men and women. Copper is so widely available in foods and through the use of copper cooking utensils that, as previously mentioned, deficiency of this mineral is thought to be rare in humans. Many believe that even a diet that is poor in other nutrients is likely to furnish sufficient copper. However, recent research suggests that the typical American diet may not contain the amount of copper it was originally thought to contain (see "Food Sources," below). In addition, there are some groups who are at particular risk of suboptimal copper intake.

Much of our understanding of copper deficiency is the result of symptoms of deficiency in animals. In animal studies and human reports, deficiency symptoms have included anemia, skeletal defects, degeneration of the nervous system, defects in the pigmentation and structure of the hair, reproductive problems, and abnormalities in the cardiovascular system. Mild copper deficiency in animals has also resulted in elevated serum cholesterol, especially when the zinc intake was high. Copper supplements have been shown to lower total cholesterol and raise HDL cholesterol (the good kind) in experimental animals and humans who have copper deficiency. Copper supplementation, along with supplementation of calcium and other minerals, has also been shown to increase bone density in postmenopausal women.

In humans, deficiency may occur in severely malnourished individuals, in which case the symptoms are anemia, impaired immunity, and bone disease. Similar symptoms have also been detected in premature infants fed a diet of only cow's milk, which is low in copper. In addition, people who suffer from sprue or celiac disease may have difficulty absorbing copper. And there is evidence that an excess of zinc may interfere with copper absorption, increasing the requirements for copper. Pregnant women may also be at risk for copper deficiency. In a study that looked at twenty-four healthy women during their pregnancy, the intake of dietary copper was far below normal, and even when supplements brought daily intake up to 2.7 milligrams, this was marginal in meeting the women's needs. This may be a cause for concern, as research has demonstrated that a copper deficiency in pregnant animals may cause birth defects in offspring.

Food Sources

Copper is widely distributed in foods, with liver, shellfish, meats, nuts, legumes, whole grain cereals, and raisins being the richest sources. Early data indicated that the average dietary intake of copper was 2 to 5 milligrams. However, more recent surveys indicate a much lower intake, often substantially below 1 milligram per day. We don't know whether this discrepancy is due to an actual decline in copper intake or differences in measuring intakes. Another factor to consider is that only 25 percent of the copper ingested is absorbed, and that many people eat highly processed, demineralized foods. Drinking water may contribute to your total daily copper intake, but this varies with the type of piping used and the hardness of the water.

Supplements

Copper is available as an individual supplement and is often included in multivitamin-mineral formulas, as well. The most common available forms of this supplement are copper gluconate and copper sulfate. Copper citrate is also available. I generally recommend copper gluconate, as it is gentler to the digestive tract. However, when taken in amounts as small as 2 milligrams, any of the forms may be well tolerated.

Optimum Daily Intake—ODI

For optimum general health, the Optimum Daily Intake for copper is:

0.52 mg for men and women

There is not enough data to permit me to make recommendations for specific conditions and concerns at this time. I recommend using the zinc-to-copper ratio to determine the amount of copper that should be consumed. For most individuals, this ratio can range from 10 to 1, to 15 to 1. For example, if you ingest 30 milligrams of zinc and 2 milligrams of copper a day, your zinc-to-copper ratio would be 15 to 1.

Remember: If you have a medical condition, please consult with your physician before taking supplements. If you suffer from Wilson's disease, please do not take a copper supplement (see "Toxicity and Adverse Effects," below).

Toxicity and Adverse Effects

In Wilson's disease, a rare hereditary disorder, copper accumulates in the liver and is then released and absorbed by other parts of the body, causing toxicity. The symptoms of this condition include hepatitis, degeneration of the lens of the eye, kidney malfunction, and neurological disorders. Acute excessive doses of copper produce nausea, vomiting, abdominal pains, diarrhea, headache, dizziness, and a metallic taste in the mouth. If untreated, this can lead to death.

27 | Manganese

MANGANESE is less abundant in the body than any of the minerals discussed in previous chapters. The human body contains between only 10 and 20 milligrams of this mineral. Most of the information now available on manganese is the result of animal experiments. When this is combined with human data, it appears that despite the relatively small amount of this mineral found in the body, manganese has many important uses.

Functions and Uses

METABOLISM

Perhaps the best-known role of manganese is its involvement in various enzyme systems. Manganese works with dozens of different enzymes that facilitate processes throughout the body, including protein, fat, and carbohydrate metabolism.

GROWTH, DEVELOPMENT, AND REPAIR

Manganese is required for normal growth and development, and for the repair of bones and connective tissue. Studies have associated low manganese levels in human infants with birth defects ranging from cleft palate to bone deformities. Manganese also appears to help maintain bone density in postmenopausal women.

THE NERVOUS SYSTEM

Another important role of manganese involves the proper functioning of the nerves. For instance, animals fed manganese-deficient diets show an increased susceptibility to convulsions. According to a study involving young human patients, insufficient manganese may also exacerbate a tendency to have epileptic seizures.

THE IMMUNE SYSTEM

Experiments have yielded evidence suggesting that manganese deficiencies may also affect the immune system. Antibody response and the activity of macrophages, granulocytes, and phagocytes—cells that protect the body from bacteria and other foreign invaders—are all stimulated by manganese. In addition, manganese is a component of the enzyme superoxide dismutase (SOD), a powerful free radical scavenger that prevents the cellular damage associated with the aging process, asthma, and cancer.

GLUCOSE TOLERANCE

Experiments indicate that manganese deficiency may also play a role in glucose tolerance. In one animal study, when glucose was given to manganese-deficient rats, their insulin output was 76 to 63 percent that of manganese-sufficient rats. It has also been reported that oral manganese supplements significantly lowered blood glucose levels in a patient who was unresponsive to insulin. This data has exciting implications for people with blood sugar problems.

RDIs and Deficiencies

The RDI for manganese is 2 milligrams for all men and women. This amount is roughly what you would consume if you were eating the typical American diet of highly refined foods. However, researchers have noted that diets high in refined carbohydrates may not supply adequate manganese. There is an especially high risk of deficiency when manganese requirements are increased, as during pregnancy or times of rapid growth. In view of the fact that manganese is poorly absorbed and is severely lacking in refined foods, many practitioners, including myself, feel that the recommendation of 2 to 5 milligrams per day is much too low.

Food Sources

Good sources of manganese include nuts and seeds (especially hazelnuts and pecans), avocados, seaweed, and whole grains such as oatmeal, buckwheat, and whole wheat. Other fruits and vegetables contain moderate amounts of this mineral. Refined grains are a poor source of manganese, as milling removes 73 percent of the manganese content, and the enrichment process does not put it back.

In general, the manganese in food is poorly absorbed in the intestines. In experimental conditions, it has been shown that phytates—present in whole grains—may interfere with manganese absorption. However, it is probable that this effect occurs to a significant degree only when extremely high amounts of fiber are eaten.

Supplements

Manganese is available in individual supplements and in some multivitamin-mineral formulas. The most common available forms of this supplement are manganese gluconate, manganese sulfate, and manganese citrate. I generally recommend the gluconate form, as it is gentler to the digestive tract.

Optimum Daily Intake—ODI

For optimum general health, the basic Optimum Daily Intake for manganese is:

15–50 mg for men and women

Based on a thorough scientific review of manganese, and on my clinical experience, the following amounts of manganese appear to be valuable for:

CONDITION	SUGGESTED DOSAGE
Cancer prevention	15–50 mg
Impaired glucose tolerance	15–50 mg
Osteo- and rheumatoid arthritis	15–50 mg
Osteoporosis	15–50 mg

Remember: If you have a medical condition, please consult with your physician before taking supplements.

Toxicity and Adverse Effects

The toxicity for manganese is low when it is ingested in the form of either manganese-rich foods or supplements. Toxicity can occur, however, when manganese is inhaled, as in the case of certain miners who are exposed to high concentrations of manganese oxide in the air. In these situations, even small doses can cause psychiatric abnormalities and nerve disorders. Manganese toxicity may also occur as a result of manganese-contaminated well water.

28 | Chromium

A S ADULTS, our bodies contain approximately 6 grams of chromium. The highest concentrations of this mineral are found in the hair, spleen, kidneys, and testes. The heart, pancreas, lungs, and brain also contain this trace mineral, but in lower concentrations.

Functions and Uses

Chromium's primary role in the body is to activate enzymes involved in the metabolism of glucose and the synthesis of proteins. Its chief functions in the body and therapeutic uses are related to this activity. As we age, many of us appear to become more and more insulin resistant—our bodies no longer respond properly to insulin. This is part of a newly recognized chronic syndrome that has come to be known as Syndrome X. It includes many age-related disorders, such as obesity, cardiovascular disease, and cancer, and eventually leads to full-blown diabetes. Chromium supplements help normalize insulin response and may play a key role in thwarting this dangerous syndrome and the downward health spiral it represents.

GLUCOSE METABOLISM DISORDERS

Commonly known as blood sugar, glucose is the fuel that our cells burn for energy. The hormone insulin regulates the amount of glucose in our blood by escorting glucose into our cells so that it can be stored for later use. This prevents our blood sugar from rising too high, as occurs in diabetes, or from falling too low, as occurs in hypoglycemia. Because chromium is the major mineral involved in insulin production, it should come as no surprise that a lack of this mineral interferes with the maintenance of healthy blood sugar levels. There is strong and growing evidence that many disorders of glucose metabolism—namely, diabetes and hypoglycemia—may, in fact, be chromium-deficiency states.

In experiments, chromium supplementation has actually been found to improve glucose tolerance in some diabetics and in people with impaired glucose tolerance. In one study, for example, ten elderly individuals were given chromium supplementation. For four of the subjects—the chromium responders—all abnormal features of the glucose-tolerance test (GTT) disappeared in a short time. These subjects previously had mild abnormalities on their GTT, while the nonresponders had more severe abnormalities. This suggests that the nonresponders might have been so severely deficient in chromium that it would have taken longer for them to show any improvement. In general, when I have recommended chromium supplements to insulin- and noninsulin-dependent diabetics, along with a diet and exercise program, their physicians were able to reduce their insulin injections or stop their oral medications. Chromium supplementation also improves the insulin resistance associated with diabetes. It is beneficial for hypoglycemics, as well.

CARDIOVASCULAR DISORDERS

Chromium depletion has also been implicated in hypercholesterolemia (high cholesterol in the blood), again because of its role in insulin production and glucose regulation. When glucose levels are elevated and insulin levels continue to rise in an attempt to clear the glucose from the blood and put it into working muscles, the body switches into a fat-storing mode. In this situation, fat tends to be deposited around the abdomen, people who have the "apple" shape are at higher risk for diabetes and heart disease. The other problem is that because of the chromium depletion, the quality of glucose is poor and the cells' receptor sites for glucose do not work optimally. This causes another problem: glucose levels remain elevated in the blood, and glucose is one of the building blocks for cholesterol. In addition to making sure you get optimum amounts of chromium, it is equally important to modify your diet and avoid white flour, sugar, and junk food. Many researchers believe that the accelerated atherosclerosis seen in diabetics may be the result of this insulin-glucose connection. In fact, studies have shown that chromium deficiency tends to decrease the liver's uptake of cholesterol and fatty acids, which could favor the accumulation of lipids in the arteries. In laboratory experiments, rats fed a chromium-deficient, high-sugar diet showed a dramatically increased accumulation of cholesterol in the arteries. On the other hand, when rats fed a high-sugar diet were supplemented with chromium, the nutrient significantly lowered their serum cholesterol levels and resulted in less accumulation of lipids in the arteries. Epidemiological evidence has borne out the results of these laboratory experiments. In several Eastern nations in which low serum cholesterol levels are common, high chromium concentrations have been found in the tissues. Moreover, studies have shown that chromium supplements increase high-density lipoproteins (HDLs, or good cholesterol) and lower low-density lipoproteins (LDLs, or bad cholesterol), in addition to lowering overall cholesterol.

BODY FAT REDUCTION

A preliminary study by Dr. Gary Evans indicated that chromium picolinate was effective in increasing lean body mass (muscle) and reducing the percentage of body fat in male athletes. There were also reports that lean body mass was increased in females on a weight-training program. A weight-reduction program appeared successful with chromium picolinate, L-carnitine, and fiber. However, much of this work is preliminary and has not yet been duplicated by other researchers. In my discussion of chromium in my book *Dare to Lose*, I say that I am not convinced that chromium in and of itself is effective for weight loss, or for increasing lean muscle or decreasing fat unless you are exercising and lowering white flour and sugar in your diet. Chromium will blunt the rise of blood sugar and insulin and prevent deposition of body fat. And, if you are carbohydrate sensitive, it is important for overall health and perhaps works synergistically with other weight-loss supplements.

RDIs and Deficiency Symptoms

The established RDI for chromium is 120 micrograms. According to long-term studies in human subjects, 200 to 290 micrograms are required daily to maintain a balance or near-balance of chromium. However, the estimated chromium intake for the average American is 50 to 100 micrograms per day. This amount is lower than the amount consumed in Italy, Egypt, South America, and India. Even a diet that is considered to be adequate in other respects may be marginal in chromium, and chromium deficiency is believed to be relatively common in the United States, with 80 percent of the population affected, according to some estimates. This is no doubt due at least in part to the refining of grains, which removes over three-quarters of the chromium. (As explained in Chapter 27, refining also removes 73 percent of the manganese. It is interesting to note that a lack of both of these minerals has been implicated in diabetes.)

It is believed that athletes may be at particular risk for marginal chromium deficiency. Strenuous running places considerable stress on the body and increases the energy requirements by seven- to twentyfold. This results in changes in hormones and other substances that function in glucose metabolism.

Food Sources

Brewer's yeast, beer, meat (especially liver), cheese, and whole grain cereals and breads are good sources of chromium. Leafy vegetables contain chromium, but in a form that is poorly absorbed. White rice and white bread—both refined products—are poor sources of this mineral. The milling of grains removes up to 83 percent of the chromium, none of which is replaced during the enrichment process.

Supplements

Chromium is available as an individual supplement and as a component of some multivitamin-mineral formulas. It is produced in several forms, including chromium chloride, GTF (glucose tolerance factor) chromium, chromium polynicotinate, chromium dinicotinate, and chromium picolinate. In GTF chromium, the mineral is generally combined with niacin, cysteine, glycine, and glutamic acid.

There appears to be some disagreement as to the true form of GTF chromium. Chromium polynicotinate is considered by some to be the true form and was discovered by Dr. Walter Mertz in 1959. Several studies have demonstrated that this form has excellent glucose-lowering properties, as well as antioxidant activity in the liver and kidneys. However, all forms of chromium have been shown to improve glucose tolerance, blood lipids, and insulin resistance.

In my clinical practice, I have found that individuals respond differently to the various types of chromium. Therefore, if you don't achieve the desired results with one chromium supplement, you should try another form.

Optimum Daily Intake—ODI

For optimum general health, the basic Optimum Daily Intake for chromium is:

200–600 mcg for men and women

Based on a thorough scientific review of chromium, and on my clinical experience, the following amounts of chromium appear to be valuable for:

CONDITION	SUGGESTED DOSAGE
Diabetes	400–1,000 mcg
High cholesterol, high LDLs, and low HDLs	400–1,000 mcg
Hypoglycemia	200–600 mcg
Impaired glucose tolerance	400–1,000 mcg

Remember: If you have a medical condition, please consult with your physician before taking supplements, especially if you have diabetes.

Toxicity and Adverse Effects

There is no known toxicity for chromium, except in the cases of chromium mining and industrial exposure, which cause chromium dust to be inhaled.

29 | Selenium

SELENIUM is present in all the tissues of the body, but is concentrated most highly in the kidneys, liver, spleen, pancreas, and testes. People do not consume enough selenium both because of the type of diet they eat and because of the low selenium content of the soil in which their food is grown. The selenium content of soil varies widely, with many areas in the United States showing serious depletion. In fact, there have been several reports of selenium deficiencies in livestock raised on selenium-depleted soil.

Functions and Uses

CANCER

Selenium's best-known and perhaps most important biological function relates to its role as an antioxidant and anticancer mineral. As we have seen in other chapters, free radicals damage our cells, possibly leading to the development of cancer and other degenerative diseases. Selenium is an activating component of the enzyme glutathione peroxidase, which protects our cells from this damage.

Many animal studies have proven that selenium deficiency increases the incidence and rate of growth of cancers in animals that are either exposed to a variety of potent carcinogens or receive transplanted tumors.

Companion studies have shown that high selenium intake protects against these cancers. For example, in one study in which rats were exposed to a potent carcinogen, only 15 percent of those who were also given selenium developed liver cancer, as compared with 90 percent of the unsupplemented rats. In another study, the occurrence of cancer was 10 percent in the supplemented group versus 80 percent in the control group. In yet another animal study, selenium supplementation reduced colon cancer incidence by more than 50 percent. In another study, selenium protected against UV-induced skin damage and cancer, retarding the onset and number of skin lesions and reducing inflammation, blistering, and pigmentation.

In humans, there is ample epidemiological evidence that high selenium is correlated with a lower incidence of many types of cancer. For instance, researchers have found that cancer risk is significantly lower in people living in areas with selenium-rich soil, in people with a high-selenium food supply, and in people with higher blood levels of selenium, when compared with people with lower intakes and blood levels. Selenium intakes in the people studied were close to 750 micrograms per day, with no toxic side effects noted. In a survey that spanned twenty-seven countries, including the United States, it was found that the cancer death rate was lower in those people whose typical diets were high in selenium. This and other cancer studies indicate that selenium is especially protective against cancer of the breast, colon, and lung. Data also suggests protection against tumors of the ovaries, cervix, rectum, bladder, esophagus, pancreas, skin, liver, and prostate, as well as against leukemia.

Since 1969, it has been known that the blood levels of cancer patients are low in selenium. In general, cancer patients with lower-than-average selenium levels have a greater number of primary tumors, more recurrences, more distant metastases (tumors that have spread to distant parts of the body), and a shortened survival time. In a study of 12,000 people conducted in Finland, the risk of fatal cancer in people with the lowest levels of serum selenium was nearly six times higher than that in people with the highest selenium concentrations.

Like other nutrients, of course, selenium cannot do its work alone. In several studies, it has been shown that selenium and vitamin E—and perhaps vitamin A, too—have a synergistic effect. For example, in one study, male smokers who died of cancer had lower levels of serum selenium, vitamin A, and vitamin E, when compared with healthy control subjects. It is well-known that vitamin E enhances the antioxidant effect of selenium. In addition, it has been found that supplementation with selenium alone and with selenium plus vitamin E in excess of the RDAs stimulates the immune system in experimental animals. This effect is particularly pronounced when the diet is high in polyunsaturated fats—a factor that has been linked to a higher incidence of certain cancers.

These studies show promise for the prevention and possible treatment of cancer with selenium supplementation. When combined with other supplements, the anticancer effect may be even greater. The National Cancer Institute is conducting ongoing chemopreventive trials of several individual nutrients, including selenium, vitamin E, and vitamin A. However, many of the human studies, including those by the National Cancer Institute, use low levels of selenium supplementation—only 200 micrograms—while population studies of people who consumed high levels of selenium through their food have shown a protective effect at levels from approximately 400–750 micrograms per day. Trials that are limited to 200 micrograms of selenium per day, are too low a dose to assess the potential protective effect of this mineral. Larger doses of selenium have been shown to be protective in animals and safe in humans. In addition, we are not sure of the extent to which selenium supplementation influences the later stages of cancer development. If its influence is strongest in the early stage, it will be very difficult for these trials to prove the connection between low selenium and cancer because of the long latency period for most cancers. (For example, it may take up to fourteen years for a single breast cancer cell to multiply and produce a tumor large enough to be detected by currently available diagnostic methods.) Finally, evidence of the synergism of nutrients has led many researchers to emphasize the need to consider several nutrients in any given diet and cancer study, instead of focusing on just one nutrient per study.

CARDIOVASCULAR DISEASE

In humans, a link has been found between selenium and heart disease. People found to have overt selenium deficiencies—alcoholics with cirrhosis of the liver and people receiving long-term intravenous feeding—have also been found to suffer from heart problems that respond to selenium supplementation. In eastern Finland, which has one of the highest mortality rates from heart disease in the world, it was found that low selenium in the blood was associated with up to a six- or sevenfold increase in the risk of death from heart disease. In addition, children in certain areas of China in which the selenium content of the soil is low are known to develop a heart disease called Keshan's disease. Their heart problems, too, respond to selenium supplementation.

OTHER FUNCTIONS

There is some evidence that selenium may also prove effective in the treatment or prevention of several other disorders. A study using 400 micrograms of selenium and approximately 25 international units of vitamin E markedly improved skin conditions such as acne and seborrheic dermatitis in the test subjects. Another study demonstrated that selenium supplementation reduces the inflammatory activity in patients suffering from autoimmune thyroiditis. This makes sense because it is likely that the severe deficiency in our soil is contributing to the increase in incidence in this condition in the first place. A Danish study examined patients with rheumatoid arthritis and found that they had lower levels of selenium. Those with the lowest levels had the more severe form of this disease. Moreover, a recent study conducted in Japan suggests that selenium and vitamin E may enhance the responsiveness of arthritis patients to conventional treatment. A fascinating study conducted in Scandinavia showed a correlation between low selenium levels and the incidence and severity of muscular dystrophy; one patient who was treated with selenium supplements showed considerable improvement after one year. Finnish researchers have also conducted a study on elderly patients who were given large doses of selenium and vitamin E for one year. After two months, researchers found an obvious improvement in their patients' mental well-being, including less fatigue, depression, and anxiety, and more mental alertness, motivation, and self-care. Finally, selenium has been shown to protect against the toxic effects of mercury, arsenic, and copper. Mercury toxicity has been recognized as a growing problem in our environment. It enters our bodies through what we eat and drink. In particular, there have been warnings about fish such as tuna and swordfish being alarmingly high in mercury.

Recently, selenium supplementation was found to reduce the severity of side effects from radiation therapy for head and neck cancer. Patients had less swelling, which translated into less discomfort and an improved ability to breath. This is just one example of how nutritional supplements—of antioxidant nutrients in particular—can lessen the severity of side effects of cancer treatment.

RDIs and Deficiency Symptoms

Selenium deficiency symptoms may include muscular weakness and discomfort. Recent studies have shown that people with celiac disease—an inborn inability to digest gluten—are at high risk for low selenium, along with other nutrients, either because their low-gluten diets are also low in selenium or because of their absorption problems. Downs syndrome patients have also been found to have low levels of selenium and other antioxidants.

In one study, refinery workers were found to have low selenium levels in spite of their dietary intake of 217 micrograms per day, which is more than three times higher than the RDI. This study indicates that because of the workers' exposure to free radicals on the job, their bodies were utilizing large amounts of selenium to produce the protective enzyme glutathione peroxidase. This suggests that exposure to toxic environmental chemicals increases the requirement for this mineral.

The RDI for selenium is 70 micrograms for all men and women.

Food Sources

There are no accurate available measurements of the selenium content of foods. However, it appears that the richest sources of selenium are seafoods, meats, and organ meats—if the animals of origin ate a diet high in selenium. Whole grains can be good sources, but, similarly, this depends on the selenium content of the soil in which they were grown. Fruits and vegetables generally contain very low amounts of selenium.

The refining process strips foods of much of their selenium content. In one study, it was found that a highly refined diet contains 61 percent less selenium than does a diet rich in unrefined foods. Cooking also reduces the content significantly, especially if the cooking water is discarded. Vitamin C seems to enhance the absorption of selenium.

Supplements

Selenium is most often available as an individual supplement. Some multivitamin-mineral formulas may include it but not necessarily in optimal doses. Check the label. You may still need to take an individual supplement for optimal doses. I recommend selenium in the form of selenomethionine, which is extracted from selenium-rich yeast or ocean plants. This form is the least toxic and appears to be the most absorbable.

Optimum Daily Intake—ODI

For optimum general health, the basic Optimum Daily Intake for selenium is:

100–400 mcg for men and women living in low-selenium areas (this includes coastal areas and glaciated areas)

100–200 mcg for men and women living in higher selenium areas

Based on a thorough scientific review of selenium, and on my clinical experience, the following amounts of selenium appear to be valuable for:

CONDITION	SUGGESTED DOSAGE
Arthritis	200–400 mcg
Cancer prevention	200–600 mcg
Heart disease	200–400 mcg
Mercury accumulation	200–600 mcg
Skin problems	200–400 mcg

Remember: If you have a medical condition, please consult with your physician before taking supplements.

Toxicity and Adverse Effects

Animal poisoning due to high-selenium soil is well known. The evidence so far seems to indicate that for toxicity to occur in humans, the intake must be very high indeed. Various studies have shown that long-term intakes of up to 500 to 750 micrograms per day have produced no signs of toxicity in humans. Data extrapolated from animal studies suggests that toxicity does not occur in humans ingesting less than 1,000 to 2,000 micrograms per day. The Food and Nutrition Board has stated that overt selenium toxicity may occur in humans ingesting 2,400 to 3,000 micrograms daily (but for some reason, the board still claims that the maximum intake of selenium should not exceed 200 micrograms).

Toxicity symptoms, which include a garlic odor in breath, urine, and sweat, have been reported among people living in high-selenium areas and among certain workers exposed to selenium. Some data, when combined with selenium's known teratogenic effect in animals, suggest that extremely high levels of selenium may also cause birth defects in humans.

30 | Iodine

OUR BODIES contain 20 to 30 milligrams of iodine. Approximately three-quarters of this is found in the thyroid gland, while the remainder is distributed throughout the body, mostly in the fluid that bathes our cells.

Functions and Uses

THE THYROID GLAND

As indicated by its high concentration in the thyroid gland, iodine is important for the proper functioning of that gland. Specifically, it is a necessary constituent of the thyroid hormones, which are used to regulate physical and mental growth, the functioning of the nervous system and muscles, circulatory activity, and the metabolism of all nutrients.

Other Uses

Recent data indicates that iodine may have functions in other parts of the body, as well. For example, the results of a study of iodine-deficient children in China suggest that hearing loss may be an iodine-deficiency disorder. In addition, iodine supplements are used in the event of a nuclear accident to prevent the absorption of radioactive iodine by the thyroid gland, protecting against thyroid damage and, possibly, thyroid cancer.

RDIs and Classic Deficiency Symptoms

The classic iodine deficiency disease is goiter, a condition in which the thyroid gland becomes enormously enlarged in an effort to compensate for insufficient hormone production. If the thyroid cannot overcome this insufficiency, hypothyroidism occurs with symptoms of listlessness, lassitude, and sluggishness appearing. Goiter may also appear in people who ingest large amounts of goitrogens—substances that decrease the production of a thyroid hormone by preventing the utilization of iodine. Goitrogenic foods include rutabagas, strawberries, peaches, peanuts, soybeans, spinach, radishes, cabbage, turnips, mustard, and cassava root. Cooking usually inactivates goitrogens.

The RDI for iodine is 150 micrograms for all men and women. The estimated intake in the United States is between 64 and 677 micrograms per day—a wide range because of widely varying soil conditions, fertilizer use, and food processing. Areas in the United States in which iodine deficiency is most common are called goiter belts, and include the Midwest, the Pacific Northwest, and the Great Lakes region. Switzerland, Central America, the mountainous regions of South America, New Zealand, and the Himalayas also suffer a high incidence of goiter owing to low-iodine soil. Simple goiter is found most often in women, especially during adolescence, pregnancy, and menopause.

Since the introduction of iodized table salt, the incidence of goiter has fallen dramatically. In the United States, it remains to be seen whether the recent efforts to reduce salt consumption will have any effect on goiter incidence.

Food Sources

The richest and most consistent food sources of iodine are seafoods, including fish, shellfish, and plants. Seaweed is extremely high in iodine, with as much as 50,000 micrograms in a three-ounce serving. Most land vegetables are rather low in iodine, unless they are grown near the seacoast or in soils enriched with iodine-containing fertilizers.

The iodine content of meat, dairy products, and eggs depends upon the iodine content of the animals' diet. Livestock destined for consumption may be encouraged to lick salt blocks that contain iodine so that their meat will be higher in this mineral. For many individuals, the most important dietary source of iodine is iodized salt, 1 gram of which supplies about 76 micrograms of iodine.

Supplements

Many individuals are supplemented with iodine through the use of iodized table salt. However, if you do not wish to increase your consumption of salt, iodine is also available in tablets as sea kelp and in concentrated liquid drops and tablets. The topical antiseptic known as tincture of iodine is not to be used orally because it is poisonous if ingested.

Optimum Daily Intake—ODI

For optimum general health, the Optimum Daily Intake for iodine is:

150–300 mcg for men and women living in low-iodine areas and consuming low-iodine diets

0–150 mcg for men and women routinely consuming iodized salt and/or seaweed products

Keep in mind that individuals who consume iodized salt or seaweed may not require iodine supplementation. However, they can safely consume the lower-range amounts usually found in multinutrient supplements.

Remember: If you have a medical condition, please consult your physician before taking supplements. If you are allergic to iodine, you may need to avoid this mineral.

Toxicity and Adverse Effects

An intake of up to 1,000 micrograms of iodine per day is considered safe. Toxicity symptoms include rash, headache, difficulty in breathing, and a metallic taste in the mouth. Very high doses—20,000 micrograms per day—can paradoxically cause a form of goiter called iodide goiter. This has been seen in certain groups of Japanese who consume great quantities of seaweed daily.

31 | Potassium

O
UR CELLS contain more potassium than any other mineral. A total of approximately 250 grams of this nutrient
can be found in the adult body.

Functions and Uses

CARDIOVASCULAR DISEASE

A growing body of evidence indicates that low levels of potassium are associated with high blood pressure, and therefore deserve more attention.
This association may be especially strong when the sodium-to-potassium
ratio is high. Some researchers feel that in certain cases, low potassium may
play a more significant role in hypertension than high sodium does. In several studies, for instance, potassium supplementation significantly lowered
blood pressure without sodium restriction. As some researchers have pointed
out, diets restricted in calories, sodium, and cholesterol are often recommended to people with cardiovascular disease. It is unfortunate that such
diets also tend to reduce nutrients such as calcium and potassium, which
may be essential for maintaining normal blood pressure.

Potassium may prove to be of value to the cardiovascular system in
other ways, as well. In one animal study, rats were given stroke-inducing
diets. The group that was supplemented with potassium suffered a 2
percent rate of fatal strokes, as compared with the 83 percent rate of the

unsupplemented group. In another animal study, potassium supplementation was able to protect against the kidney damage resulting from hypertension. In both studies, these remarkable effects occurred even when potassium did not reduce blood pressure. Studies using potassium supplementation have shown it to be effective for lowering blood pressure.

OTHER USES

Potassium is essential for maintaining the fluid balance in our cells and is required for the enzymatic reactions taking place within them. Potassium is used to convert glucose into glycogen for storage and later release. It is also used for nerve transmission, muscle contraction, hormone secretion, and other functions.

RDIs and Deficiency Symptoms

Potassium deficiency symptoms include nausea; vomiting, which can lead to further potassium losses; listlessness; feelings of apprehension; muscle weakness, muscle spasms, and cramps; tachycardia (rapid heartbeat); and, in extreme cases, heart failure.

There is no Reference Daily Intake for potassium, but it has been estimated that the average American diet contains from 2 to 6 grams per day. Potassium deficiency can result from severe malnutrition, alcoholism, anorexia nervosa, vomiting, diarrhea, or illnesses that seriously interfere with appetite. Potassium may also be depleted following severe tissue injury due to surgery or burns and during prolonged fevers. The excessive use of steroids, laxatives, and some diuretics also encourages potassium loss. If a person already has heart disease, low potassium can worsen the picture. Thus, patients with hypertension who are taking diuretics under a doctor's care are often given potassium supplements to counteract the effect.

In the body, potassium must exist in balance with sodium. Although sodium may be an important dietary determinant of blood pressure, variations in the potassium-to-sodium ratio in the diet affect blood pressure under certain circumstances. So when considering potassium levels, we must consider sodium levels as well and watch out for high-sodium foods, including canned goods, luncheon meats, sausages, and frozen foods.

Food Sources

Potassium is found in a wide range of foods. Dairy products (except for cheese, because potassium is lost in the whey), meats, poultry, and fish are all good sources. Legumes, fruits, vegetables, and whole grains are also respectable sources. People who are taking diuretics for the treatment of high blood pressure are frequently advised to eat fruits such as bananas, oranges, and tomatoes for their potassium content. However, the amount of potassium in these foods is minimal compared with the amount excreted in urine as a result of diuretic use. It would take an enormous number of bananas per day to provide the recommended amount of potassium for a patient taking diuretics. Many physicians often prescribe high-dose potassium supplements for these patients.

Bear in mind, too, that potassium is lost through cooking, although the amount of potassium lost varies according to the cooking method used. A boiled potato may have lost up to 50 percent of its original potassium content. A steamed potato, only 3 to 6 percent. Some researchers have suggested adding modest amounts of salt substitute containing potassium chloride to boiling water, as this prevents the potassium from leaching out during cooking.

Supplements

Potassium is available in tablet and liquid form. Levels above the ODI should be taken only under the advice of a professional.

Optimum Daily Intake—ODI

Since potassium is so widely available in fresh foods, you should eat more potassium-rich foods like fresh fruits and vegetables rather than use a potassium supplement. Rather, most people should be advised to reduce sodium intake so that a sodium-to-potassium ratio of 1 to 1 is achieved. If, however, you wish to take a supplement, the Optimum Daily Intake of potassium is:

99–300 mg for men and women

Your physician may suggest higher levels of potassium if you are taking certain diuretics or if you are trying to lower your blood pressure. Keep in mind, though, that high amounts of this nutrient should be taken only under professional guidance.

Remember: If you have a medical condition, please consult with your physician before taking supplements.

Toxicity and Adverse Effects

Potassium toxicity is seen when daily intakes exceed 18 grams, an amount that is unlikely to be ingested through food. Toxicity usually occurs only through the uneducated use of supplements, or when an individual has kidney failure. Excess potassium may cause muscle fatigue, irregular heartbeat, and possibly heart failure.

32 | Boron

We have known about the existence of boron, a trace mineral, for a long time. It has long been considered to be essential for plants, but only recently have we discovered the health benefits of this nutrient in humans.

Functions and Uses

THE BONES

Based on the limited data we have so far, it appears that boron has a remarkable effect on the prevention of bone loss and demineralization. In a study conducted by researchers at the United States Department of Agriculture, boron was given to postmenopausal women, who are at high risk of developing osteoporosis. The results of this study suggest that boron works very much like estrogen to prevent the loss of minerals from the bone. As a result of this and other studies, boron is considered to be an essential mineral and a useful adjunct, along with calcium and vitamin D, in the maintenance of bone health and the prevention of osteoporosis. Future studies may demonstrate boron as a safer alternative to estrogen-replacement therapy (see Chapter 21 for a more detailed discussion of osteoporosis).

THE IMMUNE SYSTEM AND INFLAMMATION

Animal research suggests that boron enhances the utilization of vitamin D_3, and modulates immune and inflammatory processes. Thus, boron may be useful in the treatment and/or prevention of osteoarthritis. In one study, subjects with osteoarthritis were given 6 milligrams of boron daily, or a placebo. A significant improvement was obtained in 50 percent of the subjects receiving the boron supplement, compared with an improvement in only 10 percent of those receiving the placebo. Other data has shown that people with arthritis have lower boron concentrations in their bones and synovial fluid than do people who do not have arthritis.

RDIs and Deficiency Symptoms

There is no established RDI for boron and no deficiency symptoms have been identified.

Food Sources

Fruits and vegetables are the best sources of boron; meat and fish are poor sources. A diet containing a variety of foods, including fruits and vegetables, supplies 1.5 to 3 milligrams of boron per day.

Supplements

Boron is available as an individual supplement and in combination with other minerals, such as calcium and magnesium.

Optimum Daily Intake—ODI

Three milligrams per day were used in the Department of Agriculture study. In general, 3 to 6 milligrams are being used by clinicians in the treatment of postmenopausal women at high risk of osteoporosis.

Remember: If you have a medical condition, please consult with your physician before taking supplements. For optimum general health, the basic ODI for boron is:

3–6 mg for men and women

Toxicity and Adverse Effects

There are no reported adverse effects with doses of 3 to 6 milligrams of boron per day.

Part 4

Beyond Vitamins and Minerals

33 | Coenzyme Q$_{10}$

COENZYME Q$_{10}$ is also known as ubiquinone, because it is ubiquitous—it exists everywhere in the body. Although coenzyme Q$_{10}$ (CoQ$_{10}$) behaves like a vitamin in that it serves as a catalyst in certain reactions, it isn't considered a true vitamin because it is synthesized in the cells. Adequate CoQ$_{10}$ is essential for optimum health, but as you will see, many people—especially those with heart problems or on certain cholesterol-lowering drugs—are at risk of CoQ$_{10}$ depletion or deficiency, sometimes with tragic consequences.

Functions and Uses

ENERGY PRODUCTION

Coenzyme Q$_{10}$ acts as a catalyst in the chain of chemical reactions that create adenosine triphosphate (ATP), a compound that yields the energy needed by cells to function. Due to CoQ$_{10}$'s role in energy production, it stands to reason that a low concentration of this substance is detrimental to health in general. Not surprisingly, CoQ$_{10}$ is most abundant in organs that require a large supply of energy, especially the heart and liver, and in the immune system.

COQ$_{10}$'s ANTIOXIDANT POWERS

Like a number of other vitamins, CoQ$_{10}$ is an antioxidant. Similar in structure to vitamin E, another antioxidant, CoQ$_{10}$ has been shown to scavenge harmful free radicals and thus may help prevent cell damage in a variety of conditions. (For more information on antioxidants, see page 33.)

CARDIOVASCULAR DISEASE

Most of the research on CoQ$_{10}$ involves the heart, since this nutrient is most concentrated in that organ. The research concerning CoQ$_{10}$'s effects in patients with heart disease is quite remarkable. For example, a number of clinical trials suggest that CoQ$_{10}$ supplements benefit people with angina, with no adverse effects. Some studies show that CoQ$_{10}$ supplementation increases the time in which people with angina are able to exercise. In another study, CoQ$_{10}$ was found to be an effective drug therapy in the actual treatment of angina. Data from many human studies indicate that this nutrient may protect the heart from damage due to heart attack. Numerous studies also suggest that CoQ$_{10}$ reduces the amount of tissue damage that occurs during open-heart surgery and, possibly, heart transplantation.

We've known as long ago as 1985 that CoQ$_{10}$ levels are low in people with cardiomyopathy—the more severe the disease, the lower the levels of this nutrient. In Japan, considerable research has been conducted on the beneficial effects of CoQ$_{10}$ supplementation for patients with congestive heart failure. This prompted the Japanese government to approve CoQ$_{10}$ in the treatment of this condition. Several large-scale studies have demonstrated that CoQ$_{10}$ is extremely effective at improving the symptoms associated with congestive heart disease, preventing a worsening of serious complications, reducing hospital admissions, and improving the overall quality of life. CoQ$_{10}$ therapy has been given both alone and with conventional medicine and no side effects have been noted in studies utilizing as much as 100 to 600 milligrams each day. One study was able to improve symptoms in patients who had not been helped by standard diuretic and digitalis therapy.

In another study, people with cardiomyopathy who were expected to die within two years under conventional therapy experienced significant clinical improvement. This suggests CoQ$_{10}$ may do more than improve quality of life of some people with this condition—it may actually prolong their lives. In another study, 87 percent of patients experienced significant and measurable improvement in heart function after six months of CoQ$_{10}$ therapy—and all of them became asymptomatic.

CoQ$_{10}$'s heart benefits do not stop there. Statin drugs are given to lower cholesterol, but they also lower CoQ$_{10}$ levels in heart, liver, and bone tissue. As explained earlier in this chapter, CoQ$_{10}$ is needed for healthy heart function, suggesting that the drugs may be helping the heart in one way and harming it in another. There is rather convincing evidence that statin drugs can cause myopathy (muscle injury), including cardiomyopathy and liver damage to as many as 1 percent of the people taking them. It is predicted that soon 36 million Americans will be taking statin drugs—putting 360,000 at risk of heart and liver damage. In addition, statin drugs have been associated with increased incidence of cataracts, cancers, nerve problems, and psychiatric problems. Deficiencies of CoQ$_{10}$ are believed to be at least partly responsible. As one researchers said, "We have studies that show statins don't cause cancer in five years. Of course, neither does smoking." No wonder that I and many other clinicians and researchers believe statin labeling should reflect this knowledge and that drug companies should be forced to put a warning on the label not to give a statin drug without also giving patients coenzyme Q$_{10}$.

The results of human and animal studies suggest that CoQ$_{10}$ also decreases irregular heartbeat (arrhythmia) even in those patients receiving psychotropic drugs, of which arrhythmia is a common side effect. CoQ$_{10}$ may also help in the treatment of mitral valve prolapse and the resulting chronic fatigue by reducing myocardial thickness, a thickening of the heart muscle that may affect heartbeat regularity.

In addition to helping people with established heart disease, CoQ$_{10}$ may also prevent disease by reducing some of the risk factors associated with heart problems. For example, human studies have demonstrated that CoQ$_{10}$ significantly protects low-density lipoproteins (LDLs, or bad cholesterol) from oxidation and lowers elevated serum cholesterol. At the same time, it raises high-density lipoproteins (HDLs)—the good cholesterol that helps protect against heart disease. Studies also suggest that CoQ$_{10}$ may lower high blood pressure. In several studies, including a controlled study of twenty hypertensive patients, 100 milligrams of CoQ$_{10}$ taken daily lowered both systolic and diastolic blood pressure.

CANCER

Certain cancer patients may benefit from CoQ_{10} supplementation, since animal studies have indicated that CoQ_{10} protects heart tissue from Adriamycin (doxorubicin hydrochloride), a cancer chemotherapy drug that is highly toxic to the heart. Several researchers have reported similar effects in humans. Yet this nutrient is rarely recommended to patients undergoing treatment with this common medication.

CoQ_{10} may also have anticancer properties of its own. In 1993, one of the researchers who used CoQ_{10} with Adriamycin reported that ten patients survived for five to fifteen years with high-dose CoQ_{10} therapy. In 1994, a Danish researcher reported on thirty-two breast cancer patients who were treated with high-dose CoQ_{10} therapy. These patients had been treated with conventional therapy, but were at high risk for recurrence. After twenty-four months on CoQ_{10} supplements, all were still alive, when at least six deaths would have been expected. Six of the women showed a partial remission of the tumor. In two women, the tumors had disappeared entirely. Patients in these studies were given 300 mg of CoQ_{10} or more per day.

CHRONIC FATIGUE AND IMMUNE DYSFUNCTION

Research has revealed that patients with chronic fatigue syndrome (CFIDS) and immune dysfunction may also benefit from CoQ_{10} supplementation. One study showed that many patients with this problem have lower levels of CoQ_{10} compared with healthy subjects. Supplementation with CoQ_{10} dramatically improved many of the symptoms associated with CFIDS, including headache, sleep disturbances, postexercise fatigue, exercise tolerance, and chronic fatigue. Patients were generally given 100 mg of CoQ_{10} per day.

OTHER USES

Coenzyme Q_{10} appears to have other uses as well. There have been extensive reports of CoQ_{10}'s effectiveness in treating many forms of muscular dystrophy and myopathy, both of which cause the weakening and wasting of skeletal muscles. The cardiac disease commonly associated with these conditions, and that may be associated with the weakened muscles, may also be improved with CoQ_{10}. This is the only known substance that safely offers improved quality of life for people with these conditions. CoQ_{10} may also help people with Parkinson's disease. In a study published in 2002, people with early Parkinson's disease were given either a placebo or CoQ$_{10}$ in dosages that ranged from 300 to 1,200 milligrams per day. At the end of the sixteen-month follow-up, researchers found that those taking the supplement developed significantly less disability and those who took the highest dose reaped the greatest benefit. Finally, some reports suggest that CoQ$_{10}$ may benefit people with periodontal disease, diabetes, and deafness. This may be linked to the fact that levels of CoQ$_{10}$ tend to decrease with age—a fact that may indicate that higher levels of the nutrient can help prevent or relieve age-related disorders.

RDIs and Deficiency Symptoms

There is no established RDI for coenzyme Q$_{10}$ and no deficiency symptoms have been identified.

Food Sources

Coenzyme Q$_{10}$ is most abundant in beef hearts, chicken hearts, and other hearts. Sardines, peanuts, and spinach are other good sources. Many plants contain a form of CoQ$_{10}$, but it may not act the same way in the body as does the form found in animal foods. Very little is known about CoQ$_{10}$ in foods, as all studies have used supplements.

Supplements

Coenzyme Q$_{10}$ is generally available in 10-, 30-, 50-, and 100-milligram capsules.

Optimum Daily Intake—ODI

There is no Optimum Daily Intake for coenzyme Q$_{10}$. Generally, 50 to 300 milligrams have been used in clinical trials and appear to be safe and effective. Some trials have used more than 600 milligrams, but this higher dose should be used only under the guidance of a professional.

Toxicity and Adverse Effects

Even in high doses, CoQ$_{10}$ results in few adverse effects. There have been some reports of gastrointestinal upset, loss of appetite, nausea, and diarrhea.

34 | Essential Fatty Acids

ALTHOUGH a low-fat diet is generally healthier than one that is higher in fat, our bodies require a certain amount of fat for proper growth and functioning. Those fats that are necessary for good health and cannot be manufactured by the body are called essential fatty acids (EFAs). They are termed essential because, like vitamins and minerals, they must be provided by the diet. This chapter focuses on the two groups of essential fatty acids that have received the most attention: omega-3 and omega-6 fatty acids.

The omega-3 family includes alpha-linolenic acid, eicosapentaenoic acid (EPA), and docosahexaenoic acid (DHA). In certain plants, omega-3 fatty acids are found in the form of alpha-linolenic acid. In the body, this fatty acid is converted to EPA, which is then converted to DHA. The oils of certain fish contain preformed EPA and DHA, which are the active and most desirable forms of the omega-3 family. Ultimately, DHA is converted to a group of anti-inflammatory prostaglandins—hormonelike substances used throughout the body. It is this final conversion to prostaglandins that is responsible for omega-3's therapeutic effects.

The omega-6 family includes cis-linoleic acid, linoleic acid, and gamma-linolenic acid (GLA). Cis-linoleic acid is found in certain plants and vegetable oils. Linoleic acid is found in most plants and vegetable oils. In the body, some cis-linoleic acid is converted to GLA, the most therapeutic form of the omega-6 family. Preformed GLA can also be found in certain plants, with evening primrose, black currant, and borage oils being the most commonly used sources. The body ultimately converts GLA to another group of anti-inflammatory prostaglandins. Again, it is this final conversion that is responsible for omega-6's therapeutic effects. However, it should be noted that cis-linoleic acid and linoleic acid can also be converted to pro-inflammatory prostaglandins.

A balance of essential fatty acids is needed for good health. Unfortunately, the average American diet does not provide a balance. Instead, because it is so high in certain vegetable oils, it provides an excess of linoleic acid, which is generally metabolized into pro-inflammatory substances, and an insufficient amount of those fatty acids that are needed to make anti-inflammatory substances. Depending on your particular needs, you may want to add omega-3 EFAs, *healthy* omega-6 EFAs, or both EFAs to your supplementation program.

Functions and Uses

As already explained, chief among the roles of the EFAs is the part they play in the body's manufacture of prostaglandins—hormonelike substances that are produced and used by all cells. Once manufactured, the prostaglandins regulate all of our body functions, including those of the cardiovascular, reproductive, immune, and nervous systems. In addition, fatty acids serve as structural parts of cell membranes and therefore help protect the cells from invading toxins, bacteria, viruses, carcinogens, and allergens. It's easy to understand why research has linked fatty acid imbalances to a variety of chronic diseases, including heart disease, cancer, diabetes, arthritis, allergies, problems related to the nervous system including behavioral problems, skin problems, and various immunological disorders. To give you an idea of how out of balance we are, over the past 100 to 150 years, the ratio of omega-6 to omega-3 fatty acids has shifted from about 2 to 1 to about 30 to 1!

CARDIOVASCULAR DISEASE

Interest in fatty acids began when researchers observed that in spite of a diet incredibly rich in fat, the Greenland Eskimos had a very low rate of heart disease, as well as a low incidence of cancer and diabetes. Intrigued by this apparent paradox, researchers studied the Eskimo diet and discovered that it was high in EPA and DHA—omega-3 fatty acids found in the cold-water fish and marine mammals that form the bulk of the Eskimo diet. Subsequent studies in Japan, Sweden, and the Netherlands confirmed that the higher the consumption of omega-3-rich fish, the lower the incidence of heart disease, and many studies continue to demonstrate that EPA protects against heart disease. For example, in 2002, results from the Nurses' Health Study confirmed that women who had a higher intake of fish or omega-3 fatty acids had a lower risk of coronary heart disease.

EPA helps prevent atherosclerosis in many ways. Platelets—the blood cells that enable our blood to clot and aggregate—can adhere to artery walls, contributing to atherosclerosis, or hardening of the arteries. EPA acts as a natural blood thinner and prevents this adhesion. It reduces damage to arterial walls, another way of inhibiting atherosclerosis. DHA and EPA have been found to improve blood lipid ratios. They lower total cholesterol, triglycerides and VLDL, while increasing the HDL. Studies with GLA have yielded results similar to those achieved with EPA. Also, studies on evening primrose oil—a rich source of GLA—as well as studies on fish oil, have demonstrated positive results in improving lipid abnormalities in certain diabetic patients, provided they received vitamin E supplementation, as well.

It is interesting to note that because aspirin thins the blood, it has been widely touted as a heart-attack preventive. Yet several studies have suggested that fish oil—whether consumed in fish or in fish-oil supplements—is superior to aspirin in preventing heart disease and is not associated with the ulcers, gastrointestinal bleeding, anemia, and other side effects that occur with aspirin use. In studies that used both aspirin and fish oil, the combination was more effective than aspirin alone. These factors, along with the fact that EPA appears to lower cholesterol and improve blood-to-fat ratios, makes fish oil a better, safer option in preventing cardiovascular disorders in people at high risk. Furthermore, there is new evidence that EPA reduces the tendency of heart arrythmias in animals and probably in humans.

EFAs also appear to be effective in the treatment of existing heart disease. There is evidence that fish oil lowers blood pressure and can reduce chest pain during exercise in people with angina. In a 2001 study, 1.5 grams of omega-3 fatty acid supplement per day reduced the progression and increased the regression of coronary artery disease. Because of its blood-thinning abilities, EPA may also be of use after bypass surgery and as an adjunct to angioplasty. In addition, GLA has been shown to reduce stress-induced hypertension in animals and to help relieve the pain of angina in humans. In a study involving 2,000 men who had survived a heart attack, those in the group who were urged to eat more fish reduced their risk of dying from all causes by 29 percent. This result is comparable to that achieved with statin drugs. I don't get it—if fish oil were a drug, most drug company reps would be touting these results relentlessly.

THE IMMUNE SYSTEM AND INFLAMMATION

Both EPA and GLA appear to have positive effects on immune function and inflammation. By blocking the pro-inflammatory prostaglandins, EPA tends to improve symptoms of asthma, chronic bronchitis, emphysema, atopic dermatitis, rheumatoid arthritis, Raynaud's disease, systemic lupus erythematosus, psoriatic arthritis, psoriasis, and gout. Fish oil supplements have been useful in treating Crohn's disease and ulcerative colitis. In a recent study using high levels of GLA (1.4 grams) from borage seed oil, patients with rheumatoid arthritis experienced a significant improvement of symptoms. In several studies, GLA relieved the symptoms of eczema and atopic dermatitis and reduced the amount of skin area that was affected. Studies using GLA have also shown clinical benefits in patients with autoimmune disorders such as lupus and multiple sclerosis. Since GLA's anti-inflammatory mechanism is slightly different from that of EPA, it appears to complement EPA's anti-inflammatory activities.

CANCER

Numerous test-tube and animal studies have shown that EPA and GLA may prevent or inhibit the growth of cancer, particularly breast cancer, in a variety of ways, suggesting the possibility of an effective yet nontoxic treatment. It appears that GLA normalizes cancer cells without harming healthy cells, stifles the growth of blood vessels that feed tumors, and inhibits growth of tumor cells. EPA has shown promise in preventing bowel cancer. Human studies have shown that EPA helps prevent metastasis—the spread of cancer—in breast cancer, colon cancer, adenocarcinoma, and lung cancer. It works alone and with conventional cancer therapy, and it appears to be beneficial as complementary therapy along with chemotherapy and radiation.

PMS AND DYSMENORRHEA

In several studies, evening primrose oil, high in GLA, has reduced symptoms of premenstrual syndrome (PMS), including depression and irritability. Researchers believe that a deficiency of GLA causes an abnormal sensitivity to the hormone prolactin, which leads to symptoms of PMS. There are also reports that GLA may be an effective treatment for fibrocystic breasts.

Supplementation with essential fatty acids also appears to be beneficial in cases of dysmenorrhea—painful menstrual periods. In a study of adolescent girls, the group that received supplements of EPA, DHA, and vitamin E experienced a marked reduction of menstrual pain after two months of supplementation. The supplements apparently prevented a buildup of the pro-inflammatory prostaglandins in the cell membranes of the uterus—a buildup that produces symptoms such as cramps, nausea, vomiting, bloating, and headaches.

OTHER USES

Fish oil and GLA may also prove to be an important component of weight-loss programs. Scientific data suggests that this nutrient enhances brown fat metabolism—a metabolically active fat that enhances metabolism, thus burning extra calories. Animal studies suggest that both fish oil and GLA may slow the progress of the kidney disease glomerulonephritis and may help patients avoid dialysis. EPA can protect against painful kidney stones. Finally, there is evidence that these essential fatty acids may be useful in the treatment of certain disorders of the central nervous system. There are reports that both fish oil and GLA affect schizophrenia. Furthermore, fish oil may help in cases of bipolar disease (manic-depressive illness), depression, and other behavioral diseases; and GLA in cases of dyslexia and attention deficit disorder (hyperactivity) in children.

RDIs and Deficiency Symptoms

There are no established RDIs for the essential fatty acids, and no deficiency symptoms have been identified, despite the fact that they are essential.

Which Fatty Acids Should You Take?

The properties of omega-3 and omega-6 fatty acids overlap to a great degree. Both enhance the body's own anti-inflammatory process, acting like cortisone, but without the undesirable side effects. Both have cardioprotective and anticancer properties. So you might be left wondering: Which one should I take? The truth of the matter is that essential fatty acid supplementation is often a case of trial and error. As a general rule of thumb, I tend to use fish oil when there is a family tendency of high cholesterol (170 or above), high triglycerides, heart arrhythmias, or other heart disease. For those with low cholesterol, I generally use GLA. For hormonal problems, I usually try GLA first. However, keep in mind that researchers and clinicians have observed individual responses to the different fatty acids, so you must be willing to experiment. Try one type of supplement for one month and then switch to the other. Compare the results and stick with whichever one is most effective. If the results are not clear-cut, you may have to use both to achieve the balance that is right for you. In fact, some practitioners suggest giving EPA/DHA and GLA supplements together, and studies have shown that EPA and GLA used together yield the best results for some purposes, such as decreasing the inflammation of rheumatoid arthritis.

Omega-3 Fatty Acids (EPA AND DHA)

FOOD SOURCES

Animals—primarily cold-water fish and seafood such as herring, salmon, tuna, cod, mackerel, and shrimp—generally have the highest levels of EPA. When possible, I like people to obtain as many nutrients as possible from food. Unfortunately, fish and seafood now have high levels of mercury and sadly, I must advise my patients to limit fish consumption. Flaxseeds and flaxseed oils are the richest sources of alpha-linolenic acid, which can be converted to EPA and DHA in the body. I prefer flaxseeds over the oil because the whole seeds contain fiber and other phytochemicals that provide additional benefits. However, many factors can inactivate this process, including smoking, environmental toxins, aging, excessive saturated fat intake, alcohol, and certain medications. Fish oil, rich in the already active forms of EPA and DHA, is the more dependable source of this essential nutrient. You can also buy eggs that come from chickens fed high omega-3 diets who pass these nutrients on to us in their eggs. There is also a food product called Liquid Eggs (Omega Pro) that is high in omega-3.

SUPPLEMENTS

It is essential that EPA and DHA supplements include vitamin E to prevent rancidity, and that supplements be taken with additional vitamin E supplements to prevent oxidation in the body. In fact, some of the conflicting results of studies using fish oil may be due to the fact that in some cases, the supplements used did not contain any vitamin E to protect them. Study results have been superior when EPA has been consumed with a vitamin E supplement.

Per capsule, fish oil supplements generally contain between 180 and 400 milligrams of EPA plus 120 to 300 milligrams of DHA. Although cod liver oil contains EPA and DHA, large doses should be avoided, because the oil contains high amounts of vitamins A and D, which, if ingested in very high amounts, could be toxic.

Optimum Daily Intake—ODI

There is no Optimum Daily Intake for omega-3 fatty acids. Population studies have generally shown that eating cold-water fish as little as two or three times a week—the equivalent of about one ounce per day—could have beneficial effects, especially regarding heart disease prevention. For people who prefer not to rely on fish as a source of EPA and DHA, I generally recommend four to six fish oil capsules (approximately 3 grams) and as many as nine to twelve capsules for autoimmune disease, Crohn's disease, colitis, skin diseases, and heart disease. Most studies used eighteen or more fish oil capsules without controlling dietary fat intake. You can achieve the same clinical benefits by eating a low-fat diet and using lower amounts (four to six capsules). Because of this nutrient's blood-thinning effect, higher amounts should be taken only under professional supervision, especially if you are also taking blood-thinning medication.

Remember: If you have a medical condition, and particularly if you are on blood-thinning medication, please consult your physician before taking supplements.

TOXICITY AND ADVERSE EFFECTS

There are no known toxic effects of EPA, DHA, or alpha-linolenic acid. Blood-clotting times do decrease with supplementation, but are still within normal range. Some of my patients have complained that high-potency EPA supplements are difficult to digest, make them burp, and leave a fishy odor and taste. Enteric-coated fish oil capsules are generally better tolerated.

Omega-6 Fatty Acids (GLA)

FOOD SOURCES

With the exception of human milk, most foods contain very little active GLA. Plants from which we extract vegetable oils generally have the highest levels of omega-6 fatty acids, with corn oil and canola oil being the most commonly used. However, oils from these plants contain mostly linoleic acid and small amounts of cis-linoleic acid, which must first be converted in our bodies to the more active, potent gamma-linolenic acid before they can be further converted to prostaglandins. This conversion—like the conversion of alpha-linolenic acid to EPA and then DHA—may be inhibited by many factors, including aging; stress; alcohol; and diets high in saturated fat, transfatty acids (found in margarine), cholesterol, sugar, and low levels of magnesium and B_6. Other vegetable oils (see below) are more potent sources of GLA, but these are not generally used as food.

SUPPLEMENTS

Both in scientific studies and in clinical practice, capsules of evening primrose oil have been the mainstay of GLA supplementation. The problem is that each evening primrose oil capsule contains only 45 milligrams of GLA along with over 100 milligrams of linoleic acid—the essential fatty acid that has inflammatory effects—exactly what you are trying to overcome with the GLA. So, you need to take a lot of primrose oil capsules to get a therapeutic amount of GLA, but at the same time you are adding even more linoleic acid to your body. However, other, richer sources of GLA have been discovered, including borage oil and black currant oil. These oils supply more GLA—240 to 300 milligrams per capsule—while containing less linoleic acid—50 milligrams per capsule. Since most of us already have an overabundance of linoleic acid in our diet, I prefer to use GLA from borage and black currant oils to correct the imbalance and obtain the desired therapeutic effect.

OPTIMUM DAILY INTAKE—ODI

There is no Optimum Daily Intake for omega-6 fatty acids. For people at risk for the conditions mentioned earlier, I generally recommend 240 milligrams of GLA as a preventive measure and 240 to 480 for therapeutic reasons. Approximately six evening primrose oil capsules per day, or one GLA capsule from borage or black currant oil will supply 240 milligrams of GLA. Higher amounts should be taken only under professional supervision to avoid upsetting the fatty acid balance in your body.

Remember: If you have a medical condition, please consult with your physician before taking supplements.

Toxicity and Adverse Effects

There are no known toxic or adverse effects for GLA.

35 | Flavonoids

FLAVONOIDS, a group of crystalline compounds found in plants, were discovered by the Nobel Prize–winning scientist Albert Szent-Györgyi in 1936. He later named this class of plant compounds vitamin P. Since his discovery, scientists have isolated more than 4,000 flavonoids. Yet even this large number may represent only a small fraction of all the flavonoids that exist in nature. These substances are responsible for the deep colors of berries and are also found in the skins of citrus fruits and in other fruits, vegetables, nuts, seeds, grains, legumes, tea, coffee, cacao, and wine. In addition, most medicinal herbs owe their therapeutic qualities to flavonoid compounds.

Flavonoids are sometimes referred to as bioflavonoids, a term often used to describe biologically active flavonoids. When purchasing vitamins that contain flavonoids, you will find that the term bioflavonoid is the one that is most frequently used. However, the terms are generally used interchangeably.

Of the thousands of these oddly-named compounds that exist, the flavonoids that have been the most studied are quercetin, rutin, naringin, hesperidin, genistein, baicalin, Pycnogenol (a product that combines several substances), catechin, and bioflavonoid complex. In this chapter, I focus on those flavonoids for which we have the greatest research thus far. No doubt we'll be learning more about these and many others of these remarkable compounds as research continues.

Functions and Uses

Recently, flavonoids have received a lot of attention because of their impressive antioxidant properties (for more information about antioxidants, see page 33). Several of these compounds appear to be even more effective than the more familiar antioxidants—vitamins C and E, for instance—in their effects, such as that of protecting low-density lipoproteins (LDLs) from oxidation. And it appears that if we are eating lots of fruits, vegetables, grains, and legumes, the consumption of flavonoids would far exceed the consumption of other antioxidants, such as vitamin C. In fact, flavonoid consumption is estimated to be between 200 and 1,000 milligrams a day.

But their contribution to health goes far beyond their antioxidant abilities. Hundreds of studies on flavonoids have demonstrated that these substances have a wide range of abilities. They may also lower cholesterol levels, offering further protection against cardiovascular disease. They also possess antiviral, anticancer, anti-inflammatory, and antihistamine activities and may therefore be useful in preventing and/or treating a wide variety of conditions. Research supports this theory.

For example, many studies—in particular, those of Dr. Chithan Kandaswami and Dr. Elliot Middleton—have demonstrated the effectiveness of a variety of flavonoids in the prevention and treatment of various cancers. These studies, which have included treatment of cancers resistant to chemotherapy, have involved both cell lines (cultures of cells grown in petri dishes) and living organisms.

In a 2002 study of 10,000 Finnish men and women, researchers discovered many specific associations between certain flavonoids in the diet and several chronic diseases. They found that: Persons with higher quercetin intakes had lower mortality from ischemic heart disease; persons with high hesperetin, kaempferol, and naringenin intakes had a lower incidence of cerebrovascular; men with higher quercetin intakes had a lower lung cancer incidence; men with higher myricetin intakes had a lower prostate cancer risk; people with higher quercetin, naringenin, and hesperetin intakes had a lower asthma incidence; and higher quercetin and myricetin intakes were associatred with a trend toward a reduction in risk of type II diabetes.

There has been considerable research performed on the antiviral activity of flavonoids, especially with viruses associated with polio, influenza, hepatitis types A and B, herpes simplex 1, human T-cell leukemia virus type I, and HIV (human immunodeficiency virus). In in vitro (test tube) conditions, for instance, baicalin and quercetin have been shown to inhibit the replication of the HIV virus by 100 percent.

It is interesting to note that many medicinal plants used for centuries contain high levels of flavonoid compounds. Examples can be found in the popular Japanese herbal medicine known as Sho-saiko-to, which is used to treat chronic liver disease. When investigators examined the ability of these herbs to inhibit the growth of cancer cells, they discovered that the combination of herbs was better at inhibiting the cancer growth than was each of the herbs when acting individually. This clearly demonstrates the synergistic effect of flavonoids.

Flavonoids that behave as phytoestrogens do not increase estrogen levels, as this name might imply. Instead, they encourage a better balance of good to bad estrogen by binding to sites for bad estrogen and helping our bodies metabolize the bad estrogen. An excess of the bad estrogen (estradiol) is implicated in breast cancer, prostate cancer, menopausal symptoms, premenstrual symptoms, endometriosis, fibrocystic breast disease, and possibly other hormonally related disorders. Flavonoids help the body convert estradiol to estriol, the safe and protective form of estrogen. In fact, estriol is the preferred form of estrogen used in Europe in hormone-replacement therapy. Rich sources of the phytoestrogens are found in soybean products and may be one reason for the lower incidence of estrogen-dependent disorders found in Eastern countries whose cuisines include soybean foods. There are even reports of flavonoids being used successfully in the treatment of osteoporosis as a safe alternative to estrogen-replacement therapy.

Considering the hundreds of studies that have been performed on flavonoids and the fact that many of the effects have been outstanding when compared with those of drug-intervention studies, it is puzzling that these substances are not used more frequently as a treatment option for HIV/AIDS, arthritis, hepatitis, and cardiovascular disease, as well as the host of other degenerative diseases that have responded in test-tube, animal, and some human experiments.

QUERCETIN

Quercetin is in many ways the most amazing flavonoid yet studied. It has been found to be active against many types of cancer, including breast, prostate, colon, gastric, head and neck, leukemia, lung, melanoma, liver, ovarian, cervical, and rhabdomyosarcoma. Although it is synergistic with various chemotherapy drugs as well as radiation, unlike these conventional forms of cancer treatment, when quercetin is used alone it damages cancer cells only. It appears to squelch cancer growth in a myriad of ways—by shutting down the growth of blood vessels that feed the cancer, by inhibiting the production of tumor-stimulating hormones and hormonelike substances; by stimulating the immune system, and through scavenging mutation-causing free radicals, to name several. Quercetin has been found to be more effective in metastatic breast cancer than is the widely touted anti-estrogen drug tamoxifen, and it is completely nontoxic.

PYCNOGENOL

The flavonoids known as proanthocyanidins are also getting a good deal of attention. Most of the research on proanthocyanidins has used Pycnogenol—a product containing proanthocyanidins and related plant flavonoids from the bark of the French Maritime pine tree—rather than grape seed extract, which also contains this type of flavonoid. There have also been a lot of studies on Activin, in particular on cancer and cardiovascular effects, as well as other highly standardized proanthocyanidins supplements such as Masquelier's OPC. Much of this research has focused on the ability of these substances to act as antioxidants, and on their beneficial effects on many types of circulation problems. Human trials have shown that these flavonoids can prevent peripheral hemorrhage, swelling of the legs due to water retention, diabetic retinopathy, and high blood pressure. Researchers have also reported success in using these substances to treat varicose veins, leg cramps, and other problems arising from insufficient blood flow. When buying this flavonoid, look for these forms and other supplements standardized to at least 20 percent proanthocyanidins.

RDIs and Deficiency Symptoms

There are no established RDIs for flavonoids, and no deficiency symptoms have been identified.

FOOD SOURCES

Flavonoids are found in fruits, vegetables, nuts, seeds, grains, and legumes (particularly soybeans and soy products), and in beverages such as tea, coffee, and wine. It is possible to obtain the basic ODI for flavonoids by eating a diet rich in these foods. Quercetin is the major flavonoid in our diet; it is estimated we eat approximately 25 milligrams per day from onions, apples, and other commonly eaten foods. Many medicinal herbs are also high in quercetin and other flavonoids.

Supplements

Supplements of many—but not all—of the various flavonoids are available individually and in combination. Those that are easiest to find include bioflavonoid complex, curcumin, hesperidin, Pycnogenol, quercetin, and rutin. Note that all flavonoids should be taken with vitamin C, as they increase vitamin C absorption and are themselves powerful antioxidants.

Optimum Daily Intake—ODI

For optimum general health, the basic Optimum Daily Intake for flavonoids—alone or in combination—is:

250–1,000 mg for men and women (to be taken with an equivalent amount of vitamin C)

For specific conditions, the following flavonoids have been found to be helpful for:

CONDITION	SUPPLEMENTS	SUGGESTED DOSAGE
Allergies, arthritis, asthma, and inflammation	quercetin	1,000–3,000 mg
Bruising and circulatory disorders, including phlebitis and varicose veins	Pycnogenol, grape seed extracts	50–300 mg
Bruising and circulatory disorders, including varicose veins	bioflavonoid complex containing rutin and hesperidin	1,000–5,000 mg
Cancer prevention and hormone imbalance	quercetin	1,500–4,500 mg (especially breast and prostate)
Viral infections, including HIV; inflammations due to arthritis and injury; and allergies	quercetin	1,500–4,500 mg

Remember: If you have a medical condition, please consult your physician before taking supplements.

Toxicity and Adverse Effects

There are no known toxicities or adverse effects for flavonoids.

36 | Other Nutrients:
Alpha-Lipoic Acid (ALA), Garlic,
Glutathione and N-Acetylcysteine (NAC),
L-Carnitine, Melatonin, and DHEA

THIS CHAPTER is devoted to those nutrients that I usually recommend only for my patients with diagnosed medical problems. Although these nutrients are not for everyone, they are effective and I do strongly recommend that you consider taking them for the uses outlined below, under professional supervision. Remember, if you take them, take them in addition to your basic optimum program of a full spectrum of vitamins and minerals—not instead of them.

Alpha-Lipoic Acid (ALA)

Alpha-lipoic acid (ALA) is a potent antioxidant in both fat- and water-soluble mediums and therefore can protect all parts of the cells of the body from free-radical damage. ALA plays another role as antioxidant helper—it can regenerate vitamin C and vitamin E after they have been "used up" neutralizing free radicals. Researchers have found ALA can also increase levels of the antioxidant enzyme glutathione and coenzyme Q_{10} in our cells. ALA appears capable of chelating certain metals, especially toxic ones like cadmium and mercury, and helps clear them out of the body. Lipoic acid has been used extensively in Germany for the treatment of diabetic neuropathy. Lipid peroxidation is believed to play a role in the development of neuropathy. ALA has been shown to significantly reduce the symptoms of neuropathy in diabetic patients. Thus, it appears lipoic acid has the potential to prevent diabetes, improve glucose control, and prevent chronic hyperglycemia-associated complications such as neuropathy.

CONDITION	SUGGESTED DOSAGE
Cataracts	300–600 mg
Glaucoma	300–600 mg
Ischemia-reperfusion injury	300–600 mg
Diabetic neuropathy	300–600 mg
Alzheimer's disease	600–1200 mg

Garlic

Garlic is a plant food used all over the world. In many ancient and modern cultures, garlic has been considered a potent medicinal herb, effective in combating heart disease, infections, and many types of cancer. Recent studies support these traditional uses for garlic, making its medicinal properties better recognized and accepted in the United States. While there is conflicting evidence as to whether garlic actually lowers cholesterol and tryglicerides in everyone, we do have strong evidence that it does lower certain other risk factors that may play an even larger role in the development and progression of heart disease. We know that garlic lowers blood pressure, thins the blood, and reduces the tendency of blood to form harmful clots (similar to aspirin). We also know that it modulates changes in the blood vessel walls related to aging and arteriosclerosis; for example, by preventing the oxidation of LDL, which damages the arterial walls and sets the stage for cholesterol build-up. Garlic—as supplements or in food—also detoxifies carcinogens.

Because garlic contains many active ingredients—including potassium, phosphorus, vitamins B and C, amino acids, germanium, selenium, and sulfur compounds—researchers are not sure which ingredient does what at this point, or if garlic's components are working alone or in combination. Some of the conflicting results in garlic studies must surely be due to the variety of forms of garlic used—everything from garlic powder (used in cooking), to raw whole garlic, and garlic capsules. Many studies showing garlic's effectiveness used standardized supplements such as Garlicin, Kwai or Kyolic, an odor-modified garlic extract.

CONDITION	SUGGESTED DOSAGE
Cardiovascular problems	600–1,200 mg; follow label directions since all have different potencies
Diabetes	600–1,200 mg
Diabetic neuropathy	300–600 mg
Insulin resistant	600–1,200 mg

Glutathione and N-Acetylcysteine (NAC)

Most people are accustomed to thinking of antioxidants as vitamins and minerals. But there are many other natural substances that function in this way. Glutathione, a powerful antioxidant enzyme produced in our bodies, is one such substance. N-acetylcysteine (NAC), an amino acid required by our bodies to produce glutathione, appears to possess particular antioxidant properties, as well. As antioxidants, these two related substances are intimately involved in the detoxification process and are important members of our defenses against environmental toxins and carcinogens. They also protect our cells from oxidative stress—damage that may occur from a variety of environmental insults. Because such damage plays a role in degenerative diseases and in the weakening of the immune system, it should come as no surprise that it is the degenerative diseases—cancer, cardiovascular disease, and arthritis, for instance—and viral infections that respond to glutathione and NAC supplementation. In general, the studies of NAC have focused on its use in the treatment of viral infections, while the studies of glutathione have concerned the treatment of cancer. However, there is considerable overlap in the function and use of these two antioxidants, and it is reasonable to assume that both work for many conditions.

CONDITION	SUGGESTED DOSAGE
Infection and immunity (including HIV)	NAC 1,200–2,400 mg plus glutathione 500–1500 mg
Detoxification Environmental pollutants, carcinogens, certain drugs	NAC 1,200–2,400 plus glutathione 500–1,500 mg
Adjuvant cancer treatment	NAC 1,200–2,400 mg plus glutathione 500–1500 mg
Pulmonary disease	NAC 1,200–2,400 mg
Neurological disease (Parkinson's/Alzheimer's)	NAC 2,400–3,800 mg

L-Carnitine

Although often called an amino acid because of its chemical makeup, L-carnitine is actually a vitaminlike nutrient, related in structure to the B vitamins. L-carnitine is the biologically active form of carnitine. It is important in the production of energy via its role in transporting fatty acids into muscles. Supplementation appears to build stamina and endurance and may therefore enhance exercise performance—particularly in people with low levels of this nutrient. L-carnitine is also often prescribed for individuals who suffer from muscle fatigue due to conditions such as fibromyalgia and chronic fatigue syndrome. Much of the research concerning L-carnitine has focused on its use in the treatment of heart disease. Approximately 60 percent of the energy for the heart muscle is supplied by fatty acids. Thus, myocardial (heart muscle) L-carnitine deficiency has been found to be associated with myopathic heart disease, aging, diabetes, diphtheria, and chronic heart failure. L-carnitine supplementation has been shown to help lessen the impairment of heart muscle function associated with these conditions.

L-Carnitine may also be important for healthy brain function, since it appears to influence the metabolism of several neurotransmitters—chemicals that facilitate the sending of signals from one nerve fiber to another. In a study involving people with Alzheimer's disease, the progression of the disease was significantly reduced in those receiving 2 grams per day of acetyl-L-carnitine—a particular form of carnitine—orally for one year. L-carnitine also seems to have some antioxidant properties, as well as the ability to help detoxify certain drugs. For example, it appears to protect the heart muscle from the damage caused by Adriamycin (doxorubicin hydrochloride), a drug used in cancer treatment.

CONDITION	SUGGESTED DOSAGE
Cardiovascular disease (heart attack, congestive heart failure, arrhythmias, and other CV conditions)	2–4 grams
Detoxification	2–4 grams
Post-exercise fatigue	2–4 grams
Chronic Fatigue Syndrome	2–4 grams
Fibromyalgia	2–4 grams

Melatonin

Although melatonin is popularly regarded as a nutritional supplement, it is really a hormone secreted by the pineal gland, a tiny aspirin-sized organ buried deep in the brain. Not to be confused with the skin pigment melanin, melatonin is a potent chemical found in every cell of every living organism. Melatonin is responsible for regulating biological rhythms both in humans and in animals.

Much of the data that has been gathered on melatonin relates to its role as timekeeper and its resulting ability to induce sleep, reduce jet lag, and untangle confused body rhythms induced by shift work. Other exciting research suggests that melatonin has a far wider range of actions. These include anticancer, antiaging, and antioxidant effects, as well as effects on fertility, sex drive, and the immune system.

Because there have been no long-term studies on melatonin supplementation, I do not recommend that healthy people use it on a long-term basis. When used in the doses recommended below it may be helpful, and it appears safe for occasional use for insomnia and jet lag. I recommend starting with .1 milligram (a tenth of a one-milligram capsule), and increasing the dose until you have corrected your sleep problem. If you are taking it for preventive purposes, I also recommend starting with the lowest dose and increasing it slowly up to 3 milligrams. Use your judgment and monitor how you feel. Even better, ask your physician to measure your melatonin level to see if it is low. Melatonin should always be taken in the evening. Do not take more than 7 milligrams per day, except under professional advice. Recent studies have shown that high doses of melatonin work synergistically with certain types of chemotherapy. In one report, melatonin improved survival times in women with breast cancer being treated with chemotherapy and lessened the side effects.

CONDITION	SUGGESTED DOSAGE
Aging-related problems	1–3 mg daily
Insomnia	1–7 mg (best if taken 1 to 2 hours before bedtime)
Jet lag	1–7 mg (best if started upon arrival at destination and continued for 5 days)

| Adjuvant cancer treatment | 10–50 mg (under professional advice) |
| Improve pituitary, thyroid and other hormone levels, and depression, in women | 3 mg |

Excess melatonin may increase the level of the hormone prolactin, which decreases sex drive in men and could theoretically accelerate the growth of prolactin-sensitive breast cancers. Some people have reported experiencing wakefulness, nightmares, morning grogginess, and headaches, or mild depression when taking melatonin. Melatonin supplements should be avoided—or taken only under professional supervision—by children, pregnant or nursing women, people trying to conceive, people with hormonal imbalances, people taking steroids, people who have severe allergies or other autoimmune disorders, and people with immune system cancers such as lymphoma or leukemia. Some researchers recommend that people with a tendency toward depression or who are on antidepressants also avoid taking this supplement. Many physicians and health professionals, including myself, suggest taking melatonin only under professional supervision.

DHEA

Like melatonin, discussed in the previous section, DHEA (dehydroepiandrosterone) is popularly viewed as a nutritional supplement, but is actually a hormone secreted by the adrenal gland. However, it is a precursor hormone—a hormone that is converted into several other hormones by the body—and for some time was thought to be less important than these metabolized end products. We now know that this hormone has many functions, including support of the immune system; repair and maintenance of tissues; reduction of allergic reactions; and, possibly, the prevention of certain forms of age-related diseases, as well as a slowing of the aging process itself. As we age, our levels of DHEA and the male and female hormones significantly decline, along with those of other hormones, including the growth hormone. It is estimated that by age sixty, DHEA levels are a third or less of those in young adults. At age eighty, people have between 80 and 90 percent less DHEA in their blood than they had at the age of twenty-five. Many researchers believe that these reduced hormone levels are closely associated with aging-related problems, such as shrinkage of muscle mass, diminished immune function, and memory loss. In fact, the majority of human studies on DHEA have focused on aging and the diseases associated with aging.

CONDITION	SUGGESTED DOSAGE
Cardiovascular disease	25–50 mg
Adjuvant cancer	50–200 mg under professional advice
Menopause	50 mg
Age-related degenerative disease (diabetes, aging, heart disease)	25–50 mg
Lupus/autoimmune disorder	50–200 under professional advice
Impotency/erectile dysfunction	50 mg

DHEA is a precursor to testosterone and estrogen, and your gender does not predict which it will be converted to. So if you have a hormonally sensitive cancer, such as a breast cancer, that has receptors for estrogen, you need to be supervised professionally and have your hormone levels measured regularly as a safeguard. Since DHEA is a hormone that can influence the production of androgens and estrogens, both other practitioners and I feel it is imperative that DHEA be used only under professional advice. Before beginning supplementation, it is best to have your physician first run a blood test of the following: DHEA; DHEAS; estradiol, estrone, and estriol, the three types of estrogen; and serum and free testosterone. Men with prostate conditions should have a physician measure their levels of dihydrotestosterone and PSA (prostate specific antigen, a marker for prostate cancer). DHEA should be used with extreme caution in men with prostate conditions, since it may raise levels of certain androgens, which are the culprits in prostate disease. The same is true of women with disorders related to excessive estrogen. Once supplementation begins, all hormone levels should be retested within three weeks to evaluate the effects of the DHEA supplement in order to adjust the dosage as necessary.

The purpose of using DHEA is to raise levels of the measured hormones so that they fall within normal ranges. You do not want to take so much DHEA that your hormone levels exceed the normal reference range.

It is best to start with low doses of DHEA—5 milligrams for women and 10 milligrams for men—and slowly increase the levels by 5 to 10 milligrams each week until the desired result is achieved. Use the lowest dosage of DHEA needed to achieve results. Serious side effects of DHEA supplementation have not been reported in human studies. Since high levels of DHEA stimulate the production of androgens, some side effects associated with high androgen levels have been reported, including acne and excessively oily skin, hair growth in women, deepening of the voice, and mood changes. Many physicians and health professionals, including myself, suggest taking DHEA only under professional advice.

Part 5

Appendixes and Notes

Summary of Vitamins, Minerals, and Other Nutrients

THE BASIC Optimum Daily Intake (ODI) is designed to enhance general health and prevent disease. Some individuals may wish to use higher levels, depending upon risk factors such as pollution, stress, and personal and family history.

Please note that for some nutrients—boron, for example—RDIs and ODIs have not yet been determined. For these nutrients, I have indicated a recommended range—in the case of boron, 3 to 6 milligrams—followed by an asterisk (*) to indicate that this dosage is not an ODI.

QUICK-REFERENCE TABLE

NUTRIENT	MAJOR USES	FOOD SOURCES	RDI	ODI
Fat-Soluble Vitamins				
Vitamin A, Beta-carotene, and other carotenoids	Antioxidant. Prevents night blindness, macular degeneration, and other eye problems. May be useful for acne and other skin disorders. Enhances immunity. Cancer prevention. May heal gastrointestinal ulcers. Protects against pollution.	Fish liver oils, animal livers, green and yellow fruits and vegetables.	5,000 IU None	5,000–25,000 IU 11,000–25,000 IU

NUTRIENT	MAJOR USES	FOOD SOURCES	RDI	ODI
Fat-Soluble Vitamins (*cont.*)				
Vitamin A Beta-carotene, and other carotenoids (*cont.*)	Needed for epithelial tissue maintenance and repair. May prevent and improve macular degeneration. May prevent prostate and other cancers.		5,000 IU (Vitamin A)	5,000–25,000 IU (Vitamin A) 11,000–25,000 IU (Beta-carotene) 10–40 mg lutein* 10–20 mg lycopene*
Vitamin D	Required for calcium and phosphorus absorption and utilization. Prevention and treatment of osteoporosis. Enhances immunity.	Fish liver oils, fatty saltwater fish, vitamin D-fortified dairy products, eggs.	400 IU	400–800 IU
Vitamin E	Antioxidant. Cancer prevention. Cardiovascular disease prevention. Improves circulation. Tissue repair. May prevent age spots. Useful in treating fibrocystic breasts. Useful in treating PMS.	Cold-pressed vegetable oils, whole grains, nuts, dark-green leafy vegetables, legumes.	30 IU	400–1,200 IU
Vitamin K	Needed for blood clotting. May play a role in bone formation. May prevent osteoporosis.	Green leafy vegetables.	80 mcg	80 mcg
Water-Soluble Vitamins				
Biotin	Needed for metabolism of protein, fats, and carbohydrates. Not enough data available, but deficiencies may be implicated in high serum cholesterol, seborrheic dermatitis, and certain nervous system disorders.	Meat, cooked egg yolk, yeast, poultry, milk, saltwater fish, soybeans, whole grains.	300 mcg	300 mcg
Choline and Inositol	Involved in metabolism of fat and cholesterol, and absorption and utilization of fat. Choline makes an important brain neurotransmitter.	Egg yolk, whole grains, vegetables, organ meats, fruits, milk.	None	25–500 mg

NUTRIENT	MAJOR USES	FOOD SOURCES	RDI	ODI
	Water-Soluble Vitamins (*cont.*)			
Choline and Inositol (*cont.*)	May be useful for panic disorders.			
Folic acid	Works closely with B_{12}. Involved in protein metabolism. Needed for healthy cell division and replication. Prevention and treatment of folic acid anemia. Stress may increase need. May be useful for depression and anxiety. May be useful in treating cervical dysplasia. Oral contraceptives may increase need. Lowers homocysteine levels.	Beef, lamb, pork, chicken liver, whole wheat, bran, green leafy vegetables, yeast.	400 mcg	400–1,200 mcg
PABA	Needed for protein metabolism. Needed for folic acid metabolism. Used topically as a sunscreen.	Liver, kidney, whole grains, molasses.	None	25–500 mg
Panto-thenic acid	Needed in fat, protein, and carbohydrate metabolism. Needed for synthesis of hormones and cholesterol. Needed for red blood cell production. Needed for nerve transmission. Vital for healthy function of the adrenal glands. May be useful for joint inflammation. May be useful for depression and anxiety. May lower cholesterol.	Eggs, saltwater fish, pork, beef, milk, whole wheat, beans, fresh vegetables.	10 mg	25–500 mg 900 mg Pantetheine
Vitamin B Complex B_1 (thiamin); B_2 (riboflavin); (riboflavin); B_3 (niacin, niacinamide); B_6 (pyridoxine)	Maintains healthy nerves, skin, hair, liver, mouth, muscle tone in gastrointestinal tract. B vitamins are coenzymes involved in energy production. Emotional or physical stress increases need. May be useful for depression or anxiety.	Unrefined whole grains, liver, green leafy vegetables, fish, poultry, eggs, meat, nuts, beans.	B_1: 1.5 mg B_2: 1.7 mg B_3: 20 mg B_6: 2.0 mg	25–300 mg

NUTRIENT	MAJOR USES	FOOD SOURCES	RDI	ODI
Water-Soluble Vitamins (*cont.*)				
	B_1: High-carbohydrate diet increases need.			
	B_2: May be useful with B_6 for treatment of carpal tunnel syndrome. May prevent cataracts. Increased need with oral contraceptives. Increased need with strenuous exercise. Antioxidant.			
	B_3: Useful for circulatory problems. May lower serum cholesterol and triglycerides and raise HDLs (1,000–2,000 mg). Certain forms cause flushing.			
	B_6: May be useful in preventing oxalate stones. May be used as mild diuretic. May be useful for PMS. Increased need with oral contraceptives. May be useful in treating asthma. P, P may be more efficacious for some people. Lowers homocysteine levels.			
Vitamin B_{12} (cobalamin)	Needed for fat and carbo-hydrate metabolism. Prevention and treatment of B_{12} anemia. Maintains proper nervous system function. May be useful for anxiety and depression.	Kidney, liver, egg, herring, mackerel, milk cheese, tofu, seafood.	6 mcg	25–500 mcg
Vitamin C (ascorbic acid)	Growth and repair of tissues. May reduce cholesterol. Antioxidant. Cancer prevention. Enhances immunity. Stress increases requirement. May reduce high blood pressure. May prevent atherosclerosis. Protects against pollution.	Green vege-tables, berries, citrus fruit.	60 mg	500–5,000 mg (higher during stress or illness)
Minerals				
Boron	Prevents bone loss. May improve bone density. Helps improve osteo-arthritis.	Fruits, vege-tables.	None	3–6 mg
Calcium	Needed for healthy bones and teeth. Needed for nerve trans-mission. Used for muscle function. May lower blood pressure. Osteoporosis prevention.	Dairy foods, green leafy vegetables, salmon, sardines, seafood.	1,000 mg	1,000–1,500 mg
Chromium	Required for glucose metabolism. May prevent diabetes. May reduce cholesterol.	Brewer's yeast, beer, meat, cheese, whole grains.	120 mcg	200–600 mcg

NUTRIENT	MAJOR USES	FOOD SOURCES	RDI	ODI
Minerals (*cont.*)				
Copper	Involved in blood formation. Needed for healthy nerves. Needed for taste sensitivity. Used in energy production. Needed for healthy bone development.	Widely distributed in foods. Also derived from copper cookware and plumbing.	2 mg	Generally available through foods: 0.5–2 mg
Iodine	Needed for healthy thyroid gland. Prevents goiter.	Iodized salts, seafood, kelp, saltwater fish.	150 mcg	150–300 mcg (0–150 mcg for those who use iodized salt)
Iron	Vital for blood formation. Needed for energy production. Required for healthy immune system.	Meat, poultry, fish, liver, eggs, green leafy vegetables, whole grain or enriched breads and cereals.	18 mg	15–25 mg men 18–30 mg women
Magnesium	Needed for healthy bones. Involved in nerve transmission. Needed for muscle function. Used in energy formation. Needed for healthy blood vessels. May lower blood pressure.	Widely distributed in foods, especially dairy foods, meat, fish, seafood.	400 mg	500–750 mg
Manganese	Needed for protein and fat metabolism. Used in energy formation. Required for normal bone growth and reproduction. Needed for healthy nerves. Needed for healthy blood sugar regulation. Needed for healthy immune system.	Nuts, seeds, whole grains, avocado, seaweed.	2 mg	15–50 mg
Phosphorus	Necessary for healthy bones. Needed for production of energy. Used as a buffering agent. Needed for utilization of protein, fats, and carbohydrates.	Available in most foods; sodas can be very high.	1,000 mg	Generally available through foods: 200–400 mg

NUTRIENT	MAJOR USES	FOOD SOURCES	RDI	ODI
Minerals (cont.)				
Potassium	May lower blood pressure. Needed for energy storage. Needed for nerve transmission, muscle contraction, and hormone secretion.	Dairy foods, meat, poultry, fish, fruit, legumes, whole grains, vegetables.	None	99–300 mg
Selenium	Cancer prevention. Heart disease prevention.	Depending on soil content, may be in grains and meat.	70 mcg	100–400 mcg (100–200 mcg for those who live in higher-selenium areas)
Zinc	Needed for wound healing. Maintains taste and smell acuity. Needed for healthy immune system. Protects liver from chemical damage.	Oysters, fish, seafood, meats, poultry, whole grains, legumes.	15 mg	22.5–50 mg
Beyond Vitamins and Minerals				
Alpha-lipoic acid	May help detoxification. May prevent cardiovascular disease. May improve diabetes. May improve diabetic neuropathy.	None	None	300–600 mg*
Coenzyme Q_{10} (CoQ)	Cell energy and metabolism. Prevents cell damage. May be useful in cardiovascular diseases such as angina, congestive heart failure, arrhythmia, and high blood pressure. May protect heart muscle and promote faster recovery from heart attack and heart surgery.	Beef hearts, chicken hearts, other hearts. Sardines, peanuts, and spinach.	None	50–300 mg*
DHEA	Antiaging properties. May strengthen immune system. May inhibit cancer.	None	None	Use only when needed 25–50 mg*

NUTRIENT	MAJOR USES	FOOD SOURCES	RDI	ODI
Beyond Vitamins and Minerals (*cont.*)				
DHEA (*cont.*)	May help prevent cardiovascular disease. May increase insulin tissue sensitivity. May help treat lupus. May relieve menopause symptoms. May improve erectile dysfunction.			
Fish oil	Prevents heart disease. May lower blood pressure. May lower triglycerides. May lower cholesterol. Prevents excess blood clotting. May relieve inflammatory and allergic reactions. May inhibit cancer. May enhance immune system. May improve bipolar disorders.	Cold-water fish.	None	1,500–3,000 mg*
Flavonoids	Antioxidant. May lower cholesterol. May prevent cardiovascular disease. May inhibit cancer. Needed to maintain healthy blood vessels. Helps fight viral infections.	Fruits, vegetables, grains, nuts, seeds, soybeans, tea, coffee, wine.	None	250–1,000 mg
Garlic	May lower blood pressure. May enhance immune system. May prevent heart disease. May lower triglycerides. May lower cholesterol. Antibacterial, antiviral, antifungal. Prevents excess blood clotting. May prevent cancer. Antioxidant.	Garlic.	None	200–1,200 mg*
GLA	May prevent heart disease. Relieves allergic reactions. Relieves eczema. Relieves arthritis. Relieves PMS symptoms. May assist in weight loss.	Evening primrose oil, borage oil, black currant oil.	None	70–240 mg*

NUTRIENT	MAJOR USES	FOOD SOURCES	RDI	ODI
Beyond Vitamins and Minerals (cont.)				
Glutathione and NAC	Antioxidant. Helps fight viral infections. May inhibit cancer. Helps maintain healthy immune system. Protects against environmental and drug toxicity. May improve Parkinson's/Alzheimer's.	Fruits, vegetables, meat.	None	Glutathione: 500–1,500 mg* NAC: 1,200–3,800 mg*
L-Carnitine	Needed for fat metabolism. May inhibit muscle fatigue diseases. May alleviate or prevent heart conditions. Helps body detoxify drugs. May improve chronic fatigue syndrome and fibromyalgia.	Animal foods.	None	2,000–4,000 mg*
Melatonin	Regulates biological rhythms. Relieves insomnia. Prevents jet lag. Has antiaging properties. Relieves some hormone-related problems. May inhibit cancer.	Found in small amounts in rice, barley, corn.	None	0.1–7 mg For short-term use, only when needed.

Drug-Induced Vitamin
and Mineral Deficiencies

MY FRIEND and colleague Dr. Jim Lavalle, pharmacist and naturopathic doctor, created the following chart to show the major interactions between many commonly taken drugs and nutrients. It is from his terrific book, *The Nutritional Cost of Prescription Drugs*, published in 2001 by Morton Publishing. If you are taking one or more of these medications, why wouldn't you take supplements to counteract the depletion of key nutrients? If your physician has not suggested that you do, show your doctor this chart. As you saw in the various chapters of this book, there are numerous studies that show that people who take both medication and certain supplements do better than people who take the drugs alone.

DRUG-NUTRIENT INTERACTION TABLE

DRUG	NUTRIENT DEPLETION
Antacids	
Aluminum hydroxide Magnesium hydroxide Magnesium oxide Magnesium sulfate Aluminum hydroxide and magnesium hydroxide Aluminum hydroxide and magnesium carbonate Aluminum hydroxide and magnesium trisilicate Aluminum hydroxide, magnesium hydroxide, and simethicone	Calcium Phosphorus
Sodium Bicarbonate	Potassium
Antibiotics	
Penicillins Cephalosporins Fluoroquinolones Macrolides Aminoglycosides	*Lactobacillus acidophilus, Bifidobacteria bifidum (bifidus)* Vitamin B$_1$ Vitamin B$_2$ Vitamin B$_3$ Vitamin B$_6$ Vitamin B$_{12}$ Biotin Inositol Vitamin K
Tetracyclines, sulfonamides	Calcium—take several hours apart from antibiotic. Magnesium Iron *Lactobacillus acidophilus, Bifidobacteria bifidum (bifidus)* Vitamin B$_1$ Vitamin B$_2$ Vitamin B$_3$ Vitamin B$_6$ Vitamin B$_{12}$ Biotin Inositol Vitamin K
Neomycin	Beta-carotene Iron Vitamin A Vitamin B$_{12}$
Co-trimoxazole	*Bifidobacteria bifidum (bifidus)* *Lactobacillus acidophilus* Folic acid

DRUG	NUTRIENT DEPLETION
Antibiotics (*cont.*)	
Isoniazid INH	Vitamin B_6 Vitamin B_3 Vitamin D
Rifampin	Vitamin D
Ethambutol	Zinc Copper
Anticonvulsants	
Barbiturates	Vitamin D Calcium Folic acid Vitamin K
Phenytoin	Biotin Vitamin D Calcium Folic acid Vitamin K Vitamin B_{12} Vitamin B_1
Carbamazepine	Folic acid Vitamin D Biotin
Primidone	Folic acid Biotin
Valproic acid	Folic acid Carnitine
Antidiabetics	
Sulfonylureas Acetohexamide Glyburide Tolazamide	Coenzyme Q_{10}
Biguanides Metformin	Vitamin B_{12}
Anti-Inflammatories	
Salicylates Aspirin Choline magnesium trisalicylate Choline salicylate	Vitamin C Folic acid Potassium Iron Sodium
Salsalate	Folic acid
Nonsteroidal Anti-Inflammatory Agents Ibuprofen, naproxen, sulindac piroxi- cam, diclofenac, diflunisal, etodolac, fenoprofen, ketoprofen, ketorolac,	Folic acid Melatonin

DRUG	NUTRIENT DEPLETION
Anti-Inflammatories (*cont.*)	
Nonsteroidal Anti-Inflammatory (cont.) meclofenamate, nabumetone, tolmetin, mefenamic acid, Celecoxib Indomethacin	Folic acid and iron
Corticosteroids Betamethasone, budesonide Cortisone, dexamethasone Flunisolide, fluticasone Hydrocortisone, mometasone Methylprednisolone Prednisone, prednisolone Triamcinolone	Calcium Vitamin D Potassium Zinc Vitamin C Magnesium Folic acid Selenium
Anti-Inflammatory Misc. Sulfasalazine	Folic acid
Antivirals	
Reverse Transcriptase Inhibitors Didanosine Lamivudine Stavudine Zalcitabine Zidovudine	Copper Zinc Vitamin B_{12} Carnitine
Non-Nucleoside Delavirdine Nevirapine	Copper Zinc Vitamin B_{12} Carnitine
Benzodiazepines	
Diazepam Alprazolam	Melatonin
Bronchodilators	
Theophylline	Vitamin B_6
Cardiovascular Drugs	
Vasodilators Hydralazine	Vitamin B_6 Coenzyme Q_{10}
Loop Diuretics Furosemide Bumetanide Ethacrynic Acid	Calcium Magnesium Vitamin B_1 Vitamin B_6 Vitamin C Potassium Zinc
Thiazide Diuretics Hydrochlorothiazide Methyclothiazide	Magnesium Potassium Zinc

DRUG	NUTRIENT DEPLETION
Cardiovascular Drugs (*cont.*)	
Indapamide Metolazone	Coenzyme Q_{10}
Potassium-Sparing Diuretics Triamterene	Calcium Folic acid Zinc
Hydrochlorothiazide & triamterene	Calcium Folic acid Zinc Vitamin B_6

ACE Inhibitors
  Captopril
  Enalopril
	Zinc

Centrally-Acting Antihypertensives
  Clonidine
  Methyldopa
	Coenzyme Q_{10}

Chlorthalidone	Zinc
Cardiac Glycosides Digoxin	Calcium Magnesium Phosphorus Vitamin B_1

Beta-Blockers
  Propranolol, metoprolol, atenolol,
  pindolol, acetutolol, betaxolol,
  bisoprolol, carteolol, carvedilol,
  esmolol, labetalol, nadolol, sotalol,
  timolol
	Coenzyme Q_{10}
	Melatonin

Cholesterol-Lowering Drugs	

HMG-CoA Reductase Inhibitors
  Atorvastatin
  Cerivastatin
  Lovastatin
  Fluvastatin
  Pravastatin
  Simvastatin
	Coenzyme Q_{10}

Bile Acid Sequestrants Cholestyramine	Vitamin A, beta-carotene, vitamin D, vitamin E, vitamin K, vitamin B_{12}, folic acid, iron, calcium, magnesium, phosphorus, zinc
Colestipol	Vitamin A, beta-carotene, vitamin D, vitamin E, vitamin B_{12}, folic acid, iron
Electolyte Replacement	
Potassium Chloride (Timed Release)	Vitamin B_{12}

DRUG	NUTRIENT DEPLETION
Female Hormones	
Oral contraceptive	Folic acid
	Tyrosine
	Vitamin B_2
	Vitamin B_6
	Vitamin B_{12}
	Vitamin C
	Magnesium
	Zinc
Estrogen Replacement (ERT) and Hormone Replacement (HRT) Therapies Estrogens, conjugated estrogens, esterified estrogens, raloxifene and medroxyprogesterone	Vitamin B_6 Magnesium Zinc
Anti-Gout Drugs	
Colchicine	Vitamin B_{12}
	Potassium
	Sodium
	Beta-carotene
Laxatives	
Mineral oil	Vitamin A
	Beta-carotene
	Vitamin D
	Vitamin E
	Vitamin K
	Calcium
Bisacodyl	Potassium
Psychotherapeutic Agents	
Tricyclic Antidepressants Amitriptyline Desipramine Nortriptyline Doxepin Desipramine	Vitamin B_2 Coenzyme Q_{10}
Phenothiazines Chlorpromazine Thioridazine Fluphenazine	Vitamin B_2 Coenzyme Q_{10}
Butyrophenones Haloperidol	Coenzyme Q_{10}

DRUG	NUTRIENT DEPLETION
Ulcer Medications	

H-2 Receptor Antagonists
  Cimetidine
  Famotidine
  Nizatadine
  Ranitidine
	Vitamin B_{12}
	Folic acid
	Calcium
	Vitamin D
	Iron
	Zinc

Proton Pump Inhibitors
  Lansoprazole
  Omeprazole
	Vitamin B_{12}

Miscellaneous	
Methotrexate	Folic acid
Penicillamine	Vitamin B_6 Magnesium Zinc Copper
Acetaminophen	Glutathione

Troubleshooting for Disorders

As you have learned in the preceding chapters, vitamins, minerals, and other nutrients cannot only help you maintain optimum health, but also allow you to control a variety of symptoms and disorders. The worksheet on page 280-281 will guide you in designing your own vitamin and mineral program to prevent ill health. This troubleshooting guide is to give you an idea of what can be done with nutritional supplements if you already have a specific disorder. (Remember: If you have a medical condition, or are pregnant or lactating, please consult with your physician before taking supplements.)

We always recommend that you take the full spectrum of antioxidants, just as we recommend taking B complex and multi-minerals. However, you will notice in this troubleshooting guide that specific nutrients are listed when the research showed that a higher level of that nutrient was therapeutic. So when we list vitamin E, perhaps you may need to take 1,200 IU total, but bear in mind that you should also be taking the other antioxidants in the ODI range.

AT-A-GLANCE NUTRITIONAL THERAPY

SYMPTOM OR DISORDER	SUGGESTED KEY NUTRIENTS
Acne	A, Beta-carotene—Natural with mixed carotenoids, Zinc
ADD/ADHD	Antioxidants, Essential fatty acids
Aging-Related Disorders	Alpha-lipoic acid, Beta-carotene, C, Coenzyme Q_{10}, DHEA, E, Glutathione, Melatonin, N-acetylcysteine
Allergies and Asthma	C, Essential fatty acids, N-acetylcysteine, Quercetin
Alzheimer's Disease	Alpha-lipoic acid, B complex, B_{12}
Anemia	B_{12}, Folic acid, Iron
Arthritis and Other Joint Problems	Essential fatty acids, Manganese, Pantothenic acid, Selenium
Autoimmune Disorders	Coenzyme Q_{10}, E, Essential fatty acids
Bipolar Disorder	Essential fatty acids
Cancer	A, Beta-carotene, C, DHEA, E, Essential fatty acids, Flavonoids, Garlic, Lycopene, Manganese, Melatonin, Selenium
Cardiovascular Disease	Alpha-lipoic acid, Beta-carotene, C, carnitine, Coenzyme Q_{10}, E, Essential fatty acids, Flavonoids, Garlic, N-acetylcysteine, Selenium
Carpal Tunnel Syndrome	B_2, B_6, Niacin
Cataracts	Alpha-lipoic acid, Beta-carotene, C, E, Lutein
Cholesterol-Related Problems	B_3, C, Chromium, Coenzyme Q_{10}, E, Garlic, Niacin, Pantethine
Circulatory Problems	B_3, E, Flavonoids
Colds and Flu	C, Zinc
Depression	B_1, B_2, B_3, B_6, B_{12}, Essential fatty acids, Folic acid, Pantothenic acid
Diabetes	Alpha-lipoic acid, Chromium, E, Essential fatty acids, Manganese
Eczema	A, Beta-carotene, E, Essential fatty acids
Fatigue, Chronic/Fibromyalgia	Carnitine, Coenzyme Q_{10}, Essential fatty acids, Iron (if deficient), Magnesium malate
Fibrocystic Breast Disease	E, Essential fatty acids
Gastrointestinal Problems	A, Beta-carotene, E, Essential fatty acids
High Blood Pressure	Calcium, Coenzyme Q_{10}, D, Essential fatty acids, Magnesium

SYMPTOM OR DISORDER	SUGGESTED KEY NUTRIENTS
HIV/AIDS	A, Beta-carotene, C, Coenzyme Q_{10}, Flavonoids, Garlic, Glutathione, N-acety-cysteine, Quercetin, Selenium, Vitamin E, Zinc
Hypoglycemia	Chromium
Immune Problems	A, Beta-carotene, C, E, Essential fatty acids, Garlic, Glutathione, N-acetylcysteine, Selenium, Zinc
Infection	C, Flavonoids, Garlic, Zinc
Insomnia	Calcium, Melatonin
Macular Degeneration	Alpha-lipoic acid, Beta-carotene, E, Lutein, Zinc
Menopause Symptoms	Calcium, E, Essential fatty acids, Magnesium
Muscle Cramps	Calcium, Magnesium
Osteoporosis	Boron, Calcium, Copper, D, Essential fatty acids, Magnesium, Manganese, Zinc
Premenstrual Syndrome	B_6, Calcium, E, Essential fatty acids, Magnesium
Prostate Conditions	Lycopene, Selenium, Zinc
Respiratory Problems	A, Beta-carotene, C, Essential fatty acids, Flavonoids, Magnesium, N-acetylcysteine
Schizophrenia	A, B_3, Beta-carotene, C, E, Essential fatty acids, Selenium
Skin Problems	A, Beta-carotene, Essential fatty acids, Zinc
Stress and Anxiety	B_1, B_2, B_3, B_6, B_{12}, C, Folic acid, Inositol, Pantothenic acid
Wound Healing	C, E, Zinc

Worksheet

How to Use the Worksheet

Begin by determining your ODIs. You may use the basic ODIs given in the following worksheet, which are in the low to middle range. These can provide many people with optimum general physical and mental health and will prevent most illnesses. Note, though, that your own ODIs may differ. Most of the ODIs given in the individual chapters on vitamins and minerals is expressed as a dosage range. Based on the information in the individual nutrient chapters and in Part One, decide whether your own ODI should be in the lower, middle, or upper level of the range. The ODI listed on the worksheet may be all you need.

Some people need to take higher amounts of certain specific nutrients. There may be factors in your life, such as your personal or family health history, that place you at a higher risk for certain diseases and disorders. If so, you may want to use supplements to provide an additional margin of safety. The worksheet illustrates and summarizes the most frequently encountered of these concerns.

For example, if cancer runs in your family, you would take higher ODIs of vitamins A, B, C, D, and E, and of manganese and selenium. If you are concerned about heart disease, your ODIs for vitamin C, vitamin E, chromium, and selenium would be higher than the basic ODIs. If you have more than one concern, do not add one specific ODI to another;

Sample Worksheet

NUTRIENT	BASIC ODI	EMOTIONAL STRESS	ENHANCE IMMUNITY	CARDIOVASCULAR DISEASE PREVENTION
Vitamin A Beta-Carotene	5,000 IU 11,000 IU		10,000–25,000 IU 25,000–50,000 IU	5,000–10,000 IU 11,000–25,000 IU
B complex	25 mg	100–500 mg	50 mg	50–100 mg
Vitamin C	500 mg	1,000–5,000 mg	1,000–5,000 mg	500–3,000 mg
Vitamin D	400 IU			
Vitamin E	400 IU			400–800 IU
Vitamin K	80 mg			
Boron	3 mg			
Calcium	1,000 mg			
Chromium	200 mcg			400 mcg
Copper	0.5 mg			
Iodine	150 mcg			
Iron	15 mg			
Magnesium	500 mg			500 mg
Manganese	15 mg			
Phosphorus	Obtained from food source			
Potassium	Obtained from food source (reduce salt)			
Selenium	100 mcg		100–200 mcg	100–400 mcg
Zinc	22.5 mg		30–50 mg	
BEYOND VITAMINS AND MINERALS				
Alpha-lipoic acid	600 mg*	600 mg	600 mg	600 mg
Coenzyme Q$_{10}$	50 mg*			50–100 mg
Fish Oil	1,500 mg		1,500–3,000 mg	1,500–3,000 mg
Flavonoids	250 mg*			500–2,000 mg
GLA	70 mg*		70–240 mg	70–240 mg
Glutathione	500 mg*			
L-Carnitine	200 mg*			200 mg
Melatonin	0.1 mg*			
N-Acetylcysteine	1,200 mg*			

*Dosage is not an ODI.

CANCER PREVENTION	SKIN PROBLEMS	DIABETES PREVENTION	OSTEOPOROSIS PREVENTION	OTHER	YOUR ODI AND DATE
10,000–50,000 IU 25,000–100,000 IU	10,000–25,000 IU 25,000–100,000 IU				
50–150 mg					
5,000–10,000 mg	3,000–5,000 mg	1,000–3,000 mg			
400–800 IU			400–800 IU		
400–800 IU		400–800 IU			
			3–6 mg		
			1,500–2,000 mg		
		400–1,000 mcg			
			500–1,000 mg		
15–50 mg		20–50 mg	15–50 mg		
			200–400 mg		
200–600 mcg	200–400 mcg				
	22.5–50 mg				
600 mg		600–1,200 mg			
100–300 mg					
1,500–3,000 mg	1,500–3,000 mg				
2,000–4,000 mg					
70–240 mg	70–240 mg				
500 mg					
10–50 mg					
1,200 mg					

simply use the upper range. For example, if you are concerned about car-diovascular disease prevention and are under great emotional stress, your ODI for vitamin C would be 5,000 milligrams, not 10,000 milligrams.

If a particular concern of yours is not listed in the worksheet, refer to the individual vitamin and mineral chapters for the ODI range and enter it in one of the columns marked "Other." For example, some women might be concerned about PMS (premenstrual syndrome).

Enter your starting ODI in the worksheet, and date it. As time goes by, evaluate the way you feel and adjust your ODIs accordingly.

Reference Abstracts for Vitamins, Minerals, and Other Nutrients

I N SOME CASES, the following abstracts provide more detailed information on the studies discussed in the chapters, and refer you to the source of the material, should you decide to read it in its entirety. In other cases, the abstracts refer to studies that are not mentioned in the chapter, but that either support the points made in the text or reveal additional benefits of the nutrient. For the sake of simplicity, in some instances we have chosen not to cite all of the studies mentioned within the chapter. If you have Web access, you can easily obtain the abstract of an article on line. Simply go to http://www.ncbi.nlm. nih.gov/PubMed. Click on "Single Citation Matcher" on the left side of the screen. Type in the information and click on "Search." When the citation comes up on the screen, click on "abstract" and the abstract will appear. If you wish, you may also subscribe to services that will allow you to order the entire article for a fee.

A note on antioxidant studies: researchers have finally understood that the magic bullet mentality doesn't apply in nutrition research, especially where antioxidants are concerned. Many of the more recent studies therefore use a combination of antioxidants. To avoid frequent repetition of references on studies that used a combination of antioxidants, we have listed these studies in Chapters 2 and 3. So, if you cannot find a particular study in the reference section of a chapter on an antioxidant nutrient, look in Chapters 2 and 3.

Chapter 1: What Are Vitamins and Minerals?

For a thorough compilation of evidence on the safety levels of a wide range of intakes of vitamins and minerals, see *Safety of Vitamins and Minerals: A Summary of the Findings of Key Nutrients* (Washington, DC: Council for Responsible Nutrition, 1991).

For a report on current evidence of the potential benefits from the regular use of vitamin and mineral supplements, see *Benefits of Nutritional Supplements* (Washington, DC: Council for Responsible Nutrition, 1993).

Chapter 2: The RDIs—The Minimum Wages of Nutrition

Marginal Vitamin Deficiencies

This editorial examines the importance of vitamin intake and notes that frank vitamin deficiency is rare in the U.S., but that there is compelling evidence that large segments of the population are consuming suboptimal levels of several micronutrients. The authors cite national surveys that show that many Americans fall far below the recommended intakes of several vitamins, and then mention evidence suggesting that such low intakes have serious health consequences, such as neural tube defects, cancer, and heart disease. They conclude that vitamin supplementation at the RDA levels may be beneficial for large segments of the population, especially elderly individuals and women of childbearing age. *Journal of American Medical Association* 270 (December 8, 1993): 2,726–2,727.

At a 1994 American College of Cardiology meeting, two-thirds of the audience of approximately 700 physicians acknowledged that they themselves took antioxidant supplements daily. *Family Practice News* (March 1, 1994): 10.

The Caveman Diet

The diet of Paleolithic humans was higher than the modern diet in many nutrients, including calcium and vitamin C. *New England Journal of Medicine* (January 31, 1985): 283–289.

Use of Supplements

This article discusses the pros and cons of supplementation. It notes that 40 percent of the population is consuming supplements, and that several economists have estimated that increasing our intake of vitamins and minerals would reduce health care costs by 25 percent for cardiovascular disease, 16 to 30 percent for a variety of cancers, and 50 percent for cataracts. *Journal of the American College of Nutrition* 13 (1994): 113–115.

Dr. Verlangieri, of the University of Mississippi, believes that everyone should take supplements, and recommends antioxidant vitamins C and E, and vitamin A or beta-carotene in excess of the RDAs. *Modern Medicine* 60 (July 1992): 15–18.

Extensive review article demonstrating that all adults should take a daily multivitamin to significantly protect against chronic disease. *Journal of the American Medical Association* 287(23) (2002): 3116–3129.

A 100-page report on the health benefits of nutritional supplementation with extensive references. Report by the Council for Responsible Nutrition (June 2002) (online version).

Myth of the Well-Balanced Diet

Article about how our food has less nutrition and more harmful chemicals than in the past. *National Catholic Reporter* (May 24, 2002) (online version).

A dietary quality index was based on foods recommended by the Food Guide Pyramid and the Dietary Guidelines, using food frequency questionnaires in a large group of women who were participating in a breast cancer detection program. After a median follow-up of 5.6 years, approximately 5 percent of the women had died. Higher diet quality scores significantly predicted lower risk of mortality, when adjusted for variables. Similar patterns were seen for cancer mortality and, to a smaller extent, for heart disease and stroke. In NHANES I Epidemiologic Follow-up Study, men and women reporting intakes of two or fewer of the food groups were 1.5 and 1.4 times as likely to die, respectively, when compared with those consuming foods from all 5 food groups. It is noted that individuals who consume a greater variety of foods are also more likely to have other healthful behaviors. Vitamin-supplement use was greater among those with higher dietary scores. It is possible that the improvement in mortality was due, in part, to the protective effect of supplement use rather than to the variety in the diet itself. It is also known that the actions of nutrients are dependent on the presence of others, and the balance of nutrition in foods is of importance. In the Dietary Approaches to Stop Hypertension Study (DASH) trial, there was a strong effect of a food-based dietary intervention on blood pressure. The DASH diet emphasized fruit, vegetables, low-fat dairy foods, and a low intake of saturated and total fat. Consumption of these food groups, with the inclusion of lean meat or meat substitutes and low-fat dairy products can have significant health benefits and reduce the risk of early mortality. *Nutrition Reviews* 59(5) (2001): 156–158.

In evaluating 4,501 female physicians from the Women Physicians' Health Study who were between 30 and 70 years of age, half of the physicians took a multivitamin-mineral supplement. Those taking supplements on a regular basis also consumed more fruits and vegetables and less fat than did occasional users or nonusers. *American Journal of Clinical Nutrition* 72 (2000): 969–975.

Antioxidants

Oxidant by-products of normal metabolism result in extensive damage to DNA, protein, and lipids. This damage is probably a major contributor to aging-related and degenerative diseases such as cancer, cardiovascular disease, immune system decline, brain dysfunction, and cataracts. Antioxidant defenses include vitamins C and E and the carotenoids. Low intakes of fruit and vegetables—rich sources of antioxidants—can double the risk of most types of cancer when compared with high intakes. Only 9 percent of the American population consumes the recommended 5 servings of fruits and vegetables each day. *Proceedings of the National Academy of Sciences* 90 (September 1993): 7,915–7,922.

This study evaluated 413 individual case-controlled pairs of individuals, and is the largest study done to date of dietary factors and lung cancer risk in nonsmokers. The results suggest that dietary beta-carotene, raw fruits and vegetables, and vitamin E supplements reduce the risk of lung cancer in nonsmokers. *Journal of the National Cancer Institute* 86 (January 5, 1994): 33–38.

The Alliance for Aging recommends supplements of C, E, and beta-carotene far in excess of the RDA to prevent many conditions associated with aging. This article also quotes Jeffrey Blumberg, M.D., of Tufts University, who believes that we know enough at this time to make recommendations about supplementation. *Medical Tribune* 1 (March 24, 1994).

In a double-blind placebo-controlled study on the effect of vitamin E supplementation on the immune response of healthy elderly individuals, the majority of subjects who received 800 international units of vitamin E showed significant enhancement of their immune system. *Nutrient Modulation of the Immune Response* (New York: Marcel Drecker, 1993), 223–238.

The risk of cataract was 45 percent lower among women who used vitamin C supplements for 10 or more years. *British Medical Journal* (August 8, 1992): 335–339.

In a study of 30,000 people living in a single province of China, the overall death rate from cancer was less in the groups that took vitamin supplements than it was in groups that took "dummy" pills. *Journal of the National Cancer Institute* (September 1993): 1,446–1,447.

Chapter 3: The Optimum Daily Intakes (ODIs)

Antioxidant Supplementation and Cancer

What follows is a sampling of the many articles published on the potential benefit of antioxidant supplements. For a fuller discussion of free radical damage and the role of antioxidants, see Nancy Bruning, *The Natural Health Guide to Antioxidants* (New York: Bantam, 1994).

Healthy subjects were supplemented with 15 milligrams of beta-carotene (25,000 international units), 30 milligrams of vitamin C, and 15 milligrams of vitamin E. These amounts stimulated free radical–scavenging activity. This study confirmed the well-known antioxidant effects of these vitamins, with maximum protection occurring after 30 days. This type of supplementation would be an easy and rapid way to increase the oxidative stress defenses in various diseases in which free radicals occur. *The Annals of Pharmacotherapy* 27 (November 1993): 1,349–1,350.

Gladys Block has written many articles that support the role of antioxidants in reducing cancer risk. In this review article, Dr. Block argues that based on all of the available scientific literature, antioxidants do in fact demonstrate a protective defense against cancer in studies looking at food consumption and supplementation. For example, of approximately 130 studies that examined supplemental vitamin C, beta-carotene, or vitamin E, or their rich food sources, 120 have found statistically significant reduced risks of cancer of the lung, larynx, esophagus, oral cavity, pancreas, stomach, cervix, rectum, colon, ovary, endometrium, breast, and bladder. The level of intake is determined in part by the level of oxidative stress. Individuals, or populations, vary in the level of such stressors, which include nitrosamines, smoking, alcohol, ozone, and other environmental pollutants; infections; vigorous exercise; chronic disease; and sunlight exposure. No single level of intake is "right" at all times. *Nutrition Reviews* 50 (July 1992): 207–213.

In Linxian, China, approximately 30,000 adults, ages 49 to 69, received a daily vitamin and mineral supplement at dose ranges one to two times the RDA. There was significantly lower mortality in those receiving supplementation with the antioxidants beta-carotene, vitamin E, and selenium. The reduction was mainly due to lower cancer rates, especially stomach cancer, with reduced risk beginning to arise one to two years after supplements were started. *Journal of the National Cancer Institute* 18 (September 25, 1993): 1,492–1,498.

More than 12,000 women and men between 35 and 60 years of age and 45 and 60 years of age, respectively, were followed for up to 8 years starting in 1994. A subgroup of 1,000 subjects for 2 years took a daily multivitamin supplement containing 6,000 micrograms of beta-carotene, 120 milligrams of vitamin C, 30 milligrams of vitamin E, 100 micrograms of selenium as selenium-enriched yeast, and 20 milligrams of zinc gluconate daily. Results showed that vitamin and mineral levels rose to levels that are consistent with having a positive benefit. The values that were found for beta-carotene and vitamin E in the supplemented group after 2 years of supplementation were levels associated with lower risk of cancer in observational studies. *Cancer Detection and Prevention* 25(5) (2001): 479–485.

Antioxidants and Cardiovascular Disease

This article reviews the relationship of antioxidants and atherosclerosis. It discusses evidence to support the theory that oxidative stress and inflammation lead to this condition, and the various roles of antioxidant nutrients vitamins C and E, beta-carotene, and the glutathione system. *Heart Disease and Stroke* 3 (1994): 52–57.

These two Harvard School of Public Health studies showed a reduced risk of heart disease for both men and women who took beta-carotene and vitamin E supplements. *New England Journal of Medicine* 20 (May 20, 1993): 1,444–1,487. (See also Chapters 6 and 8.)

In studying 468 men and women who were between 66 and 75 years of age, it was found that after adjusting for variables, a 20 percent higher plasma vitamin C level and a 20 percent higher beta-carotene level was associated with a significantly smaller intima-media thickness in men. Those with low blood concentrations of these vitamins were 2.5 times as likely to have carotid stenosis of >30 percent. *American Journal of Clinical Nutrition* 74 (2001): 402–408.

In 21 consecutive chronic heart failure (CHF) patients compared with controls, plasma alpha-tocopherol and retinol were within the normal range, but vitamin C and beta-carotene were lower in the CHF subjects. This study showed that antioxidant status is altered in patients with CHF, and selenium may play a role in the severity of the disease, rather than in the degree of left ventricular function. *European Journal of Heart Failure* 3 (2001): 661–669.

Other Antioxidant Studies

Exercise: Antioxidant supplementation has been shown to reduce oxidative stress and speed recovery from muscle soreness after exercise. In one study, subjects took supplements containing 592 milligrams of vitamin E, 1,000 milligrams of vitamin C, and 30 milligrams of beta-carotene. These supplements significantly reduced exercise-induced oxidative stress. *Journal of Applied Physiology* 74 (1993): 965–969.

In evaluating 20 well-trained sportsmen, all athletes, runners, and cyclists, who were used to participating in duathlonlike competitions, subjects trained approximately 14 hours per week. The effects of 90 days' supplementation with placebo or an antioxidant cocktail of vitamin E at 500 milligrams/day and beta-carotene at 30 milligrams/day, with the addition of vitamin C at 1 gram/day during the last 15 days on sportsmen's antioxidant defenses were studied. This study showed that antioxidant supplementation enhanced the antioxidant enzyme activity of superoxide dismutase and catalase in neutrophils and could protect neutrophils against auto-oxidation by free radicals. Theoretically, high doses of antioxidants could prevent muscle injury and soreness and enhance muscle repair after exercise-induced damage. *European Journal of Physiology* 443 (2002): 791–797.

A dose of vitamin E may ease that stiff ache some of us feel after a bout of exercise, according to the results of a study on healthy men. The study's authors believe the vitamin acts as an antioxidant, mopping up the damaging by-products of a strenuous workout. If you are one to experience a great deal of soreness and fatigue after a workout, vitamin E might be of benefit to help combat soreness and exercise-induced stress.

Infection and Cataracts: Two Canadian studies showed lower rates of infectious disease and cataracts among elderly people who took antioxidant vitamins. *Medical Tribune* (March 24, 1994): 1.

Life Span: This study showed that men who consume 300 milligrams of vitamin C daily (through food and supplements) had a 40-percent lower death rate from heart disease and other causes than those whose intake was less than 50 milligrams. *Epidemiology* 3 (1992): 194–202.

Overall Health: In this study, people who ingested less than 100 milligrams of vitamin C per day experienced the greatest number of clinical signs and symptoms, while those who ingested 200 milligrams per day had the least symptoms. Moreover, 50-year-olds who consumed the highest levels of vitamin C were clinically similar to 40-year-olds. *Journal of Advancement in Medicine* 7 (Spring 1994): 31–34.

Eye Disorders: This article reviews the role of nutrition in eye disorders. In the Nurses' Health Study, for example, women in the highest fifth of total carotene intake (14,500 international units per day) had a lower risk of cataracts compared with those in the lowest fifth. Vitamin C supplementation for over 10 years reduced the risk of cataracts by 45 percent. Regarding the intake of antioxidants vitamin C, vitamin E, beta-carotene, and riboflavin, those who were in the highest fifth had a 40-percent lower risk of cataracts. The carotenoid family in general was associated with a highly significant reduced risk of macular degeneration. The recommended amounts of antioxidants to achieve this protection are in considerable excess of the RDIs. *Journal of Nutritional Biochemistry* 5 (February 1994): 66–76.

Other

Supplementation with antioxidants may prevent neuronal injury (injury to brain cells) in schizophrenia. Membrane phospholipids can be corrected by omega-3 fatty acids. The authors suggest that vitamins E, C, and A; beta carotene, CoQ_{10}, flavonoid compounds, as well as other antioxidants are therapeutic, along with omega-3 fatty acids. Since the oxidative stress exists before the onset of psychosis, the use of antioxidants and fatty acids from the very onset may reduce the oxidative injury and dramatically improve the outcome of illness. *Neuropsychopharmacology, Biology and Psychiatry* 25(3) (2001): 463–93.

Graves' disease: In a study of 56 hyperthyroid patients, subjects were treated either with the methimazole alone, or with an antioxidant mixture of vitamin E at 200 milligrams, beta-carotene at 3 milligrams, vitamin C at 250 milligrams, copper at 1 milligram, zinc at 7.5 milligrams, manganese at 1.5 milligrams, and selenium at 15 micrograms, or with a combination of the medication and the antioxidants. Improvement was found at 8 weeks in the methimazole group and at four weeks in the antioxidant group alone or in combination with the methimazole. The hyperthyroid patients had increased malondialdehyde content and superoxide dismutase activity and a reduction in catalase activity, compared to the control subjects. The authors suggest that these signs and symptoms of Graves' disease may be related to increased free radicals, and antioxidants may be a therapeutic tool to reduce the symptoms. *International Union of Biochemistry and Molecular Biology* 51 (2001): 105–109.

Diets containing high levels of antioxidants such as vitamins C and E seem able to reduce the risk of suffering age-related immune dysfunction and arteriosclerosis. Diet supplementation with these antioxidants may protect the mitochondria against respiration-linked oxygen stress, with preservation of the genomic and structural integrity of these energy-producing organelles and concomitant increase in functional life span. *Annals of the New York Academy of Sciences* Articles 959 (April 2002): 508–516.

Multinutrient Studies

Many studies have examined the effects of several nutrients at once. Many of these looked at antioxidant nutrients in particular. The following is a selection of the most significant of these multinutrient studies.

Cancer

This article reviews the use of vitamin and mineral supplementation in cancer treatment. It discusses the benefits of folic acid, folinic acid, vitamin K, and multivitamin and -mineral supplements in enhancing the effects of chemotherapy and radiation, as well as the possible antitumor effects of the nutrients themselves. It also discusses a study that evaluated 65 patients with bladder cancer, in a randomized comparison of BCG therapy along with multivitamins in the RDA range versus the same RDA-multivitamin plus megavitamin therapy. The megavitamin therapy included 4,000 international units of vitamin A, 100 milligrams of B_6, 2,000 milligrams of C, 400 international units of E, and 90 milligrams of zinc. BCG therapy did not significantly reduce tumor recurrence. Recurrence after 10 months was markedly reduced in patients receiving the megadose vitamins. The 5-year estimates of tumor recurrence were 91 percent in the RDA group, and 41 percent in the megadose group. Overall recurrence was 24 of 30 patients in the RDA group and 14 of 35 in the megavitamin group. *Adjuvant Nutrition in Cancer Treatment,* 1992 Symposium Proceedings. Patrick Quillin, Ph.D., R.D., R. Michael Williams, M.D., Ph.D., editors, Cancer Treatment Research Foundation, Arlington Heights, IL, 1992.

This article gives a general overview of the randomized controlled large-scale worldwide prevention and treatment trials with respect to cancer. Daily dose ranges in these trials for vitamin A are approximately 25,000 international units; beta-carotene, 30 to 180 milligrams; vitamin C, 1,000 milligrams; vitamin E, 400 milligrams; calcium, 1,200 milligrams; and omega-3 fatty acids, 10 grams. *Annals of Medicine* 26 (1994): 73–78.

Premenstrual Syndrome

A double-blind, randomized study on 44 women with PMS was conducted assessing the efficacy of a nutritional supplement. Subjects received 6 tablets of the supplement, 12 tablets of the supplement, or a placebo. Significant treatment effects were noted in three subgroups of the 6-tablet group and in all four subgroups of the 12-tablet group. The results of this study suggest that this nutritional supplement may play a role in the management of PMS. *American Journal of Clinical Nutrition* 10 (1991): 494–499.

Skin

This article reviews the role of nutrients in skin disorders. Vitamin A may help prevent the development of chemical and UV light–induced skin cancers in animals. Oral retinoids may provide some benefit in patients with some types of skin cancers. Vitamin A supplementation at 25,000 international units in seriously injured patients enhanced wound healing and resistance to infection. Selenium is useful in protecting against UV-induced tanning, sunburn, and skin and other cancers. Vitamin C may be beneficial in the prevention of UV skin damage. Melanoma cell growth inhibition has been seen with vitamin B_6, C, D, and E. For the severely ill patient, 1 to 2 grams of vitamin C daily are recommended to enhance recovery. Topical zinc may be used for acne; fish oil, evening primrose oil, and Chinese herbal teas may be useful in atopic dermatitis. Vitamins A and D may be useful in the treatment of psoriasis. *Journal of the American Academy of Dermatology* 29 (1993): 447–461.

Life Span
Antioxidant defenses are sufficient to allow a life span of 70 to 100 years. The amounts required of antioxidants to achieve these protective effects are in considerable excess of the RDI. The author recommends daily supplements of 200 to 400 international units of vitamin E, 100 to 250 milligrams of vitamin C, and 25 milligrams of beta-carotene. *Journal of Nutritional Biochemistry* 5 (February 1994): 66–76.

Homocysteine
The Methylation Miracle, by Paul Frankel, Ph.D., and Nancy Bruning (New York: St. Martin's Press, 1999).

If We All Took Supplements
A 100-page report on the health benefits of nutritional supplementation with extensive references. Report by the Council for Responsible Nutrition (June 2002) (online version).

The Double Standard
Reports have come to light that many medical journals have been allowing drug firms to influence editorial content. This article suggests ways to limit drug firms' influence (September 9, 2001) (online version).

Reports have surfaced that some scientists are unscrupulously taking money for papers that are actually written by a drug company. *The Guardian* (February 7, 2002) (Online version).

Reports have surfaced that since drug companies fund research studies that "positive outcomes" are part of the deal. *New England Journal of Medicine* 342(20) (2000).

87% of the doctors who are involved in setting national guidelines on disease treatment have a relationship with drug companies, and 38% serve as employees or consultants for pharmaceutical companies. *Journal of the American Medical Association* 287 (2002): 612–617.

Most advisory panels to the FDA have ties to manufacturers of the drug they are evaluating. The Alliance for Human Research Protection (2002) (online version).

Ninety-six percent of peer-reviewed articles had financial ties to the drug they were studying. *New England Journal of Medicine* 338(2) (1998): 101–106.

Chapter 4: How to Design Your Own Nutritional Supplement Program
A researcher with the National Institute on Aging discusses research studies on the relationship between free radicals and longevity. *Antioxidants: Chemical, Physiological, Nutritional and Toxicological Aspects* (Princeton, NJ: Princeton Scientific, 1993), 151–161.

A University of California at Los Angeles researcher studied nearly 12,000 people, ages 25 to 74, for 10 years. The men who took an average 300 milligrams of vitamin C per day in food and supplements experienced a 42 percent lower death rate from heart disease and other causes than did the men whose intake was less than 50 milligrams. The women in the study did not see similar benefits. *Epidemiology* 3 (1992): 194, 202.

Chapter 5: Your Total Health Plan

This excellent, comprehensive article reviews the effects of the protective factors found in plant foods such as fruits and vegetables. These include beta-carotenes, vitamin C, sulfur-containing compounds, protease inhibitors, and many others. *Nutrition Action Health Letter* 21 (April 1994): 7–13.

In evaluating over 200 studies for the relationship between fruit and vegetable consumption and cancer, it was found that there was a significant protective effect in 128 of the 156 dietary studies. Low fruit and vegetable intake resulted in twice the risk of most cancers compared with high intake. *Nutrition and Cancer* 18 (1992): 1–29.

Chapter 6: Vitamin A and Carotenoids

See also references on "Antoioxdants" for Chapters 2 and 3.

Infections and Immunity

In this study, 24 nonsmoking healthy males, ages 19 to 39, received 30 milligrams of beta-carotene per day or a placebo while on a low-carotenoid diet. Subjects received 12 exposures to UV-A/B light over 16 days. Follow-up was continued for 28 days. Delayed hypersensitivity test responses were significantly suppressed in the placebo group. There was no significant suppression in the beta-carotene group. The authors conclude that beta-carotene protects against photosuppression of immune function. *American Journal of Clinical Nutrition* 56 (1992): 684–690.

Cardiovascular Disease

The predominant antioxidants protecting the LDL molecule against oxidative stress (free radicals) are vitamin E, vitamin A, and beta-carotene. Vitamin C is the first line of defense and also regenerates vitamin E. Antioxidants appear to protect the LDL molecule from increased lipid peroxidation, and thereby slow the atherosclerotic process. *Archives of Internal Medicine* 155 (1995): 241–246.

As part of the ongoing Physicians' Health Study, a group of 333 men with a history of cardiovascular disease were studied. Those who took 50 milligrams (85,000 international units) of beta-carotene every other day had half as many heart attacks, strokes, and deaths related to heart disease as those who did not take supplements. *Circulation* 82 (1992): Suppl. III: 202.

This article reviewed literature with respect to beta-carotene and vitamin E supplementation in men who smoke or consume alcohol. In one study, the highest carotene intake resulted in a 29-percent reduction in the risk of developing coronary heart disease. Among smokers, men with the highest carotene intake had a 70-percent reduction in coronary risk. *Nutrition Report* 11 (1993): 73, 80.

In studying 468 patients, it was found that after adjusting for variables, a 20 percent higher beta-carotene and a 20 percent higher plasma vitamin C level were also associated with a significantly smaller intima-media thickness in men. Compared with men with high blood concentrations of beta-carotene or cholesterol-adjusted vitamin E, those with low blood concentrations of these vitamins were 2.5 times as likely to have carotid stenosis of >30 percent. *American Journal of Clinical Nutrition* 74 (2002): 402–408.

Ulcers

In a 4-week study of 40 patients with chronic gastric ulcers, the number of patients whose ulcers completely healed or shrank was highest in the group that received 150,000 international units of vitamin A daily. The authors suggest that since gastric ulcers may be thought of as a precancerous condition, vitamin A may have a role in the prevention of cancer from gastric ulcers. *Lancet* (October 16, 1982): 876.

Cancer Prevention

Many studies show a correlation between high consumption of beta-carotene and/or higher vitamin A (retinol) blood levels, and lowered incidence of these cancers: lung, endometrium, bronchus, bladder, breast, cervix, rectum, and the skin cancer melanoma. Such studies have been conducted all over the world including the United States, England, Finland, Japan, Norway, and Poland. What follows is a representative sampling.

Designer food programs are underway to include food protective phytochemicals in food products. Diet supplementation with nontoxic doses of vitamin A and carotene may help prevent breast cancer. Three different carotenoids that may prevent breast cancer include beta-carotene, apo-carotenal, and canthaxanthin. Carotenoids appear to be the most active in preventing the activation of chemical carcinogens, while retinoids alter the promotional stage of carcinogenesis. The role of phytoestrogens, flavonoids, fiber, and other compounds are also reviewed. *Primary Care and Cancer* 14 (February 1994): 10–11.

In a 5-year study, 8,278 Norwegian men showed a threefold decrease in lung cancer with an increase in vitamin A consumption. Beta-carotene was the major source of this vitamin. *International Journal of Cancer* 15 (1975): 561–565.

This study was the largest study to date of dietary factors and lung cancer risk in nonsmokers. The results suggest that dietary beta-carotene, raw fruits and vegetables, and vitamin E supplements reduce the risk of lung cancer in nonsmokers. *Journal of the National Cancer Institute* 86 (January 5, 1994): 33–38.

In evaluating 549 cases of ovarian cancer compared with 516 controls, utilizing dietary questionnaires, it was found that intakes of carotene, especially alpha-carotene, from food and supplements were significantly and inversely associated with risk of ovarian cancer, especially in postmenopausal females. Lycopene intake was significantly and inversely associated with risk for ovarian cancer, especially in premenopausal women. The foods most strongly related to a reduction in risk of ovarian cancer were raw carrots and tomato sauce. Consumption of fruits, vegetables, and food items high in carotene and lycopene may reduce the risk of ovarian cancer. *International Journal of Cancer* 94 (2001): 128–134.

Lycopene is an antioxidant that has the ability to quench singlet oxygen. The most compelling evidence for lycopene and protection against disease exists for prostate cancer. Protective effects of lycopene have been reported for oral cavity, esophagus, breast, and skin cancer. *Journal of Nutraceuticals, Functional & Medical Foods* 3(2) (2001): 9–23.

Supplementation as Cancer Treatment

Some studies on animals and humans suggest that vitamin A or beta-carotene can affect the course of an already established cancer or precancer. These include the following:

This article reviews the potential benefit of beta-carotene and vitamin A derivatives in the treatment and prevention of oral leukoplakia and cervical cancer. High-dose vitamin A derivatives have resulted in a 50 percent to 90 percent regression of oral lesions; however, therapy is limited due to toxicity. Similar studies conducted using beta-carotene resulted in a 71-percent response and no toxicity. Topical application of vitamin A derivatives to the cervix has resulted in a 50 percent regression of lesions. Beta-carotene appears to have similar benefit with no toxicity. *Drug Therapy* (July 1992): 55–60. See also *The Female Patient* 17 (February 1992): 120–125.

In this study, 20 patients diagnosed with colon cancer were given 30 milligrams a day of beta-carotene for 6 months after surgery. Cancer cell proliferation was inhibited by 44 percent after 4 weeks of supplementation, and by 57 percent after 9 weeks of supplementation. It remained low for 6 months after supplementation was discontinued. *Cancer Research* 53 (1993): 3,723–3,725.

In this controlled, randomized study of 307 surgically-treated lung cancer patients, one group of subjects was given 300,000 international units of vitamin A daily for 12 months. After a year, 37 percent of the supplemented group and 48 percent of the control group developed new primary tumors. Second primary tumors developed in 19 supplemented patients, but 29 of the control patients. *Journal of Clinical Oncology* 11 (1993): 1,216–1,222.

This review article states that all 13 of the published studies show a cancer-protective effect from the intake of carotenoids. Of these, 5 studies used beta-carotene alone. A recent multi-center study achieved a 55 percent response rate with beta-carotene, which was comparable to that achieved with the more toxic vitamin A. The author states, "In those that had an early primary head and neck cancer that was considered cured, the prevention of a second cancer may be accomplished with nontoxic agents such as vitamin E and beta-carotene." *The Nutrition Report* (October 1994) 12(10): 73–80.

High-dose vitamin A therapy (300,000 international units daily for 12 months) was tested on 307 patients whose lung cancer was removed surgically. After a year, 37 percent of the patients who received the supplement experienced a recurrence or new primary tumor, compared with 48 percent of the control group—a statistically significant difference. *Journal of Clinical Oncology* (July 1993) 11(7): 1,204–1,207.

Supplementation as Complementary Cancer Treatment

In this Finnish study, researchers gave cancer patients a wide variety of vitamin and mineral supplements, including 15,000 to 40,000 international units of vitamin A and 10,000 to 20,000 international units of beta-carotene, along with their chemotherapy and radiation treatments. The supplemented group lived longer and suffered fewer side effects than did those who were unsupplemented. *Anticancer Research* 12 (May–June 1992): 599–606.

Female patients who were older than 18 years of age with biopsy-proven cervical intraepithelial neoplasia (CIN) 2 or CIN 3 within 3 months of enrollment into this study; subjects were randomized to receive either 30 milligrams daily of beta-carotene or a placebo. The response rate with beta-carotene was highest in women with no HPV at 61 percent, 30 percent for those who were indeterminate/low-risk, and 18 percent for those at high-risk. It is also noted that no harm was found to women who supplemented with beta-carotene, with regard to the progression of cervical intraepithelial neoplasia after 24 months of therapy. *Cancer Epidemiology, Biomarkers & Prevention* 10 (2001): 1029–1035.

Skin

In this review article, the authors point out that vitamin A has been used to treat acne since the early 1940s. In one series, 100 patients were given 100,000 international units per day. Of these, 97 were "cured or almost cured." A 1981 report indicated that doses of 50,000 to 100,000 international units were ineffective, but that intake of 300,000 international units daily for 3 to 4 months was highly efficacious. The researchers postulated that the risk of toxicity at the higher dosage range was exaggerated. *Drugs* 27 (1984): 148–170.

This is an extensive review of the protective effects of oral and topical antioxidant therapy as a defense against UV light exposure. The antioxidants reviewed include vitamin E, coenzyme Q_{10}, glutathione, vitamin C, and carotenoids. The reviewers feel that prophylactic antioxidant administration should start early and be used throughout the year to provide optimum conditions for protection. I. Emerit Basel, ed., *Free Radicals and Aging* (Switzerland: Birkhauser Verlag, 1992), 328–340.

This article reviews the role of nutrients and skin disorders. Vitamin A may help prevent the development of chemical and UV light–induced skin cancers in animals. Oral retinoids may provide some benefit in patients with some types of skin cancers. Vitamin A supplementation at 25,000 international units in seriously injured patients enhanced wound healing and resistance to infection. *Journal of the American Academy of Dermatology* 29 (1993): 447–461.

A statistically significant inverse relationship was found between the risk of skin cancer and a high intake of fish, vegetables, cruciferous vegetables, beta-carotene, and vitamin C-containing foods. Those subjects who developed skin cancer had lower beta-carotene and vitamin A levels than did the control subjects. Nutrition and Cancer 18 (1992): 237–244.

HIV Infection and AIDS

In this study, 21 HIV-infected patients, most of whom were taking AZT, were given either 180 milligrams per day of beta-carotene or a placebo for 4 weeks in a crossover trial. Patients on beta-carotene had average elevations in their CD4 cells of approximately 17 percent, as well as improved levels of CD4 helper cells, in many cases. Total white blood cell counts increased only on beta-carotene. The vitamin therapy had no side effects. Medical Tribune 4 (February 25, 1993): 1.

Dr. Gregg Coodley and colleagues conducted a double-blind, placebo-controlled, crossover clinical study by giving participants either 180 milligrams per day (300,000 international units) of beta-carotene or a placebo. Beta-carotene supplementation was associated with an increase of total white blood cell count, of CD4 count, and of CD4/CD8 ratio. Journal of Acquired Immune Deficiency Syndrome 6 (1993): 272–276.

Vision

In this study, researchers interviewed 112 subjects regarding their dietary and supplement intake, and measured plasma levels of beta-carotene. Those with the lowest plasma levels had 5 times the risk of developing cataracts of those with high levels. Supplement to the American Journal of Clinical Nutrition 53 (1991): 352S.

Dietary intake of beta-carotene was inversely associated with acute macular degeneration in patients ages 55 to 80. High vitamin C intake was associated with a marginal but significant decrease in developing acute macular degeneration. The authors conclude that increased intakes of antioxidants, beta-carotene, and vitamin C might decrease the risk of macular degeneration. Investigative Ophthalmology and Visual Science 34 (December 1993): 1,134.

Fourteen male patients 61 to 79 years of age receiving rather low levels of dark-green leafy vegetables each day were placed on an additional portion of 5 ounces sauteed spinach 4 to 7 times per week or lutein-based antioxidant (3 patients). Patients demonstrated short-term positive effects in visual function in one or both eyes with this mild therapeutic approach. Journal of the American Optometry Association 70(1) (1991): 24036.

Participants completed a 26-week program of lutein supplementation (40 milligrams/day for 9 weeks, 20 milligrams/day thereafter); 10 participants also took 500 milligrams docosahexaenoic acid (DHA)/day, vitamin B complex, and digestive enzymes. Participants self-tested their visual acuity on their computer screen and their central visual-field extent on a wall chart weekly for 14 weeks, biweekly thereafter. Short-term vision improvements after lutein supplementation previously reported in age-related macular degeneration also occured in retinosa pigmentosa, especially in blue-eyed individuals. Also, vitamin A may increase visual field benefits. Optometry 71(3) (2000): 147–164.

In a study of almost 5,000 people, funded in part by the National Eye Institute, a mixture of 500 milligrams of vitamin C, 400 international units of vitamin E, and 15 milligrams of beta-carotene reduced the risk of vision loss by 10 percent. A mixture of 80 milligrams of zinc and 2 milligrams of copper reduced the risk by 11 percent. Nutrition Week 31(40) (2001): 7.

Bioavailability

In this study, 38 women randomly received 12 milligrams of beta-carotene from food (raw carrots or carrot juice) or from purified beta-carotene capsules after receiving a low carotenoid diet prior to and during the study. After 12 weeks, both groups had significant increases in their blood levels of beta-carotene, with the beta-carotene-capsule group having the greatest response. Nutrition Research 16 (1996): 565–575.

Chapter 7: Vitamin D

In this study of 3,000 elderly females, half were given 1,200 milligrams of calcium plus 800 international units of vitamin D, and half were given a placebo. The supplemented group had a 30 percent lower incidence of nonvertebral fractures and a 41-percent lower incidence of hip fractures compared with that of the placebo group. *Nutrition Reviews* 51 (1993): 183–185.

Cancer Prevention

The third NHANES found that vitamin D deficiency is a major unrecognized epidemic in adult women of childbearing age. Vitamin D is not only important to bone health, it regulates immune function and controls cellular proliferation. There is an inverse association of increased risk of dying from breast, colon, ovarian, and prostate cancer in people living further away from the equator. Children receiving vitamin D supplements from age 1 year on have an 80 percent decreased risk of developing Type I diabetes. Adults have a 50 percent decreased risk of developing colon cancer later in life when their serum levels of D are equal to or greater than 50 nanomoles/liter. The author asserts that the recommendations by the Institute of Medicine for vitamin D (400 international units for middle-aged adults, 600 international units for older adults) are too low. The safe upper limit of vitamin D for ages 1 and above is 2,000 international units per day. *American Journal of Clinical Nutrition* 76 (2002): 3–4.

It is noted that humans evolved at equatorial latitudes, without modern clothing and shelter, so their vitamin D supply would have been equivalent to at least 100 micrograms/day (4,000 units/day). The modern-day human level vitamin D is approximately half of that level. The level of vitamin D used in clinical trials has been small but has shown some benefit. Vitamin D supplementation at 20 micrograms/day (800 international units/day) is noted for preventing bone loss, reducing fracture risk, lowering blood pressure, and lowering circulating parathyroid hormone concentrations. Greater vitamin D nutrition levels may be involved in reducing the occurrence of breast, prostate, and bowel cancers and autoimmune conditions such as multiple sclerosis and insulin-dependent diabetes mellitus. Supplementation with at least 25 micrograms/day of vitamin D (1,000 international units/day) not just during the winter, but all year long, may be warranted, since it is safe, inexpensive, and, with calcium, can prevent bone loss. *Journal of Nutrition and Environmental Medicine* 11 (2001): 275–291.

Blood Pressure/Cardovascular Disease

Women who take vitamin D supplements lower their risk of death from heart disease by one-third. A research team analyzed data from nearly 10,000 women over the age of 65 who were enrolled in a study of how often osteoporosis causes broken bones. Of these, more than 4,200 women reported that they took vitamin D supplements at the time of the study, and another 733 reported a prior history of supplement use. After following the women for an average of nearly 11 years, researchers found that the risk of heart disease death was 31 percent lower in those women who were taking vitamin D at the time of the study. The researchers note that calcium supplements, education, self-reported health status, or health-related behaviors had no effect on the protection afforded by vitamin D. 42nd annual conference on Cardiovascular Disease and Epidemiology Prevention in Honolulu, Hawaii (April 23, 2002).

In this study of over 300 women, younger women who consumed at least 400 international units of vitamin D per day had lower systolic blood pressure. (They also had significantly higher calcium and potassium intakes.) In older women, systolic blood pressure was significantly lower in those who consumed at least the RDAs of both calcium and vitamin D. The authors point out that this is the first report of a significant relationship between vitamin D and blood pressure, and that 50 to 75 percent of the women in the study had estimated vitamin D intakes of less than the RDA. *American Journal of Clinical Nutrition* 42 (July 1985): 135–142.

Other Uses
The authors found that small oral doses and topical treatment of vitamin D improved symptoms of psoriasis, and that the lower the levels of vitamin D in the body, the more severe the disease. *Archives of Dermatology* 125 (1989): 231–234.

Chapter 8: Vitamin E
See also references on "Antioxidants" for Chapters 2 and 3.

Overview
A prominent researcher discusses the clinical relevance of vitamin E and concludes that vitamin E has equivocal benefits in intermittent claudication, cutaneous ulcers, burns, wound healing, tardive dyskinesia, epilepsy, hemolytic anemia, and adult respiratory distress syndrome. Studies on its effect on platelets and LDL cholesterol oxidation support the benefits of vitamin E and cardiovascular disease. Regarding cancer, larger trials with higher doses of vitamin E are needed to determine its effect on cancer. Studies on vitamin E and immunity, especially in the elderly, are promising. *Lancet* 345 (January 21, 1995): 170–175.

This article discusses the popularity of vitamin E due to its role in preventing aging, cancer, heart disease, infertility, and chronic disease. The author estimates savings of $8 billion if Americans took vitamin E supplements. *Hippocrates* (November/December 1994): 46–53.

Natural vitamin E includes four tocopherols and four tocotrienols. RRR-alpha-tocopherol is the most abundant form in nature and has the highest biological activity. Although vitamin E is the main lipid-soluble antioxidant in the body, not all its properties can be assigned to this action. As antioxidant, vitamin E acts in cell membranes where it prevents the propagation of free-radical reactions, although it has also been shown to have pro-oxidant activity. Although we already have substantial information on the action, effects, and metabolism of vitamin E, there are still several questions open. The most intriguing is its interaction with other antioxidants, which may explain how foods containing small amounts of vitamin E provide greater benefits than larger doses of vitamin E alone. *Journal of Physiology and Biochemistry* 57(2) (2001): 43–56.

Tocotrienols have vitamin E antioxidant activity, but can also inhibit cholesterol synthesis by suppressing HMG-CoA reductase. In this study, 13 hypercholesterolemic subjects received placebo, 13 received alpha-tocotrienyl acetate, 12 received gamma-tocotrienyl acetate, and 13 received delta-tocotrienyl acetate at 250 milligrams/day. Subjects followed the American Heart Association Step 1 Diet for 12 weeks and, after the first 4 weeks, began taking the supplements with their evening meal for 8 weeks. Alpha-tocotrienyl acetate increased in vitro LDL oxidative resistance and reduced its rate of oxidation. Tocotrienyl acetate supplements are hydrolyzed, absorbed, and can be measured in human plasma. Tocotrienyl acetate supplements do not lower cholesterol in hypercholesterolemic individuals who are already on low-fat diets. Alpha-tocotrienyl can significantly reduce LDL oxidizability. *Free Radical Biology & Medicine* 29(9) (2000): 834–845.

In the last 10 years, precise cellular functions of alpha-tocopherol, some of which are independent of its antioxidant/radical-scavenging ability, have been revealed. Alpha-tocopherol also inhibits cell proliferation, platelet aggregation, monocyte adhesion, and the oxygen burst in neutrophils. Other antioxidants, such as beta-tocopherol and probucol, do not mimic these effects, suggesting a nonantioxidant, alpha-tocopherol–specific molecular mechanism. *Journal of Nutrition* 130(7) (2000): 1649–1652.

Several studies have indicated potential roles for dietary antioxidants in the reduction of degenerative disease such as vascular dementia, cardiovascular disease, and cancer. In support of epidemiological studies, the researchers' studies indicate that the antioxidant properties of vitamin E and polyphenols contribute to reducing the risk of cardiovascular disease. Researchers demonstrated that these dietary antioxidants may have a preventive role in cancer, potentially through the suppression of angiogenesis. These findings concur with epidemiologic, clinical, and animal studies, suggesting that the consumption of green tea and vitamin E is associated with a reduced risk of cardiovascular disease and cancer, the leading causes of morbidity and mortality among the elderly. *Annals of the New York Academy of Sciences* 928 (2001): 226–235.

Antioxidant Powers
In this study, animals fed heated vegetable oil showed a 38- to 97-percent decrease of vitamin E levels in their blood and tissues. *Nutrition Reports International* 32 (November 1985): 1,179–1,186.

In this study of 100 healthy elderly people, higher levels of peroxides were found in those with lower levels of vitamins C and E. In people supplemented daily with 400 milligrams of C and/or 400 milligrams of E, peroxide levels decreased. The authors conclude that long-term supplementation of vitamins C and E can protect against free radical damage, which is thought to play a role in the aging processes and degenerative diseases. *Annals of Nutrition and Metabolism* 28 (May–June 1984): 186–191.

Cancer Prevention and Treatment
This study, conducted by the U.S. National Cancer Institute and Finland's Public Health Institute, involved 29,000 males, one group of which took supplements, including vitamin E. It was found that 50 milligrams of vitamin E per day reduced prostate cancer by 34 percent and colorectal cancer by 16 percent. However, it did not reduce lung cancer in smokers, as was hoped. *New England Journal of Medicine* 330 (April 14, 1994): 1,029–1,035.

Low vitamin E intake may enhance the effect of selenium deficiency, which is associated with increased risk of fatal cancer. *British Medical Journal* 290 (February 9, 1985): 417–420.

Researchers found that the D-alpha tocopherol succinate form of vitamin E inhibits the proliferation of estrogen receptor-positive and estrogen receptor-negative human breast cancer cell lines in a dose-dependent manner *in vitro*. *Nutrition and Cancer* 19 (1993): 225–229.

Vitamin E was found to reduce the free-radical damage in experimental animals given anticancer chemotherapy. The authors conclude that this provides strong evidence for the protective use of vitamin E in cancer-free animals. They further suggest that its use during anticancer therapy is theoretically advisable because it may reduce the toxicity of some drugs, without reducing the drugs' effectiveness. The authors cite several other studies that report the benefits of large doses of vitamin E and other antioxidant vitamins to cancer patients. *Anticancer Research* 3 (1983): 59–62.

Researchers found that adding vitamin E to prostate cancer cells inhibits the production of a receptor for testosterone, called the androgen receptor (AR), which is needed in order for the cancer to grow and develop. The fewer ARs there are in a prostate cancer cell, the less capable the remaining ARs, no matter how they are activated, are to turn on the genes that stimulate prostate cancer growth and progression. Previous research has shown that vitamin E can protect against the development of prostate cancer, reducing risk from 18 percent to 12 percent among male smokers. Vitamin E inhibits the expression in prostate cancer cells of prostate-specific antigen. Vitamin E can prevent cells from making androgen receptors. This is the first study to show how an agent can, in fact, specifically inhibit a prostate cancer cell's ability to manufacture AR. Vitamin E might work best when administered with other natural treatments that also appear to protect against prostate cancer, such as vitamin D and selenium. Proceedings of the National Academy of Sciences 99 (2002): 7408–7413.

Selenium and alpha-tocopherol, the major form of vitamin E in supplements, appear to have a protective effect against prostate cancer. Gamma-tocopherol is a major component of vitamin E in the U.S. diet and the second most common tocopherol in human serum. In a study of 10,456 men, the risk of prostate cancer declined with increasing concentrations of alpha-tocopherol. For gamma-tocopherol, men in the highest fifth of the distribution had a fivefold reduction in the risk of developing prostate cancer than men in the lowest fifth. Selenium levels and prostate cancer risk was in the protective direction with individuals in the top four-fifths of the distribution having a reduced risk of prostate cancer compared with individuals in the bottom fifth. Statistically significant protective associations for high levels of selenium and alpha-tocopherol were observed only when gamma-tocopherol concentrations were high. The use of combined alpha- and gamma-tocopherol supplements should be considered in upcoming prostate cancer prevention trials. *Journal of the National Cancer Institute* 92(24) (2002): 2018.

In one study, researchers looked at the antioxidant effect of alpha-tocopherol vs. mixed tocopherols. The mixed tocopherol was much more potent in inhibiting lipid peroxidation than alpha-tocopherol alone. *Journal of Cardiovascular Pharmacology* 39(5) (2002): 714–21.

Alpha-tocopheryl succinate (alpha-TOS), a redox-inactive analogue of vitamin E, is a strong inducer of apoptosis, whereas alpha-tocopherol (alpha-TOH) lacks apoptogenic activity. The potential of alpha-TOS as an antitumor agent was investigated using nude mice with colon cancer xenografts; it was found that alpha-TOH exerted modest antitumor activity and acted by inhibiting tumor cell proliferation. In contrast, alpha-TOS showed a more profound antitumor effect, at both the level of inhibition of proliferation and induction of tumor cell apoptosis. Alpha-TOS was nontoxic to normal cells and tissues, and exerted a cooperative proapoptotic activity. Finally, alpha-TOS suppressed tumor growth in vivo. Vitamin E succinate is thus a potent and highly specific anticancer agent and/or adjuvant of considerable therapeutic potential. *Clinical Cancer Research* 8(3) (2002): 863–9.

Cardiovascular Disease

Two landmark studies suggested vitamin E supplementation reduces the rate of heart disease in women and men by 40 percent. Data from these two studies—the Nurses' Health Study and the Physicians' Health Study—were published in *New England Journal of Medicine* 328 (May 20, 1993), 1,444–1,456 and 1,487–1,489.

Another landmark study, from the Center of Human Nutrition of the University of Texas Southwestern Medical Center, found that only groups of subjects who received at least 400 international units per day of vitamin E experienced a decrease of the susceptibility of LDL cholesterol to oxidation from free radicals. *Arteriosclerosis, Thrombosis and Vascular Biology.* 15 (1995): 190–198.

This article reviewed literature with respect to beta-carotene and vitamin E supplementation in men who smoke or consume alcohol. In one study of 40,000 men, those taking at least 100 international units of vitamin E per day for two or more years had a 40-percent reduction in the risk of coronary heart disease compared with men not taking supplements. *Nutrition Report* 11 (1993): 73, 80.

These letters to the editors argue that it is not premature to recommend vitamin E supplementation for the prevention of coronary artery disease, and that the reasons for withholding vitamin E therapy are not convincing. A substantial number of physicians in the United States are taking vitamin E supplements themselves. The authors question, "If vitamin E is good enough for physicians, why is it not good enough for their patients?" *New England Journal of Medicine* (November 4, 1993): 1,424.

In this study by prominent researcher Dr. Jialal, subjects were given 800 international units of vitamin E, 1,000 milligrams of C, and 30 milligrams of beta-carotene per day, and experienced a 40-percent decrease in the oxidation rate of blood lipids. A group that received 800 international units of vitamin E alone experienced similar results, leading the researchers to conclude that combining the three antioxidants was no better than using vitamin E alone. However, it should be noted that the amounts of the other two antioxidants may have been too low to exert any noticeable effect. *Circulation* 88 (December 1993): 2,780–2,786. See also *Journal of the American College of Nutrition* 12 (1993): 631-637.

Consumption of vitamin E reduces the risk of cardiovascular disease and cancer along with other antioxidants as well. Vitamin E suppresses angiogenesis, thereby having a preventive role in cancer. Meydani, M. "Nutrition interventions in aging and age-associated diseases." *Annals of the New York Academy of Science* 928 (2001): 226–235.

Cardiovascular disease is the leading cause of morbidity and mortality in the Western world. Antioxidants, especially alpha-tocopherol, have beneficial effects on cell functions that are pivotal in atherogenesis. It inhibits platelet aggregation and pro-inflammatory activation of monocytes and macrophage function—collectively preventing damage to arteries. *Nutrition Reviews* 60(1) (2002): 8–14.

Wound Healing/Skin Conditions

The authors note that daily doses of 800 to 2,000 international units of vitamin E are recommended by some physicians to prevent postoperative problems in women who have undergone breast augmentation. *Plastic and Reconstructive Surgery* 69 (June 1982): 2,029–1,030.

Topical vitamin E is one of the natural treatments reviewed for nonsurgical scar revision. Chang, C.W., and W. R. Ries. "Nonoperative techniques for scar management and revision." *Facial Plastic Surgery* 17(4) (2001): 283–288.

Subjects with a history of atopic dermatitis (AD) received either 400 international units of Vitamin E (d-alpha-tocopherol) daily or a placebo for 8 months. A significant number of subjects in the vitamin E group showed great improvement compared to the placebo group, and there was almost complete remission of AD in several of the vitamin E group subjects. Those who showed greatest improvement and who experienced near remission demonstrated a 62 percent decrease in serum IgE levels compared to baseline while there was a 34.4 percent reduction in the placebo group. Elevated serum IgE has been considered a predictor for the prognosis of AD treatment and these results suggest that an addition of 400 milligram of vitamin E per day, along with elimination of identified allergens (including food) may be a cost-effective tool in the management of AD. *International Journal of Dermatology* 41 (2001): 146–150.

The Immune System

In this study, 5 discoid lupus erythematosus patients given 800 to 2,000 international units of vitamin E daily made an excellent recovery, with no side effects. This disease is normally treated with thalidomide and immunosuppressants, which have considerable side effects. The author concludes that treatment of autoimmune diseases such as DLE with vitamin E would seem preferable to the use of potentially hazardous drugs. *British Journal of Dermatology* III (July 1984): 125–126 (letter).

Patients receiving 900 to 1,600 international units of vitamin E per day showed complete or almost complete clearing of lupus symptoms. Lower dosages of 300 international units had no benefit. *Cutis* 21 (1978): 321–325.

In this study, 7 rheumatoid arthritis patients who no longer responded to conventional therapy alone were also given 400 international units of vitamin E and 350 micrograms of selenium. In 4 of these patients, joint pain disappeared; in the remaining 3, pain lessened and joint mobility markedly increased. *Biological Trace Element Research* 7 (May–June 1985): 195-198.

Patients with osteoarthritis of the hip or knee were treated for three weeks with vitamin E (d-alpha-tocopheryl acetate) 400 milligrams 3 times per day; equivalent to approximately 600 international units 3 times per day of diclofenac (50 milligrams 3 times per day). Both treatments appeared to be equally effective in reducing the circumference of knee joints and walking time and in increasing joint mobility. This vitamin has been reported to have anti-inflammatory activity and may also inhibit prostaglandin synthesis. In addition, vitamin E may help stabilize lysosomal membranes, thereby inhibiting the release of enzymes believed to play a role in the pathogenesis of osteoarthritic joint damage. *Zeitschrift fur Rheumatologie* 49 (1990): 369–373.

Neurological Disorders

Vitamin E intake in food and supplements may help slow the decline in mental functioning among older people. It may counteract the damage to brain cells by free radicals. Previous research showed that people who consume more vitamin E to retain mental function are less likely to develop Alzheimer's disease. According to the findings, over 60 percent of the nearly 3,000 participants showed some decline in their mental function, while 39 percent had no decline or improved. The group reporting the highest intake of vitamin E had the slowest decline in mental function compared to the lowest intake group. Those with the highest intake of vitamin E had a 32 percent reduction in their rate of mental decline. But the number of people taking the vitamin E during the study doubled—otherwise an even greater effect may have been noted. High intake of vitamin E was linked to a 70 percent reduction in developing Alzheimer's during a 4-year period. *Archives of Neurology* 59 (2002): 1125–1132.

In a study of 5,395 participants after a mean follow-up of 6 years, 197 subjects developed dementia, of which 146 had Alzheimer's disease. After adjusting specific variables, high intake of vitamin C and vitamin E was associated with a lower risk of Alzheimer's disease. Among current smokers, this relationship was most and also present for intake of beta-carotene and flavonoids. This trial suggests that higher intakes of vitamin C and vitamin E from food is associated with decreased risk of Alzheimer's disease. *Journal of the American Medical Association* 287 (2002): 3223–3229.

Alzheimer's disease is a chronic and progressive neurodegenerative disorder characterized by cognitive and functional deficit and by behavior disturbance. Donepezil, new cholinesterase inhibitors, and vitamin E have proved effective in delaying the progression of Alzheimer's disease. *Tex Med* 97(12) (Dec 2001): 50–58.

Women's Health

Fibrocystic Breast Disease

In a study of 26 women with breast disease and 8 controls, 85 percent (22 women) of those who received daily supplementation of 600 international units of vitamin E for 8 weeks responded to the treatment. In 10 women, there was a total disappearance of cystic lesions and breast tenderness, and in 12 women, lesions decreased in number and size. The authors suggest that vitamin E supplementation may be an inexpensive and safe way of treating this disorder. *Nutrition Research* 2 (1982): 243-247.

Menstrual Disorders/Menopause

Vulvovaginitis improved with vitamin E treatment. It has been suggested that vitamin E, through its ability to improve the blood supply to muscles or by promoting a greater utilization of oxygen, relieved ischemia that was causing intermittent claudication. In girls given vitamin E tablets at a dose of 50 milligrams 3 times daily, improvement during the menstrual phase was shown in 76 percent of the treatment group and only in 29 percent of a control group. Fifty-nine percent of the treated individuals improved in 2 stages, compared with 14 percent of controls. This study showed the potential benefit of vitamin E in the treatment of spasmodic dysmenorrhea. *Lancet* (1955): 844–847.

In evaluating 100 girls with primary dysmenorrhea, 50 took five 100-unit tablets of vitamin E daily compared with 50 (mean age of 16.9 years) who took 5 placebo tablets per day. The treatment started 2 days before the beginning of menstruation and continued through the first 3 days of bleeding for 2 consecutive menstrual periods. It was found that the severity of pain was reduced in both groups, but the reduction was greater in the group treated with vitamin E. Br J Obstet Gynaecol 108 (November 2001): 1181–1183.

It is suggested that vitamin E, among other natural products, be tried for management of hot flashes in breast cancer survivors and in men taking hormonal blockade therapy for prostate cancer. While there is some debate about the safety of soy phytoestrogens, vitamin E is completely safe to use in these patients. Lancet Oncology 2(4) (2001): 199–204.

Contraceptives

The authors administered 100 milligrams of vitamin E every other day to 51 women who suffered excessive menstrual bleeding after insertion of an IUD. In almost every subject, blood loss was reduced to normal. International Journal of Fertility 28 (1983): 55–56.

Breakthrough bleeding occurs in a significant number of Norplant users. Blood concentrations of lipid peroxide from Norplant users and depo-medroxyprogesterone acetate users who had bleeding problems were significantly higher than normal menstrual controls. It is believed that in progestin-only contraceptive users, higher lipid peroxide and lower vitamin E levels may cause endometrial cell damage and reduce the endometrial angiogenic response. This study suggests that vitamin E supplementation might counteract the adverse consequences of this increased oxidative stress due to Norplant and progestins. Hum Reproduction 15(Suppl. 3) (2000): 18–23.

Other Uses

Diabetes

In a study of 30 elderly patients with angina, daily supplementation with 900 international units of vitamin E for 4 months lowered fasting plasma insulin concentrations and triglycerides. The researchers conclude that high doses of vitamin E might be useful therapy for elderly insulin-resistant patients with coronary heart disease. American Journal of Clinical Nutrition 61 (1995): 848–852. A previous study with similar results was published by the same author in American Journal of Clinical Nutrition 57 (May 1993): 650–656.

Vitamin E supplementation has been shown to inhibit platelet aggregation in normal, non–vitamin E deficient subjects. Oral vitamin E is relatively nontoxic. In two double-blind, crossover trials, the first showed a decreased platelet thromboxane production in 22 Type I diabetics who received 400 milligrams of DL-alpha-tocopherol acetate daily for 4 weeks, and similar results were found in a second study of 9 insulin-dependent patients receiving 1,000 milligrams of vitamin E daily for 5 weeks. Vitamin E at 500 international units has been shown to increase HDL cholesterol over a 3-month treatment. In diabetic patients with hypercholesterolemia, plasma cholesterol levels have been reported to fall significantly after 16 weeks with vitamin E supplementation. A reduction in plasma peroxide levels has also been observed. Prostaglandins Leukotrienes and Essential Fatty Acids 40 (1990): 169–176.

Vitamin E supplementation can improve insulin efficiency and glycemic equilibrium, as shown by the decrease of glycaemia, glycated haemoglobin, and fructosamine values. In addition, this kind of supplementation lowers plasma lipid peroxidation and oxidizability of low density lipoproteins, which is involved in the atherogenesis process. Moreover, it helps to fight against complications such as retinopathy. Journal de la Societe de biologie. 195(4) (2001): 391–398.

Vision

In comparing vitamin E effects on cataract prevention, there was a 56-percent decrease in cataract risk in subjects who took vitamin E supplements compared with those who didn't take supplements. American Journal of Clinical Nutrition (1991 Supplement) 53: 346S–351S.

In a study of almost 5,000 people funded in part by the National Eye Institute, a mixture of 500 milligrams of vitamin C, 400 international units of vitamin E, and 15 milligrams of beta-carotene reduced the risk of vision loss by 10 percent. A mixture of 80 milligrams of zinc and 2 milligrams of copper reduced the risk by 11 percent. *Nutrition Week* 31(40) (2001): 7.

Exercise and Muscle Damage

In this double-blind study, subjects who took 800 international units of vitamin E exercised at 75 percent of their maximum heart rate for 45 minutes. When they were compared with those who took a placebo, the supplemented subjects experienced less oxidative stress to their tissues after the exercise. The authors conclude that vitamin E may provide protection against oxidative injury after exercise. *The Nutrition Report* 264 (1993): R992–R998.

In this study, researchers from the USDA supplemented 23 men with either 800 international units of vitamin E or a placebo daily for 7 weeks. Vitamin E reduced exercise-induced oxidative damage in both young and old subjects. The researchers discovered that vitamin E blunted the immune signals that trigger inflammation. *Food Chemical News* 34 (September 28, 1992): 52.

Toxicity and Absorbability

In a review of the literature, the authors found that vitamin E is not mutagenic, carcinogenic, or teratogenic. Very few side effects have been reported in humans even at doses of 3,200 milligrams per day. Side effects have been uncommon in other large trials. The adverse reaction reports have been mostly individual case reports or uncontrolled studies. *American Journal of Clinical Nutrition* 48 (September 1988): 612–619.

Natural vitamin E has been found to be more bioavailable than synthetic forms. *American Journal of Clinical Nutrition* 60 (1994): 397–402.

Review Articles

Gamma-tocopherol is the major form of vitamin E in many plant seeds and in the U.S. diet, but has drawn little attention compared with alpha-tocopherol, the predominant form of vitamin E in tissues and the primary form in supplements. However, recent studies indicate that gamma-tocopherol may be important to human health and that it possesses unique features that distinguish it from alpha-tocopherol. Gamma-tocopherol appears to be a more effective trap for lipophilic electrophiles than alpha-tocopherol. Gamma-tocopherol is well absorbed and accumulates to a significant degree in some human tissues. Some of its metabolites are different from that of other tocopherols and may be of physiologic importance. Gamma-tocopherol, but not alpha-tocopherol, inhibits cyclooxygenase activity and thus possesses anti-inflammatory properties. Some human and animal studies indicate that plasma concentrations of gamma-tocopherol are inversely associated with the incidence of cardiovascular disease and prostate cancer. These distinguishing features of gamma-tocopherol and its metabolite suggest that gamma-tocopherol may contribute significantly to human health in ways not recognized previously. This possibility should be further evaluated, especially considering that high doses of alpha-tocopherol deplete plasma and tissue gamma-tocopherol, in contrast with supplementation with gamma-tocopherol, which increases both. This review is on the bioavailability, metabolism, chemistry, and nonantioxidant activities of gamma-tocopherol and epidemiologic data concerning the relation between gamma-tocopherol and cardiovascular disease and cancer. *American Journal of Clinical Nutrition* 74(6) (2001): 714–722.

At least 8 vitamin E isoforms with biological activity have been isolated from plant sources. Since its discovery, mainly antioxidant and recently also cell-signaling aspects of tocopherols and tocotrienols have been studied. Although the antioxidant activity of tocotrienols is higher than that of tocopherols, tocotrienols have a lower bioavailability after oral ingestion. Tocotrienols penetrate rapidly through skin and efficiently combat oxidative stress induced by UV rays or the ozone. Tocotrienols have beneficial effects in cardiovascular diseases both by inhibiting LDL oxidation and by down-regulating HMG CoA reductase, a key enzyme regulating cholesterol synthesis. Important novel antiproliferative and neuroprotective effects of tocotrienols, which may be independent of their antioxidant activity, have also been described. Tocotrienols make up a considerable portion of total vitamin E in many food sources. In vitro, they have been shown to exhibit enhanced antioxidant properties compared with tocopherols. In addition, they have been shown to have cholesterol-lowering, anticarcinogenic, and neuroprotective properties, which may not be related to their antioxidant function. After oral ingestion, however, they have a short half life, which accounts for their low bioavailability. A promising approach to utilize tocotrienols may be the topical application onto the skin. In this scenario, uptake and distribution within the skin do not depend on transfer proteins, thereby allowing active concentrations to be reached in skin after topical supplementation. *Journal of Nutrition* 131 (2001): 369S–373S.

Chapter 9: Vitamin K
In evaluating dietary vitamin K intake in residents of a nursing home and free-living subjects who attended a day-care center, vitamin K intake level was much lower in the nursing home residents than in the free-living subjects. There were many more cases of the intake being below the recommended daily intake for vitamin K in the nursing home residents than in the control population at 86.0 vs. 11.4 percent, respectively. Elderly nursing home subjects in this study generally had a poor dietary vitamin K intake and might be at risk for osteoporosis. Green leafy vegetable consumption, which is a rich source of vitamin K, is encouraged. *Asia Pacific Journal of Clinical Nutrition* 11(1) (2002): 62–65.

Behavior
Vitamin K-deficient animals became less active and suffered from general malaise. These results suggest that vitamin K deficiency may contribute to physical and psychiatric symptoms. *Physiology and Behavior* 34 (May 1985): 727–734.

Cancer
Anticoagulant drugs have been demonstrated to reduce metastasis and improve survival in cancer patients. Since vitamin K is involved in coagulation, one would think it is contraindicated in cancer patients. However, vitamin K has unique antineoplastic properties alone, and also augments patient survival when used in conjunction with radiation therapy. Paradoxically, vitamin K also increases the antimetastatic capacity of anticoagulant therapy. *Adjuvant Nutrition in Cancer Treatment,* 1992 Symposium Proceedings, eds. Patrick Quillin, Ph.D., R.D.; R. Michael Williams, M.D., Ph.D. (Arlington Heights, IL: Cancer Treatment Foundation, 1992).

Cardiovascular Disease
In studying 600 men who were 50 to 70 years of age and were asymptomatic for atherosclerosis, subjects underwent coronary artery calcium burden via electron-beam computed tomography, along with measuring their percent of undercarboxylated serum osteocalcin, which is a biochemical index of vitamin K cofactor activity. Poor vitamin K status was 1 of 5 significant risk factors for severe coronary artery calcification. After adjusting for variables, poor vitamin K status was associated with a 2.7-fold increased risk of severe coronary artery calcification, which was comparable with the risk attributed to being a current smoker. Subclinical vitamin K deficiency has been suspected to play a role in vascular calcification, bone metabolism, and increased hip fracture risk in the elderly. There was concern from the audience regarding the role of warfarin, which is one of the most commonly prescribed medications in the United States, with large numbers of individuals with valvular disease taking warfarin to prevent strokes. If warfarin worsens vitamin K status, this might increase coronary artery calcification, which may be doing

more harm than good when this anticoagulant is prescribed. *Family Practice News* 32(1) (2002): 1–2.

Chapter 10: Vitamin B Complex

The Elderly

B_{12} deficiencies in the elderly can result in neuropsychiatric disorders such as depression, personality changes, mood swings, cognitive impairment, memory loss, gait abnormalities, orthostatic hypotension, and optic and peripheral neuropathies. Folic acid deficiency may result in reduced DNA formation, failure of cell proliferation, demyelinization, and degeneration of the central nervous system. Hyperhomocysteinemia is more prevalent in the elderly due to subclinical deficiencies of B_6, B_{12}, and folic acid, and is a risk factor for heart attack. Hyperhomocysteinemia is treatable with these vitamins. Considering the high cost of treatment in a long-term care facility, the authors suggest it is both efficient and cost effective to assess the levels of these vitamins periodically. *Clinical Laboratory Sciences* 6 (September/October 1993): 272–274.

In a randomized, placebo-controlled, double-blind study, 14 geriatric patients suffering from depression were given antidepressant treatment with 10 milligrams each of B_1, B_2, and B_6. Within 4 weeks, supplemented patients demonstrated improved B-vitamin status and improved scores on ratings of depression and cognitive function, compared with the placebo group. The levels of B vitamins used in this study were 5 to 8 times the RDA. *Journal of the American College of Nutrition* 11 (1992): 159–163.

HIV Infection

In a study of 296 HIV-infected men, those who took a multivitamin supplement were one-third less likely to develop full-blown AIDS, compared with those who did not take supplements. Those who had higher-than-average intakes of vitamins A, B_1, B_2, or niacin had higher CD4 counts. *Medical Tribune* (March 24, 1994): 18.

Chapter 11: Vitamin B₁ (Thiamin)

Surgery

Elderly patients experienced a significant lowering of thiamin levels in the blood after surgery. The authors suggested that thiamin deficiency may be one factor in postoperative mental confusion and overall deterioration in this population, and that more attention should be paid to assessing their thiamin status. *Age and Aging* 11 (1982): 101–107.

Thiamin Intake and Absorption

Although the classic signs of beriberi were absent, 28 percent of study subjects had low thiamin levels. This subclinical condition may not be a vitamin deficiency disease per se, but rather may be due to a high calorie intake that overtaxes the oxidative metabolism. High calorie diets with disproportionately low intakes of vitamins and minerals may be the source of widespread marginal malnutrition that is not being sufficiently recognized by physicians. *Journal of the American College of Nutrition* 7 (1988): 61–67.

Severe disease increasingly interferes with the dietary intake of thiamin, and alcoholism interferes with the absorption of thiamin in a major fashion. *American Journal of Clinical Nutrition* 36 (November 1982): 1,067–1,082.

Healthy volunteers underwent a 4-day adaption phase, in which the carbohydrate intake was 55 percent of total energy intake, followed by an intervention period in which the carbohydrate intake was 65 percent of total energy for 4 days, and then 75 percent for another 4 days. It was found that during the intervention periods, thiamin decreased significantly in the plasma as well as the urine. This study showed that an increase of dietary carbohydrate intake from 55 percent to 65 percent and 75 percent, respectively, of total caloric intake for 4 days per period resulted in a reduction in plasma and urine levels.

High carbohydrate diets may require more thiamin. *International Journal of Vitamin and Nutrition Research* 71(4) (2001): 217–221.

Because exercise stresses metabolic pathways that depend on thiamin, riboflavin, and vitamin B_6, the requirements for these vitamins may be increased in athletes and active individuals. On the basis of metabolic studies, the riboflavin status of young and older women who exercise moderately appears to be poorer in periods of exercise, dieting, and dieting plus exercise than during control periods. Exercise appears to decrease nutrient status even further in active individuals with preexisting marginal vitamin intakes or marginal body stores. Thus, active individuals who restrict their energy intake or make poor dietary choices are at greatest risk for poor thiamin, riboflavin, and vitamin B_6 status. *Amercian Journal of Clinical Nutrition* 72(2 Suppl) (2000): 598S–606S.

Despite modern pharmacologic agents in the therapy of heart failure, the prevalence of heart failure is increasing worldwide. Two new studies confirmed that all diuretics lead to increased urinary thiamin excretion depending on the urinary flow rate. In at-risk patients such as an elderly person, chronic diuretic treatment may lead to a subclinical thiamin deficiency, which may influence prevalence and/or severity of heart failure. *Nutrition Reviews* 58(10) (2000): 319–323.

Immunity
In this study, thiamin-deficient experimental animals showed less response to immunization vaccinations. *Proceedings of the Society of Experimental Biology and Medicine* 77 (1951): 526–530.

Psychiatric Disease
In a study of psychiatric patients, schizophrenics, and alcoholics, as a group, these subjects were significantly overrepresented in low-thiamin patients. *British Journal of Psychiatry* 141 (1982): 271.

A survey of 172 unselected psychiatric patients showed 30 percent to be biochemically deficient in thiamin, although only 1 of these had clinical symptoms of deficiency. An inadequate intake of vitamins, particularly B_1, can result in mental illness. *Clinical Neurorpharmacology* 8 (July–September 1985): 286–293.

Thiamin-dependent processes are diminished in brains of patients with several neurodegenerative diseases. The decline in thiamin-dependent enzymes can be readily linked to the symptoms and pathology of the disorders. The interactions of thiamin with oxidative processes may be part of a spiral of events that lead to neurodegeneration. The reversal of the effects of thiamin deficiency by antioxidants, and amelioration of other forms of oxidative stress by thiamin, suggest that thiamin may act as a site-directed antioxidant. The data indicate that the interactions of thiamin-dependent processes with oxidative stress are critical in neurodegenerative processes. *Neurochemistry International* 40(6) (2002): 493–504.

Cancer
The authors speculate that thiamin supplementation (in this study, 100 milligrams per day) could help prevent cell damage, fibrinogenesis, and collagen breakdown in cancer patients. *Journal of Nutrition, Growth and Cancer* 1 (July–December 1984): 207–210.

Menstrual Problems
In a trial of girls who had moderate to severe spasmodic dysmenorrhea, 100 milligrams of thiamin hydrochloride/day was given orally daily for 90 days. Results showed 87 percent were cured, 8 percent were relieved to where the pain was almost nonexistent, and 5 percent showed no effect in the 3 different groups of varying intensities of dysmenorrhea. Adolescent females are known to be deficient in vitamins B_1, B_2 and B_6. *Medical Research* 103 (1996): 227–231.

Toxicity

Toxicity of thiamin was seen only in cases in which doses were thousands of times larger than normal. There have been no toxic effects of thiamin administered by mouth reported in humans. Robert S. Goodhart and Maurice E. Shils, *Modern Nutrition in Health and Disease*, 6th ed. (Philadelphia: Lea and Febiger, 1980).

Chapter 12: Vitamin B₂ (Riboflavin)

Anemia

Riboflavin administered with iron-enhanced recovery from microcytic anemia in men and children. *Human Nutrition. Clinical Nutrition* 37C (1983): 413–425.

Esophageal Cancer

In this animal study, nearly half the subjects fed a riboflavin-free diet developed precancerous or cancerous tumors of the esophagus. The authors concluded that riboflavin helps to maintain the lining of the mouth and esophagus, and that its deficiency may increase the susceptibility of these tissues to carcinogens. *Journal of the National Cancer Institute* 72 (April 1984): 941–948.

Cataracts

Riboflavin deficiency has been linked to cataract formation in some studies. Low riboflavin intake or impaired riboflavin utilization could lead to an increase in cataract formation. *American Journal of Clinical Nutrition* 34 (May 1981): 861–863.

Carpal Tunnel Syndrome

A man with carpal tunnel syndrome was given 50 milligrams of riboflavin and 500 milligrams of pyridoxine (B₆) daily for a total of eight months. All of his CTS symptoms disappeared. *Proceedings of the National Academy of Science* 81 (November 1984): 7,076–7,078.

Exercise

Riboflavin plays a role in energy production. The daily allowance for riboflavin is proportional to energy needs. Regular exercise has been shown to increase the daily needs of riboflavin. Mild deficiencies have been shown in athletes undergoing strenuous daily exercise. *Nutrition Research* 4 (1984): 201–208.

Weight-reducing women require more than the RDA of riboflavin during both periods of nonexercise and periods of exercise. *American Journal of Clinical Nutrition* 41 (February 1985): 270–277.

Oral Contraceptives

In this study, riboflavin deficiency was found to be more prevalent in women taking oral contraceptives than in women who were not. *American Journal of Clinical Nutrition* 35 (March 1982): 495–501.

Detecting and Alleviating Deficiencies

In an Indian study, 4 milligrams of riboflavin (the RDA) failed to correct deficiencies in half the subjects. *Nutrition Research* 2 (1982): 147–153.

The authors studied 42 adolescent boys with no clinical symptoms of riboflavin deficiency. Biochemical testing showed that 38 percent were deficient in this nutrient. *American Journal of Clinical Nutrition* 39 (May 1984): 787–791.

Chapter 13: Vitamin B₃ (Niacin and Niacinamide)

Cardiovascular Disease

When subjects were given 100 milligrams per deciliter of niacin and 200 milligrams per deciliter of chromium for 4 weeks, it significantly lowered their serum cholesterol. Supplementation for 4 months resulted in a further decrease in serum cholesterol. *Journal of Family Practice* 27 (December 1988): 603–606.

In evaluating 139 patients who participated in a double-blind, placebo-controlled trial, subjects randomly received either gemfibrozil or extended-released niacin, which was initially started at 375 milligrams and was increased weekly to 2,000 milligrams. The extended-release niacin had a greater effect on raising HDL cholesterol and apolipoprotein A-1 levels than did gemfibrozil. Increasing apolipoprotein A-1 (a cardioprotective subfraction of HDL) is an additional benefit by which niacin has an antiatherogenic effect. *Arteriosclerosis, Thrombosis and Vascular Biology* 21 (2001): 1783–1789.

Subjects took simvastatin plus niacin at an average dose of 3.2 grams/day. There was nearly a 70 percent drop in the incidence of death, nonfatal myocardial infarction, stroke, and hospitalizations for cardiovascular disease during a 3-year follow-up. The niacin-statin regimen resulted in substantial reductions in coronary disease progression, measured by coronary angiography. The niacin dose was gradually increased to achieve a 10-milligrams/deciliter increase in serum HDL levels. With the combined treatment, there was an average increase in HDL of 30 percent. *Family Practice News* (January 1, 2001): 7.

Efficacy, safety, and tolerability of once-daily niacin for the treatment of dyslipidemia associated with Type II diabetes given 1,000 or 1,500 milligrams of niacin per day or placebo. Only niacin significantly increased HDL-C and reduced triglyeride levels and significantly improved total cholesterol to HDL-C ratio. In both ER niacin groups, there was an initial increase in fasting blood sugar (FBG) levels between weeks 4 and 8 but this value returned to baseline levels by week 16. *Arch Intern Med* 162 (2002): 1568–1576.

Niacin favorably alters all major lipid subfractions at pharmacologic doses. Alone or in combination with drugs, it promotes regression of coronary artery disease, decreases coronary events, stroke, and total mortality. Major recent progress in niacin is in 4 areas. First, recent data indicate that it increases high-density lipoprotein (HDL) and lowers triglycerides and low-density lipoprotein (LDL) by mechanisms different from drugs and that when given together have synergistic effects. New data on an extended-release preparation of niacin given once nightly indicates that it is as effective and has greater tolerability than immediate-release niacin. Finally, emerging evidence indicates that niacin can be used effectively and safely in patients with Type II diabetes mellitus, who often have low HDL levels. *Current Atherosclerosis Reports* 3(1) (2001): 74–82.

Cancer

In this animal study, only 14 percent of the subjects that were given niacinamide along with a potent carcinogen developed pancreatic cancer, as compared with 43 percent of those that were given the carcinogen alone. The authors concluded from this and previous research that niacinamide inhibits cancer at several sites, and that since niacin has low toxicity, it may be useful in cancer prevention. *Journal of the National Cancer Institute* 73 (September 1984): 767–770.

In mice with laboratory-induced breast cancer, the effectiveness of radiation therapy with or without the administration of niacin was assessed. The average size of the tumor in mice given niacinamide with radiation was decreased by 86 percent 2 weeks after treatment, and remained 79 percent lower after 4 weeks. The authors suggest that niacin sensitizes tissues to the effects of radiation and may have a role in the treatment of malignant tumors. *Cancer Research* 45 (August 1985): 3,609–3,614.

Supplements

In this study, 120 patients with severe intermittent claudication received either 2,000 milligrams of IHN or a placebo. After 3 months, the IHN group had significantly larger changes in claudication times and in number of free-walking paces compared with the placebo group. In the whole patient population, IHN gave improvements in subjective and functional assessments of intermittent claudication that were statistically significantly greater than the placebo. The improvement was particularly marked in smokers. *British Journal of Clinical Practice* 42 (1988): 377–383.

In this study, 15 patients with Raynaud's disease were given 1 gram of IHN 4 times each day for 9 months. At the end of the trial, the Reactive Thermal Gradient was found to be significantly improved when compared with baseline values. Subjective ratings of cold, numbness, and pain significantly improved. General tolerance to IHN at this dosage was good; no side effects or adverse reactions were found. *Journal of International Medical Research* 9 (1981): 393–400.

Toxicity
This article reviews four cases of niacin-induced hepatotoxicity. All patients were using sustained-release niacin preparations in a dose of at least 2.6 grams per day. *Southern Medical Journal* 30 (January 1994): 30–32.

Chapter 14: Vitamin B$_6$ (Pyridoxine)
Overview
A deficiency in vitamin B$_6$ results in skin and nervous system disorders, kidney disorders, depression of immune responses, anemia, and carpal tunnel syndrome. Studies have shown deficiencies of and/or an increased need for B$_6$ in oral contraceptive users and alcoholics; during certain situations such as exposure to radiation; and from certain drugs, cardiac failure, pregnancy, and lactation. *American Journal of Medical Technology* 49:1 (1983): 17–21.

Emotional Illness
In 15 chronic schizophrenic patients, pyridoxine was added to their previous drug regimen at a dose of 50 milligrams 3 times daily. After 4 to 6 weeks of this therapy, 8 patients reported a certain degree of subjective improvement. The patients stated they felt more alert and responsive, more active mentally and physically. After the therapy continued for 8 to 10 weeks, there was slow but continued improvement, which became more apparent. The third month of therapy eliminated the lack of drive and motivation and the blunted affect in 8 patients and was replaced by feelings of well-being, and the patients agreed to be referred either to occupational therapy or to a vocational and rehabilitation program. *British Journal of Psychiatry* 122 (1973): 240.

Of the psychiatric patients admitted to the hospital in this study, 53 percent were deficient in at least one of the following: B$_6$, thiamin, or riboflavin. B$_6$ is associated with depression and other emotional disorders, and the authors suggest that along with riboflavin, B$_6$ deficiency has a primary role in the cause of emotional disorder. *British Journal of Psychiatry* 141 (1982): 271–272.

The authors describe how 500 milligrams of B$_6$ were effective in treating an acutely schizophrenic patient who did not respond to other psychotropic medications. They recommend that B$_6$ be considered as an alternative treatment for this disorder. *Biological Psychiatry* 18:11 (1983): 1,321–1,328.

Carpal Tunnel Syndrome
A patient with carpal tunnel syndrome (CTS) who was given 500 milligrams of B$_6$ and 50 milligrams of riboflavin supplements experienced complete disappearance of his symptoms. *Proceedings of the National Academy of Sciences* 81 (November 1984): 7,076–7,078.

In this small study, 4 out of 6 CTS patients claimed some partial relief after B$_6$ supplementation. The authors note that a number of recent studies report that patients with CTS respond to pyridoxine treatment, but that a large double-blind controlled study is necessary to fully test the efficacy of this treatment. *Annals of Neurology* 15 (January 1984): 104–107.

Childhood Epilepsy and Autism

Pyridoxine-dependent seizures (PDS) in infants, which should be suspected in every infant with convulsions before 18 months of age, were controlled by administration of B_6. Failure to treat PDS with B_6 promptly results in severe mental retardation or death. *Annals of Neurology* 17 (February 1985): 117–120.

Many forms of infant and childhood epilepsy respond to B_6 treatment. All infants with refractory epileptic seizure must be given an adequate trial of B_6. *Archives of Disease in Childhood* 58 (1983): 1,034–1,036 (letter).

The effects of vitamin B_6 and magnesium supplementation on 60 autistic children were examined in a double-blind trial. The combination resulted in a significant improvement in many aspects of autistic behavior. *Biological Psychiatry* 20 (May 1985): 467–478.

Premenstrual Syndrome

The researchers report overwhelming evidence in both their study and others that 100 milligrams per day of B_6 appears to have a 60 to 80 percent success rate in the treatment of PMS. B_6 has been effective in cases in which progesterone has failed. Owing to the low toxicity of B_6, it is the authors' opinion that it should be tried as the first line of treatment in PMS. *The Practitioner* 228 (April 1984): 425–427.

The author has used amino acid–chelated magnesium and vitamin B_6 together at doses of 100 milligrams each, every 2 hours, during menses and 4 times a day. There was a progressive reduction in the intensity and duration of menstrual cramps with vitamin B_6 and magnesium supplementation over a 4- to 6-month period. Vitamin B_6 increases the influx of magnesium ion into the myometrial cell, and the magnesium ion has an antispasmodic effect. Vitamin B_6 supplementation alone between 200–800 milligrams/day has a wide variety of effects, which include decreased appetite with less craving for sweets; increased energy for work; sedation and better sleep patterns; improvement of mastalgia and breast congestion; a reduction in urgency and frequency of urination, with increased volume of urine, suggesting an increased bladder capacity; control of premenstrual weight gain; midcycle leukorrhea, suggesting increased secretion of cervical mucus; a reduction in susceptibility to stress and improved ability to deal with stress; and regulation of the menstrual cycle and duration of menses in oligomenorrheic and hypermenorrheic patients. *Clinical Obstetrics and Gynecology* 21(1) (1978): 139–145.

Pregnancy and Breastfeeding

In a study of 24 mothers and their infants, only those who received supplements of 10 to 20 milligrams of B_6 daily produced milk that met the American Academy of Pediatrics recommended concentration of B_6. *American Journal of Clinical Nutrition* 41 (January 1985): 21–31.

In this double-blind trial, 52 pregnant women were given pyridoxine supplements. Those who received 7.5 to 20 milligrams per day delivered babies whose Apgar scores were significantly higher than those of infants of mothers who received only 2.6 milligrams. *Journal of Nutrition* 114 (May 1984): 977–988.

Cardiovascular Disease

After a 6-week run-in period in which there were no lipid-lowering medications given, hyperlipidemic subjects participated in a randomized, double-blind, crossover trial. Subjects received either fenofibrate at 200 milligrams/day plus placebo or 200 milligrams of fenofibrate with 650 micrograms of folic acid, 50 micrograms of vitamin B_{12} and 5 milligrams of vitamin B_6. After the fenofibrate-plus-placebo therapy, there was a significant increase in homocysteine concentration by 44 percent. When fenofibrate was given with the vitamins, there was only a 13 percent increase. It may be that the increase in homocysteine from the fenofibrate treatment may counteract the cardioprotective effect of the lipid-lowering effects. This study recommends the routine use of folic acid, vitamin B_6 and vitamin B_{12} with fenofibrate therapy. *Atherosclerosis* 158 (2001): 161–164

Five healthy, white, male volunteers without elevated homocysteine levels received each of the following series of oral B vitamin supplements: Series 1 consisted of 1 milligram of folic acid, 10 milligrams of vitamin B_6 and 0.4 milligram of vitamin B_{12}; series 2 contained 5 milligrams of folic acid, 10 milligrams of vitamin B_6 and 0.4 milligram of vitamin B_{12}; and series 3 contained 5 milligrams of folic acid, 100 milligrams of vitamin B_6 and 0.4 milligram of vitamin B_{12}. Each series of vitamins was consumed daily for a period of 6 days. In series 3, the daily dose of vitamin B_6 was 100 milligrams, and serum pyridoxal 5^1-phosphate levels increased, while serum cystathionine levels decreased for the first time. In this third series, total homocysteine levels were significantly lowered, which did not happen in the second or first series. In this study, only the higher level of vitamin B_6 at 100 milligrams/day lowered total homocysteine levels and raised P5P levels. There was a statistically significant decrease in cystathionine noted with the 100 milligrams vitamin B_6 supplementation. It has been shown that supplementation of vitamin B_6 alone is associated with a reduction in serum folate levels. *Clinical Chemistry and Laboratory Medicine* 39(8) (2001): 768–771.

In this double-blind, placebo-controlled trial, treatment with a combination of folic acid, vitamin B_{12}, and pyridoxine significantly reduced homocysteine levels and decreased the rate of restenosis and the need for revascularization of the target lesion after coronary angioplasty. This inexpensive treatment, which has minimal side effects, should be considered as adjunctive therapy for patients undergoing coronary angioplasty. *New England Journal of Medicine* 345(22) (2001): 1593–1600.

Asthma
In this study, 15 adult asthmatics had significantly lower pyridoxine levels than did 16 healthy controls. Those subjects who took 50 milligrams of B_6 daily reported a dramatic decrease in the frequency and severity of wheezing or asthmatic attacks while taking the supplement. *American Journal of Clinical Nutrition* 41 (1985): 684–688.

Sickle Cell Anemia
In this study, 16 patients with sickle cell anemia had pyridoxine levels significantly lower than those of 16 healthy controls. B_6 has been shown to have anti-sickling properties, and these studies suggest that pyridoxine supplementation may have therapeutic benefits. *American Journal of Clinical Nutrition* 40 (August 1984): 235–239.

Chinese Restaurant Syndrome
This study shows that the symptoms of Chinese Restaurant Syndrome caused by monosodium glutamate sensitivity fail to recur after treatment with 50 to 200 milligrams of pyridoxine. *Hoppe-Seyler's Zeitschrift fur Physiologishe Chemie* 365:3 (1984): 405–414.

Kidney Disease
In this study, the administration of 25 to 200 milligrams of B_6 daily led to decreased oxalate secretion in patients with a form of hereditary kidney disorder. (Excess oxalate may lead to calcium deposits in the kidney, which may in turn lead to kidney failure and death.) *New England Journal of Medicine* 312 (April 11, 1985): 953–957.

In a group of 22 patients with oxalate kidney stones, a dose of 250 to 500 milligrams of B_6 was found to be an effective treatment. *Canadian Medical Association Journal* 131 (July 1984): 14.

Melanoma
In animal experiments, topical injections of B_6 retarded the growth of malignant melanoma. In one study, the tumors of the treated mice weighed 62 percent less than

those in untreated controls. In another, tumor growth was inhibited by 39 percent. *Nutrition and Cancer* 7 (January–June 1985): 43–52.

The Immune System

In this overview, the authors point out that pyridoxine deficiencies cause more profound effects on immune system function than do deficiencies of any other B vitamin. Both human and animal studies have shown B_6 to be involved in a wide variety of organs and processes of the immune system. *American Journal of Clinical Nutrition* (Supplement) 35 (February 1982): 418–421.

In laboratory animals, vitamin B_6 deficiency impaired the immune response and increased the animals' susceptibility to a cancer-causing virus. *Journal of Nutrition* 114 (May 1984): 938–945.

Bioavailability

The authors studied the bioavailability of B_6 from several foods and found that the amount of B_6 in foods does not necessarily represent the amount of the vitamin available to humans. In fact, the bioavailability of B_6 from natural sources is limited. *Journal of Nutrition* 113 (1983): 2,412–2,420.

Toxicity and Utilization

The authors report 7 cases of neurotoxicity resulting from massive intakes (2 to 6 grams per day) of B_6. Symptoms of toxicity include unsteady gait, numb feet, and numbness and clumsiness of the hands. In most of the cases, B_6 was the only nutritional supplement used by the patient. All patients improved substantially following withdrawal of B_6. *New England Journal of Medicine* (August 25, 1983): 445–448.

In this study, a group of 22 patients received doses of 250 to 500 milligrams of pyridoxine with no ill effects, and the authors concluded that these amounts are safe for long periods (up to 6 years). *Canadian Medical Association Journal* 131 (July 1984): 14.

There are many reports stressing the absence of toxic side effects of vitamin B_6 at doses up to 500 milligrams. In the strictly scientific sense, no causal relationship between pyridoxine and neuropathy has been demonstrated. It would appear that long-term administration of up to 200 milligrams daily may still be considered safe. *International Journal for Vitamin and Nutrition Research* 58 (1988): 105–118.

An extensive review article on pyridoxine and P5P. Some individuals have an enzymatic deficiency of inhibition of pyridoxal kinase making conversion of pyridoxine to P5P inefficient or inadequate. If a patient does not improve with B_6 supplementation, they may however improve with P5P supplementation such as in sideroblastic anemia, carpal tunnel syndrome, PMS, and homocysteinemia. *Alternative Medicine Review* 6(1) (2001): 87–92.

Chapter 15: Vitamin B$_{12}$ (Cobalamin)

Subclinical Anemia

Even slightly decreased B_{12} levels are often important even though the classic hematological hallmarks may be absent. Of patients with pernicious anemia, only 64 percent had very low B_{12} levels, suggesting the need to pay close attention to all low B_{12} levels. *Archives of Internal Medicine* 148 (August 1988): 1,712–1,714.

The Nervous System

The authors of this review recommend that the patient who fails to respond to treatment of any psychiatric symptom complex should be evaluated for B_{12} deficiency. *Biological Psychiatry* 16 (1981): 197–205.

Vitamin B_{12} and folate levels were analyzed in patients with major depression and psychotic depression. The authors confirm previous findings that low B_{12} is associated with mental disturbance. Low B_{12} levels may predispose the development of psychotic symptoms during a depressive episode. *British Journal of Psychiatry* 153 (August 1988): 266–267.

Dementia that is caused by vitamin B_{12} deficiency may not be accompanied by anemia if serum cobalamin levels are inadequate. Homocysteine and methylmalonic tests should be done to confirm cobalamin deficiency. Vitamin B_{12} deficiency can result in demyelination and cognitive changes. Elevated homocysteine levels have been associated with poor word recall in the elderly and, an increased risk of atherosclerosis, thrombosis, and stroke. Increased homocysteine levels increase the risk of silent brain infarction in the elderly and are associated with vascular dementia. *Neurology* 57(1 of 2) (2001): 1742.

Cardiovascular Effects

After a 6-week run-in period in which there were no lipid-lowering medications given, hyperlipidemic subjects participated in a randomized, double-blind, crossover trial. Subjects received either fenofibrate at 200 milligrams/day plus placebo or 200 milligrams of fenofibrate with 650 micrograms of folic acid, 50 micrograms of vitamin B_{12} and 5 milligrams of vitamin B_6. After the fenofibrate plus placebo therapy, there was a significant increase in homocysteine concentration by 44 percent. When fenofibrate was given with the vitamins, there was only a 13 percent increase. It may be that the increase in homocysteine from the fenofibrate treatment may counteract the cardioprotective effect of the lipid-lowering effects. This study recommends the routine use of folic acid, vitamin B_6 and vitamin B_{12} with fenofibrate therapy. *Atherosclerosis* 158 (2001): 161–164.

In this double-blind, placebo-controlled trial, treatment with a combination of folic acid, vitamin B_{12}, and pyridoxine significantly reduced homocysteine levels and decreased the rate of restenosis and the need for revascularization after coronary angioplasty. This inexpensive treatment, which has minimal side effects, should be considered as adjunctive therapy for patients undergoing coronary angioplasty. *New England Journal of Medicine* 345(22) (2001): 1593–1600.

Cancer Prevention

In this animal study, mice were implanted with tumor cells. Only 2 of the 50 that received B_{12} and ascorbic acid developed tumors, while all 50 of the untreated mice developed tumors. Vitamin B_{12} and vitamin C given separately in the same doses did not have the same effect. *IRCS Medical Science* 12 (September 1984): 813.

Smokers—especially smokers with precancerous changes in the bronchial tissues—were found to have low circulating levels of B_{12} and folate. Supplementation decreased the number of patients with atypical cells, suggesting that this may be an effective form of early intervention. *Journal of the American Medical Association* 259 (March 11, 1988): 1,525–1,530.

Chapter 16: Folic Acid

Cervical Dysplasia and Cancer

Oral contraceptives may cause localized rather than systemic folate deficiency, which could alter the susceptibility of cervical cells to cancer-causing substances. In this controlled study of oral contraceptive users with mild to moderate cervical dysplasia, those women supplemented with 10 milligrams of folic acid daily showed significant improvement over those who were unsupplemented. The authors concluded that localized changes in folate metabolism may be misdiagnosed as cervical dysplasia, or that these changes are an integral part of the condition and that dysplasia may be arrested or reversed with folic acid supplementation. *American Journal of Clinical Nutrition* 35 (1982): 73–82.

The author cites studies that suggest that folic acid supplementation may help reduce the risk of cervical cancer in women taking combination oral contraceptives. One study involved 89 women with mild to moderate cervical neoplasia who had been taking combination oral contraceptives for 6 months or longer. This double-blind random study concluded that folate (10 milligrams per day for 3 months) had a substantial beneficial effect on cervical epithelium. There was no change among the women in the placebo group. *Journal of the American Medical Association* 244:7 (1980): 633–634.

Pregnancy and Birth Defects

Mothers of children born with harelip received 10 milligrams of folic acid plus a multivitamin daily prior to or during the first trimester of their subsequent pregnancies. Only 1 of the supplemented mothers gave birth to another child with harelip; 15 of the unsupplemented group had children with this birth defect. The authors state that the results are highly suggestive that moderate supplementation may reduce the rate of recurrence of some birth defects. *Lancet* (July 24, 1982): 217.

In a randomized controlled trial, 2,104 women who received multivitamin supplementation with trace minerals were compared with 2,052 women who received trace element supplements only. The multivitamin supplement contained 12 nutrients, including .8 milligram of folic acid, 4 minerals, and 3 trace elements. The trace element supplement contained copper, manganese, zinc, and low-dose vitamin C. The group that received the multivitamin plus trace element supplements had a significant decrease in the incidence of infants born with neural tube defects. *New England Journal of Medicine* 327 (December 24, 1992): 1,832–1,835.

This is an editorial responding to the study cited above. The author notes that vitamin supplements containing both a multivitamin and trace elements supplement were used, so that one cannot be sure that the preventive effect was due to folic acid alone or to an association with other nutrients. *New England Journal of Medicine* 327 (December 24, 1992): 1,875–1,877.

This Irish study of more than 56,000 pregnant women demonstrated that the maternal levels of folic acid and B_{12} associated with neural tube defects were not those usually associated with deficiency. The authors note that since food fortification has been made to include both B_{12} and folic acid, the prevalence of neural tube defects has fallen from 4.7 to 1.3 per 1,000 individuals. *Quarterly Journal of Medicine* 87 (1993): 703–708.

Depression

In this review article, the authors point out that depression is a common manifestation of severe folate deficiency. Depressed patients with folate deficiency had more severe illness and responded less well to conventional antidepressant therapy than those without this deficiency. In addition, those in whom the deficiency was treated made better recoveries than those with untreated folate deficiency. *The Lancet II* (July 28, 1984): 196–198.

A consistent finding in major depression has been a low plasma and red cell folate, which has also been linked to poor response to antidepressants. The present investigation was designed to investigate whether the co-administration of folic acid would enhance the antidepressant action of fluoxetine. Patients were randomly assigned to receive either 500 micrograms of folic acid or an identical-looking placebo in addition to 20 milligrams fluoxetine daily. Overall, there was a significantly greater improvement in the fluoxetine plus folic acid group. The Hamilton Rating Scale score improved most significantly in women as did decreases in homocysteine levels. Folic acid is a simple method of greatly improving the antidepressant action of fluoxetine and probably other antidepressants. Folic acid should be given in doses sufficient to decrease plasma homocysteine. Men require a higher dose of folic acid to achieve this than women, but more work is required to ascertain the optimum dose of folic acid. *Journal of Affective Disorders* 60(2) (Nov 2000): 121–130.

Previous studies suggest that folate deficiency may occur in up to one-third of patients with severe depression, and that treatment with the vitamin may enhance recovery of the mental state. Total plasma homocysteine is a more sensitive measure of functional folate (and vitamin B_{12}) deficiency. This study analyzed the blood chemistries of patients with severe depression and compared it to controls. A biological subgroup of depression with folate deficiency, impaired methylation, and monoamine neurotransmitter metabolism has been identified. Detection of this subgroup, which will not be achieved by routine blood counts, is important in view of the potential benefit of vitamin replacement. *Journal of Neurology, Neurosurgery and Psychiatry* 69(2) (August 2000): 228–232.

Mental Retardation

Large doses of folic acid (2 milligrams three times a day) have been reported to improve the behavior of adults with a chromosomal abnormality linked with mental retardation. Female carriers of the syndrome, who are apt to be mildly retarded, might also benefit from folate supplementation. *American Journal of Medicine* 77 (October 1984): 602–611.

Cardiovascular Effects

A Boston University and Tufts University study of more than 1,000 older adults found that subjects with high blood levels of homocysteine were twice as likely to develop Alzheimer's disease as those with low or normal levels. An animal study conducted at the National Institute on Aging found feeding folic acid to mice with Alzheimer's-like damage to the brain cells were able to repair themselves. The mice fed the folate-deficient diet were not. *Alternative Medicine* (August 2000): 20.

Men who were hyperlipidemic, after a 6–week run-in period in which there were no lipid-lowering medications given, received either fenofibrate at 200 milligrams/day plus placebo or 200 milligrams of fenofibrate with 650 micrograms of folic acid, 50 micrograms of vitamin B_{12} and 5 milligrams of vitamin B_6. There was a 6-week treatment period, followed by an 8-week washout period, which was then followed by the second treatment for another 6 weeks. After the fenofibrate-plus-placebo therapy, there was a significant increase in homocysteine concentration by 44 percent. When fenofibrate was given with the vitamins, there was a 13 percent increase, which was significantly lower than without the vitamins. It may be that the increase in homocysteine from the fenofibrate treatment may counteract the cardioprotective effect of the lipid-lowering effects. These nutrients may help reduce most of the risk that occurs during fenofibrate therapy by minimizing the increase in homocysteine. This study recommends the routine use of folic acid, vitamin B_6, and vitamin B_{12} with fenofibrate therapy. *Atherosclerosis* 158 (2001): 161–164.

Male volunteers without elevated homocysteine levels received each of the following series of oral B vitamin supplements: Series 1 consisted of 1 milligram of folic acid, 10 milligrams of vitamin B_6 and 0.4 milligram of vitamin B_{12}; series 2 contained 5 milligrams of folic acid, 10 milligrams of vitamin B_6 and 0.4 milligram of vitamin B_{12}; and series 3 contained 5 milligrams of folic acid, 100 milligrams of vitamin B_6 and 0.4 milligram of vitamin B_{12}. In this third series, total homocysteine levels were significantly lowered, which did not happen in the second series. This study showed that the combined supplementation with vitamin B_6, folic acid, and vitamin B_{12} is superior to folic acid alone in lowering total homocysteine levels. In these studies, only the higher level of vitamin B_6 at 100 milligrams/day lowered total homocysteine levels, while the dose of folic acid was unaltered. There appears to be an interaction between vitamin B_6 and folic acid, which suggests that they should be given together to avoid depletion of one of them. It has been shown that supplementation of vitamin B_6 alone is associated with a reduction in serum folate levels. *Clinical Chemistry and Laboratory Medicine* 39(8) (2001): 768–771.

In this double-blind, placebo-controlled trial, treatment with a combination of folic acid, vitamin B_{12}, and pyridoxine significantly reduced homocysteine levels and decreased the rate of restenosis and the need for revascularization of the target lesion after coronary angioplasty. This inexpensive treatment, which has minimal side effects, should be considered as adjunctive therapy for patients undergoing coronary angioplasty. *New England Journal of Medicine* 345(22) (2001): 1593–1600.

The Immune System

This overview cites studies indicating that deficiencies of folic acid lead to a reduction in the resistance to disease in humans and animals. Both antibody and white cell production are affected. *American Journal of Clinical Nutrition* (Supplement) 35 (February 1982): 421.

Associations of plasma homocyteine (tHcy) with risk factors for cervical neoplasia (CIN) and 24–h intakes and biochemical indices of nutrients were examined in subjects with CIN and control subjects. Folate, vitamin B_{12}, copper, and severity of dysplasia are associated with tHcy. Folate supplementation significantly lowers tHcy even in folate-replete subjects. *Nutrition* 16(6) (2000): 411–416.

Researchers found that some women who have a defect in the gene encoding the enzyme methylenetetrhydrofolate (MTFHR) combined with a low folic acid intake have an increased risk of cervical cancer. Those exposed to human papilloma virus also have an increased risk of precancerous tissue, particularly in those women with an abnormal MTFHR. *Cancer Epidemiology Biomarkers & Prevention* 10(12) (2001): 1275–1280.

Impaired Absorption and Metabolism of Folic Acid

Anticonvulsants and sulfasalazine (prescribed for inflammatory bowel disease) may interfere with folate absorption. Gastric surgery and intestinal conditions can also interfere. There is some evidence that the physiological process of aging influences the intestinal absorption of folate. *American Journal of Clinical Nutrition* 36 (November 1982): 1,060–1,066.

In this study, blood levels of folate in a healthy woman fell by 29 percent when she received therapeutic doses of aspirin. (However, the authors point out that it is not known whether tissue stores were affected.) *Journal of Laboratory and Clinical Medicine* 103 (June 1984): 944–948.

Adverse Effects

Oral supplementation of folic acid lowers the plasma zinc levels and increases zinc excretion. Therefore, women with cervical dysplasia undergoing folic acid treatment may be particularly prone to zinc deficiency. This may be a hazard—especially in users of oral contraceptives, because this medication may also lower zinc levels. *Journal of the National Cancer Institute* 74 (January 1985): 263 (letter).

Chapter 17: Pantothenic Acid

Emotional and Physical Stress

Exercise

In this overview, the authors discuss why pantothenic acid has long been considered an antistress vitamin. They cite several studies of pantothenic supplementation, including: laboratory rats who showed a significant improvement in exercise tolerance and resistance to radiation-induced injury; humans who better withstood cold water stress; and the delay in the onset of fatigue. Human subjects consuming 10 grams of pantothenic acid per day significantly increased tolerance to cold water stress. Another study, testing a B-complex vitamin on exercise fatigue, concluded that 30 milligrams of pantothenic acid daily may act to delay the onset of fatigue. Only one study in the literature reported negative results with 20 milligrams per day. In the study conducted by the reviewers, 1 gram of pantothenic acid daily did enhance exercise endurance. *Journal of Sports Medicine* 24 (1984): 26–29.

The Nervous System

The authors point out that homopantothenic acid (HOPA), a naturally occurring substance, is now in widespread clinical use as a potent agent to improve epilepsy, postencephalitic sequelae, mental retardation, and mental and physical disorders in children. *Tohoku Journal of Experimental Medicine* 140 (1983): 45–51.

The Immune System

In human and animal studies, pantothenic acid deficiencies depress antibody responsiveness to antigens. *American Journal of Clinical Nutrition* (Supplement) 35 (February 1982): 421.

In this overview, the authors point out that lower blood levels of pantothenic acid are associated with arthritis. They cite studies showing that pantothenic acid supplements have helped alleviate symptoms of this disease, and urge that further trials are indicated. *The Practitioner* 224 (February 1980): 208–211.

In this study, 30 out of 37 patients with chronic discoid lupus improved with massive doses of pantothenic acid (6 to 10 grams), followed by lower maintenance levels of 2 to 4 grams per day. *Journal of Investigative Dermatology* 15 (1950): 291.

Cardiovascular Disease

In this study, 24 patients with Types IIA, IIB, or IV hyperlipidemia received pantethine in doses of 300 milligrams, 3 times daily. After 1 year, there was a significant decrease in serum cholesterol and triglyceride levels. *Clinical Therapies* 8 (1986): 537.

Pantethine was as effective as fenofibrate in lowering total and LDL cholesterol without the side effects of fenofibrate in hypercholesterolemic patients. These results suggest it is the therapy of choice for hypercholesterolemia. *Current Therapeutic Research* 38 (1985): 386–395.

Supplementation of pantethine resulted in normal serum values in 83 percent of hypercholesterolemic patients and 35.7 percent of hypertriglyceridemic patients. *Current Therapeutic Research* 34 (1983): 383–390.

Supplementation with pantethine in doses of 300 milligrams, 4 times daily, in hyperlipidemic patients demonstrated inhibition of platelet aggregation and thromboxane production. *Current Therapeutic Research* 35 (1984): 700.

Chapter 18: Biotin

Those with abnormal microflora (bacterial overgrowth) or "leaky gut syndrome," where micronutrient absorption is compromised, such as in autoimmune diseases, skin diseases, ulcerative colitis, cancer, and irritable bowel syndrome, may be at risk for inadequate biotin nutrition. Biotin deficiency is a potent teratogen in some animals and there is evidence of marginal, asymptomatic biotin deficiency as a common occurrence in human pregnancy. Inadequate biotin nutrition may be more common than we think. *American Journal of Clinical Nutrition* 75 (2002): 179–180.

The Nervous System

In this study, 8 patients experienced marked improvement in their hemodialysis-related neurologic disorders with daily supplementation of 10 milligrams of biotin. The authors conclude that biotin supplementation is effective in preventing and treating the neurological disorders that can result from chronic hemodialysis. They recommend that biotin therapy be started in patients with advanced renal failure before severe symptoms appear. *Nephron* 36 (1984): 183–186.

Dermatitis

Treatment of the mothers of breast-fed infants with seborrheic dermatitis by injection of pharmacologic doses of biotin has been reported to have beneficial effects. *Nutrition in Health and Disease*, 6th ed. (Philadelphia: Lea and Febiger, 1980), 274–279.

Chapter 19: Choline, Inositol, and PABA

Cardiovascular Disease

Atherosclerosis

In this study, 9 men and 9 women with high triglycerides and cholesterol were given lecithin. Triglycerides, cholesterol, and platelet aggregation were all significantly decreased, and HDL cholesterol was increased. The authors conclude that lecithin may be a useful adjunct in the treatment of atherosclerosis. *Biochemical and Medical Metabolism and Biology* (January–February 1986): 31–39.

Cholesterol Levels

This study reports on over 153 patients with hyperlipidemia treated with inositol hexaniacinate at dosages from 600 to 1,800 milligrams per deciliter without reports of side effects or adverse reactions. The researchers concluded that inositol hexaniacinate is superior to nicotinic acid as an oral therapeutic agent. *International Record of Medicine* 174 (1961): 9–15. See also *Nutrition Reports International* 28 (1983): 899–911 and *British Journal of Clinical Practice* 42 (1988): 719–722.

In 10 Alzheimer's patients, extremely high doses of lecithin (35 grams daily) significantly lowered total cholesterol and LDL cholesterol and raised HDL cholesterol after 2 to 3 months in a double-blind crossover study. *American Journal of Psychiatry* 139 (1982): 1,633–1,634.

Neurotransmitters

The rates at which neurons synthesize neurotransmitters such as serotonin, acetylcholine, and the catecholamines—norepinephrine and dopamine—depend on the availability of the precursors: tryptophan, choline, and tyrosine, respectively. The concentrations of precursors in the circulation and in neurons change rapidly after food consumption, depending upon what is eaten. Nutrient intake normally influences the synthesis of these neurotransmitters. These neurotransmitters participate in the control of a number of bodily functions and behaviors, such as hunger, food choice, sleep, alertness, sensitivity to environmental stimuli, and disease states. Dietary manipulations—or the consumption of individual nutrients—can thus be used as adjunctive tools in the treatment of some diseases of these neurons. *Journal of Neural Transmitters* 15 (1979): S69–S79.

Learning Disabilities

This article reviews 2 case reports of young children with multiple neurodevelopmental delays. Both were followed from age 4 to age 8. At age 4, one child was given 2,400 milligrams of choline as a thick oil form of lecithin with noted results. Treatment was not continued. At age 5, treatment was resumed, first with 500 milligrams of choline, and then with an increased dose of 3,000 milligrams twice a day. Significant improvement was seen. He was also given fish oil for treatment of Raynaud's disease. The other child was also treated with choline. At age 4, the dose was 500 milligrams. This was increased to 1,000 milligrams over time. There was significant improvement. *Journal of the American College of Nutrition* 12 (1993): 239–245.

Chapter 20: Vitamin C (Ascorbic Acid)

Antioxidant Powers

In a study of 100 elderly people, in those who were supplemented with 400 milligrams of vitamin C and/or 200 milligrams of vitamin E, serum lipid peroxides declined to as little as 74 percent of initial levels after one year. The authors conclude that long-term supplementation of moderate amounts of these nutrients presumably protects against free radical damage, which may play a role in aging and the development of degenerative diseases. *Annals of Nutrition and Metabolism* 28 (May–June 1984): 186–191.

In studying nonsmoking men, individuals limited their fruit and vegetable intake to ≤3 servings/day and consumed a multivitamin and mineral supplement daily. Subjects consumed vitamin C starting at 250 milligrams at weeks 3 to 4 and increasing to 500 milligrams, 1,000 milligrams and 2,000 milligrams at weeks 5 to 6, 7 to 8 and 9 to 10, respectively, and other subjects consumed a placebo tablet. Plasma vitamin C levels rose 55 percent in vitamin C–supplemented subjects by the end of the tenth week of treatment, and measures of oxidative stress decreased by 60 to 90 percent. There were significant reductions in indicators of oxidative stress at the 500-milligram, 1,000-milligram and 2,000-milligram doses versus placebo. The antioxidant protection was similar at the 1,000-milligram and 2,000-milligram dose. *Journal of the American College of Nutrition* 20(6) (2001): 623–627.

Stress

Forty-five participants in the 1999 Comrades 90-kilometer marathon were divided into 3 equal groups. Group 1 received 500 milligrams of vitamin C daily, group 2 received 1,500 milligrams of vitamin C daily, and group 3 received a placebo for 7 days before the race and for 2 days following completion. The study demonstrated that the group receiving the 1,500 milligrams of vitamin C daily had an attenuation of the adrenal stress hormone and anti-inflammatory polypeptide response to prolonged exercise compared to the lower dose of vitamin C or the placebo. Adrenaline levels and cortisol levels were significantly lower in the 1,500-milligram–vitamin C group compared with the other 2 groups, demonstrating an attenuation of the stress response and perhaps less inflammation due to the prolonged exercise. *International Journal of Sports Medicine* 22(7) (2001): 537–543.

One thousand milligrams of vitamin C or a placebo was given to subjects 3 times daily and then they underwent stressful testing. Study results showed beneficial effects for people receiving the vitamin C under stress compared to placebo. The findings indicate that individuals with high blood levels of ascorbic acid exhibit fewer physical and mental signs of stress when subjected to acute psychological stressors than do subjects with lower levels of vitamin C. They recovered from a stressful situation faster and cortisol levels and blood pressure were lower in the vitamin C group only. Since high-dose vitamin C supplements were used, the researchers caution, ". . . this is different vitamin C than you get from oranges, or even the general powder forms . . . I'm not sure you would get the same results from natural vitamin C." *Psychopharmacology* 159 (2002): 319–324.

The Immune System

Vitamin C has been shown to reduce symptoms experienced by asthmatics challenged with histamine or methacholine. Vitamin C significantly reduced airway reactivity to methacholine aerosol. *American Review of Respiratory Disease* 127 (February 1983): 143–147.

Vitamin C levels in serum and body tissues lower with age. Vitamin C enhanced the immune responsiveness in subjects who received doses of 500 milligrams. The authors conclude that vitamin C should be considered as a possibly successful nontoxic and inexpensive substance that may have some application in improving immune competence of the aging. *Gerontology* 29 (1983): 305–310.

This article reviews the 21 placebo-controlled trials that have been conducted since 1971 to evaluate vitamin C's effect on the common cold. Doses ranged from 1 to 4 grams per day, and in each of the studies, vitamin C reduced the duration of the cold and the severity of its symptoms by an average of 23 percent. The author concludes that it is reasonable to use vitamin C during a cold. *Scandinavian Journal of Infectious Diseases* 26 (1994): 1–6.

In this trial of 3 matched groups of 46 subjects, 1 group of marathon runners took 600 milligrams of vitamin C daily 21 days before a marathon, a sedentary control group also took vitamin C, and another group of runners took a placebo. The results suggest that vitamin C supplementation may enhance resistance to post-race upper respiratory infection, and that it may reduce the severity of infection in sedentary people. *American Journal Clinical Nutrition* 57 (1993): 170–174.

Life Span

This study showed that men who consumed 300 milligrams of vitamin C daily, through food and supplements, had a 40 percent lower death rate from heart disease and other causes than did those whose intake was less than 50 milligrams. *Epidemiology* 3 (1992): 194–202.

Tissue Repair and Wound Healing

In this review article, the authors conclude that clinical studies provide evidence that wound healing in subjects judged not deficient in vitamin C can be significantly accelerated with supplements in daily dosages of 500 to 3,000 milligrams. The subjects of the studies reviewed included those recovering from surgery and other injuries, pressure sores, and leg ulcers. *Oral Surgery* (March 1982): 231–236.

Cancer

In this famous study by Cameron and Pauling, 100 advanced cancer patients who received large supplemental doses of ascorbic acid lived from 4.2 to 20 times longer than the controls. The authors conclude that ascorbic acid is of definite value in the treatment of patients with advanced cancer. *Proceedings of the National Academy of Sciences* 73:10 (October 1976): 3,685–3,689.

In this follow-up study by Hoffer and Pauling, high-dose vitamin C (12 grams per day) was given with other nutrients to 101 cancer patients, and the results were compared with 31 cancer patients who did not receive supplements. Among the 80 percent of "good responders" in the supplemented group, the mean survival time was 122 months for patients with cancer of the breast, uterus, ovaries, and cervix, and 72 months for those with other types of cancer. By way of contrast, the mean survival time was only 5.7 months for patients who did not receive supplements. *Journal of Orthomolecular Medicine* 5 (1990) 3: 143–154.

In a controlled study, high levels of vitamin C reduced the risk of cervical cancer by 60 percent. *Journal of the National Cancer Institute* 80 (June 15, 1988): 580–585.

A statistically significant inverse relationship was found between the risk of skin cancer and a high intake of fish, vegetables, cruciferous vegetables, beta-carotene, and vitamin C-containing foods. *Nutrition and Cancer* 18 (1992): 237–244.

In an animal model, it was found that infusion of ascorbic acid before radiation therapy significantly protected healthy tissue against fatal radiation syndrome and the destruction of skin layers. The researchers discovered that much more radiation was required to produce the ill effects of radiation in the ascorbic acid-treated animals. The ascorbic acid did not protect the tumor or interfere with the radiation therapy in an adverse way. Extrapolating this to a human model, one might suggest that high-dose vitamin C therapy prior to radiation treatment might allow for the dose to be increased with an expected increase in tumor response, without increasing complications. *American Journal of Clinical Nutrition* 54 (1991): S1281–S1283.

Researchers developed a topical vitamin C solution that protects the skin against UV light exposure. It can deliver 20 times the amount of vitamin C normally found in skin, and it cannot be washed off. It is protective for as long as 3 days, and it is effective against UV-A and UV-B oxidative damage. The researchers note that if vitamin C levels are enhanced in the skin, premature aging, wrinkles, and even skin cancer may be prevented. *Journal of the National Cancer Institute* 83 (1991): 847–850.

In a trial of subjects with colon polyps, 19 received ascorbic acid at 3 grams daily, and 17 received placebo. In the vitamin C group compared with the placebo group, there was a reduction in polyp area at 9 months of follow-up, and there was a trend toward reduction in both number and area of rectal polyps during the middle of the trial. These data suggest that vitamin C temporarily influenced polyp growth or turnover. *Cancer* 50 (1982): 1434–1439.

Vitamin C's role in the prevention of disease and malignancy has been studied over the last several decades. Vitamin C intake has been shown to have an inverse relationship with gastric cancer. Recent follow-up studies on high-risk populations suggest that ascorbic acid, the reduced form of vitamin C, protects against gastric cancer, for which H. pylori is a significant risk factor. In populations infected with H. pylori, there is a reduction in gastric juice ascorbic acid concentration. This article reviews the risk factors for gastric cancer and the role of vitamin C in prevention of the disease. *Nutrition Reviews* 60(1) (2002): 34–36.

Cardiovascular Disease

In this review article, the author discusses studies of the beneficial effects of vitamin C on veins and arteries. In one study, the deep vein thrombosis rate was lowered by 50 percent in surgical patients given 1,000 milligrams of vitamin C daily. In another clinical trial, atherosclerotic patients given vitamin C could walk farther without feeling pain or breathlessness. Vitamin C may help to prevent cholesterol deposits by preventing and repairing damaged arterial walls and moving cholesterol away from the arterial wall to the liver. The author suggests that atherosclerosis is a long-term deficiency of vitamin C. *American Heart Journal* 88:3 (1974): 387–388.

High intakes of vitamin C or fruits and of green vegetables that are high in vitamin C have been related to lowered mortality from stroke and heart disease. The author suggests that ascorbic acid has a preventive effect on hypertension. *International Journal for Vitamin and Nutrition Research* 54 (1984): 343–347.

Two studies show that when people with high cholesterol were given 300 to 1,000 milligrams of vitamin C daily, their cholesterol levels dropped. *Lancet* (October 20, 1984): 907.

Correlations between serum HDL cholesterol and vitamin C intake were positive and significant in women. In men, high levels of HDLs seem to be associated with very high vitamin C intakes. If an adequate supply of vitamin C is necessary for the maintenance of optimal HDL levels, then perhaps the requirements of men are substantially higher than those of women. *American Journal of Clinical Nutrition* 40 (December 1984): 1,334–1,338.

Lipoprotein(a) is an independent risk factor for coronary heart disease. In 1989, Drs. Rath and Pauling discovered that lipoprotein(a) is a surrogate for vitamin C, and that optimal vitamin C intake prevents the deposition of lipoprotein(a) in the vascular wall. Linus Pauling Institute for Science and Medicine Newsletter (March 1992): 2.

In studying men and women it was found that after adjusting for variables, a 20 percent higher plasma vitamin C level and 20 percent higher beta-carotene levels were associated with significantly smaller intima-media thickness in men. Compared with men with high blood concentrations of beta-carotene or cholesterol-adjusted vitamin E, those with low blood concentrations of these vitamins were 2.5 times as likely to have carotid stenosis of >30 percent. *American Journal of Clinical Nutrition* 74 (2001): 402–408.

HIV Infection and AIDS

This study reviews the synergistic effects of NAC and vitamin C on HIV suppression. NAC caused approximately a 2-fold inhibition of HIV reverse transcriptase activity and had a synergistic effect when tested simultaneously with ascorbic acid. The continuous presence of ascorbic acid was necessary for HIV suppression. These results support the potent antiviral effects of ascorbic acid and suggest its synergistic effect with compounds such as NAC. *American Journal of Clinical Nutrition* 54 (1991): S1231–S1235.

An evaluation of the micronutrient intake of 108 HIV-positive patients found that the highest levels of total intake of vitamin C, B_1, and niacin were associated with a significant decreased progression rate to AIDS. *American Journal of Epidemiology* 138 (1993): 937–951.

Taking vitamin C to bowel tolerance (40 to 100 grams daily) is reported to put AIDS into extended clinical remission. The author recommends that all at risk for AIDS take vitamin C to bowel tolerance. *Mental Hypothesis* 14 (August 1984): 423–433.

Smoking

This study revealed that smokers have lower bloodstream levels of vitamin C than do nonsmokers. Two to four times as many smokers as nonsmokers had vitamin C deficiencies in the near-scurvy range. Smokers have a special need for vitamin C, and a normal dietary intake may not adequately keep their vitamin C level within a normal range. *Federation Proceedings* 43 (1984): 861.

Eye Disorders

In a study of almost 5,000 people funded in part by the National Eye Institute, a mixture of 500 milligrams of vitamin C, 400 international units of vitamin E, and 15 milligrams of beta-carotene reduced the risk of vision loss by 10 percent. A mixture of 80 milligrams of zinc and 2 milligrams of copper reduced the risk by 11 percent. *Nutrition Week* 31 (40) (2001): 7.

Dementia and Alzheimer's Disease

After a mean follow-up of 6 years of 5,395 participants, 197 subjects developed dementia, of which 146 had Alzheimer's disease. After adjusting certain variables, high intake of vitamin C and vitamin E was associated with a lower risk of Alzheimer's disease. Among current smokers, this relationship was most and also present for intake of beta-carotene and flavonoids. The possible contribution of free-radical damage to the etiology of Alzheimer's disease has been discussed in the literature for years. This trial suggests that higher intakes of vitamin C and vitamin E from food are associated with a decreased risk of Alzheimer's disease. *Journal of the American Medical Association* 287 (2002): 3223–3229.

Other Uses

Pregnancy Complications

In a study of 87 pregnant women, 74 percent of those with abruptio placentae had significantly lower blood levels of vitamin C than did those without this complication. The authors concluded that a deficiency of vitamin C could result in symptoms observed in this complication of pregnancy. *Human Nutrition and Clinical Nutrition* 39C (May–June 1985): 233–238.

Male Infertility

Infertile men with lowered sperm counts were given 1,000 milligrams of vitamin C daily. Throughout the several weeks of the study, there was a continuous rise in the percentage of normal sperm, sperm viability, and sperm motility. *Journal of the American Medical Association* 249 (May 27, 1983): 2,747–2,748.

Schizophrenia

This article reviews several clinical studies in which ascorbic acid supplementation improved symptoms in schizophrenic patients. One gram per day of ascorbic acid supplementation significantly improved depressive, manic, and paranoid symptoms; 8 grams per day improved 10 out of 13 patients on stable neuroleptic regimens; 2 grams of ascorbic acid plus haloperidol was more beneficial than haloperidol alone; 2 to 6 grams per day improved patients on medications while 1 patient achieved full remission within one week. *The Nutrition Report* 8 (September 1990): 65, 72.

The Elderly

Vitamin C therapy of 1,000 milligrams per day given to institutionalized elderly led to an improvement of their nutritional status and a reduction in petechial hemorrhages (pin-sized red dots under the skin). *American Journal of Clinical Nutrition* 34 (1981): 871–876.

Hospital Patients

The vitamin C levels of 199 elderly hospital patients were measured upon admission. Those with low vitamin C levels had a mortality rate of 45 percent during the study, but only 27 percent of those with higher vitamin C levels died, although the severity of illness was the same in both groups. In addition, half were given 200 milligrams of vitamin C daily; half were given a placebo. Those with low initial levels of vitamin C who received the supplement tended to improve more than did those given the placebo. The authors conclude that supplementation of patients who have low vitamin C levels may improve their prognosis. *International Journal for Vitamin and Nutrition Research* 54 (January–March 1984): 65–74.

Lung Protection
In this study of 2,526 adults, those with a higher intake of vitamin C had better lung function. The authors conclude that vitamin C protects the lungs. This effect was not limited to smokers, but was more evident in asthmatic and bronchitis patients. *American Journal of Clinical Nutrition* 59 (1994): 110–114.

Optimum Vitamin C Intake
The author arrived at an estimated body pool of vitamin C of 5,000 milligrams for a 70-kilogram person. An intake of 200 milligrams daily would maintain this level. This refers to people who are free from stress. Individuals who have high levels of physical activity or who experience strain from pregnancy, mental stress, diabetes, injury, infection, cancer, atherosclerosis, pollution, or medications may require much higher dosages. *Nutrition and Health* 1 (1981): 66–77.

Human beings are genetically programmed to consume the diet that was available to our ancient hunter-gatherer ancestors, who evolved 40,000 years ago. The authors estimate that these people consumed a diet containing almost 400 milligrams of vitamin C each day. *New England Journal of Medicine* 312 (January 31, 1985): 283–289.

In a study of adolescent boys, the group that was given 70 milligrams of vitamin C daily improved their aerobic work capacity by 10 percent. The authors conclude that the optimal intake of vitamin C is 80 to 100 milligrams a day. *International Journal for Vitamin and Nutrition Research* 54 (January–March 1984): 55–60.

Rats maintain a vitamin C body pool that is 5 times greater than the pool calculated for humans. *Journal of Biological Chemistry* 230 (1958): 923.

The author reviews data concerning the synthesis of vitamin C in animals and the ingestion of vitamin C in nonvitamin C–producing animals, both under normal conditions and under stress. He concludes that this data suggests that the optimum daily intake of vitamin C for humans is between 250 and 4,000 milligrams. *Proceedings of the National Academy of Sciences* 71:11 (1974): 4,442–4,446.

The author notes that most animals produce their own vitamin C at the rate of up to 275 milligrams per kilogram daily, and that this is much higher than the RDA for humans, which is .9 milligram per kilogram. In animals that must obtain vitamin C from the diet, about 10 times this amount, necessary to prevent scurvy, was needed to maintain health, and up to 40 milligrams per kilogram was needed to survive the stresses of long-term captivity. Research suggests that the amount of vitamin C necessary to prevent scurvy is less than that required for maximal enzyme activity. *New England Journal of Medicine* 314 (April 3, 1986): 892–902.

An in-hospital depletion-repletion study was conducted on 7 healthy volunteers for a period of 4 to 6 months. Participants consumed a diet containing under 5 milligrams of vitamin C daily. The authors looked at bioavailability, plasma saturation, and neutrophil, monocyte, and lymphocyte saturation of varying amounts of vitamin C. Based on the data from this study, the researchers conclude that the RDA of 60 milligrams should be increased to 200 milligrams. *Proceedings of the National Academy of Science* 93 (1996): 3,704–3,709.

This study compared the vitamin C content of reconstituted frozen orange juice to that of ready-to-drink orange juices purchased 4 to 5 weeks before their expiration date. The orange juices from frozen concentrates contained 86 milligrams of reduced vitamin C per fluid cup at the first evaluation and 39 to 46 milligrams per cup after 4 weeks of storage. The ready-to-drink juices averaged significantly lower reduced vitamin C at 27 to 65 milligrams per cup upon the first evaluation and 0 to 25 milligrams per cup at expiration 4 weeks later. The ready-to-drink orange juice had two- to three-fold higher concentrations of oxidized vitamin C versus the orange juices reconstituted from frozen. The decompensation rate of reduced vitamin C was similar for all juices at 2 percent per day once the orange juice was opened. This study showed that ready-to-drink orange juice should be purchased 3 to 4 weeks prior to the expiration date and consumed within 1 week of opening. *Journal of the American Dietetic Association* 102(4) (2002): 525–529.

Toxicity and Adverse Effects
Based on 2 studies in which adults were supplemented with 3,000 to 10,000 milligrams of vitamin C daily, the authors conclude that the probability of oxalate stone formation due to ingestion of vitamin C is very small. *International Journal for Vitamin and Nutrition Research* 54 (April–September 1984): 245–249.

Previous studies have suggested that high doses of vitamin C destroy B_{12} in the body. More recent studies, using superior techniques, have shown no significant evidence of destruction of B_{12} body stores with up to 2,000 milligrams of vitamin C. *Scottish Medical Journal* 27 (1982): 240–243.

The authors reviewed human and animal studies and found that the few case reports of possible rebound scurvy are anecdotal and not well-founded. They conclude that there is no basis for the belief that high-dose vitamin C consumption leads to rebound scurvy in humans. *Nutrition Research* 8 (1988): 1,327–1,332.

When comparing kits used by physicians to determine oxalate levels in the urine, the authors of this study found that ascorbic acid interferes with those kits using oxidase, but less so with those using decarboxylase. *Clinical Biochemistry* 26(2) (April 1993): 93–96.

Chapter 21: Calcium
Overview
This article discusses those who may be at risk for inadequate calcium intake from poor diet, problems with absorption and utilization such as age, physical activity, estrogen deficiency, phosphorus-calcium balance, and diets high in protein, fat, and fiber. It is suggested that calcium balance can be maintained either by estrogen replacement therapy or by increased calcium intake. *American Journal of Clinical Nutrition* 36 (November 1982): 986–1013.

Cardiovascular Effects
The postmenopausal women in the trial, all of whom had not regularly used estrogens for the year prior to the start of the study, consumed 910 milligrams of dietary calcium on average at the beginning of the study. They were then assigned to take 1,000 milligrams of calcium (as calcium citrate) or a placebo, as two 200 milligram tablets before breakfast and then three 200 milligram tablets in the evening. By the end of a year, the women supplementing with calcium citrate showed a significant—7 percent—increase in HDL. This magnitude of increase parallels that seen with statin drugs, and is associated with a 20 to 30 percent reduction in cardiovascular events. LDL cholesterol dropped by 6 percent in the same women. No significant changes occurred in those receiving the placebo. *American Journal of Medicine* 112(5) (2002): 343–347.

This review article discusses various epidemiological and clinical studies correlating high calcium intakes with low blood pressure in men and in pregnant and nonpregnant women. For example, in one clinical trial, 1,000 milligrams of calcium given daily to hypertensives produced a 48 percent reduction in systolic blood pressure. *Nutrition Reviews* 42:6 (1984): 205–213.

In a controlled, double-blind, randomized study, 48 hypertensives were given 1,000 milligrams of calcium per day for 8 weeks. Of these, 21 (44 percent) achieved a therapeutically meaningful reduction in their blood pressure. Of the responders, 14 had previously required therapy with antihypertensive drugs to achieve similar results. Oral calcium therapy was remarkably well tolerated. *Annals of Intestinal Medicine* 103:6 (1985): 825–831.

During a 4-year controlled study of 81 women, half of them were given 1,500 milligrams of calcium per day. Of the hypertensive women, those who took the supplement experienced a significant reduction in systolic blood pressure. In the unsupplemented women, systolic blood pressure continued to rise, even though they were given hypertensive medication. *American Journal of Clinical Nutrition* 42 (July 1985): 12–17.

In this study, the diets of over 10,000 adults were examined. Of the 17 nutrients examined, low calcium was most consistently associated with high blood pressure. Intakes of potassium, sodium, and vitamins A and C were also lower in people with higher blood pressure, while cholesterol intake was not consistently different. The authors concluded that diets that restrict the intake of calories, sodium, or cholesterol may also reduce the intake of calcium and other nutrients that may be protective against hypertension. *Science* 224 (June 29, 1984): 1,392–1,398.

In this study, 12 normal men consumed a high-salt diet (6.6 grams per day) for 2 weeks. They experienced an increase in excretion of calcium and phosphorus. Those who consumed a low-calcium diet also excreted more phosphorus. Men with the higher calcium intake had lower blood pressure. The authors suggest that sodium intake may influence blood pressure through its effects on calcium and potassium excretion, and that these effects may be more pronounced in people with low calcium intake. *American Journal of Clinical Nutrition* 41 (January 1985): 52–60.

Oral calcium supplementation can lower blood pressure in hypertensive individuals. It appears that salt-sensitive hypertensives may benefit the most. *Journal of Nutrition* 117 (1987): 1,806–1,808.

Cancer

This article reviews several studies of the relationship between vitamin D, calcium, and colon cancer. The incidence of colon cancer in Scandinavian countries was correlated with the intake of milk. In Southern California, where there is high exposure to sunlight and milk is fortified with vitamin D, an association was found between high milk consumption and a lowered risk of colon cancer. Yogurt has been shown to explicitly convey colonic bacterial flora that inhibits the effects of known colonic carcinogens. *Nutrition Reviews* 43:6 (1985): 170–172.

Researchers examined the cells lining the colons of 10 patients with family histories of colon cancer, and found that they had a proliferation pattern characteristic of high-risk individuals. After supplementation with calcium, the cells were less proliferative and were almost the same as those in people at low risk for colon cancer. *New England Journal of Medicine* 313 (1985): 1,381–1,384.

A group of nearly 2,000 men was followed for 19 years. Those who developed colorectal cancer were found to have consumed significantly less calcium and vitamin D than those who did not. Men with the lowest intake had 2.7 times the risk of those with the highest intake. The authors concluded that both vitamin D and calcium may have anticancer activity. *Lancet* (February 9, 1985): 307–309.

A study that evaluated 2,591 Dutch adults, ages 40 to 65, found that women with the lowest calcium intake had an increased risk of gastrointestinal cancer. Both men and women with a lower-than-average intake of calcium had a higher risk of colorectal mortality. *International Journal of Cancer* 54 (1993): 20–25.

Osteoporosis

Women of all ages should be encouraged to maintain a daily calcium intake of 1,000 to 1,500 milligrams and to participate in weight-bearing exercise for 30 minutes 3 times weekly to reduce their risk of falls and fractures. Persons at risk should avoid medications known to compromise bone density such as glucorticoids, thyroid hormones, and chronic heparin therapy. *American Family Physician* 63(6) (2001): 1121–1128.

Calcium supplements of 1,000 milligrams per day were given to 14 postmenopausal women. The results of this study led the authors to conclude that calcium therapy, which has no serious side effects, decreases bone resorption in cases of postmenopausal osteoporosis. Previous studies have shown that 1,000 to 2,500 milligrams of calcium per day reduce the incidence of vertebral fracture by 50 percent, and that 1,000 milligrams of calcium daily protect healthy menopausal women against osteoporosis. *American Journal of Clinical Nutrition* 39 (June 1984): 857–859.

In a study of 26 healthy women ages 47 to 66, bone density increased with calcium supplementation with or without estrogen therapy. *New York State Journal of Medicine* 75 (1975): 326–336.

The author of this article suggests that the only rational approach to osteoporosis is prevention. Current data indicates that osteoporotic patients consume less calcium, require more dietary calcium to achieve calcium balance, lose more bone mass per day, and have lower vitamin D hormone levels than do controls. According to one study, postmenopausal women with osteoporosis require 1,500 milligrams per day of calcium to attain calcium balance, compared with 1,000 milligrams in premenopausal controls. *Nutrition Reviews* 41:3 (1983): 83–85.

Calcium intake was found to be lower in both men and women with subsequent hip fracture than in those without hip fracture. A daily intake of over 765 milligrams of calcium was associated with a 60 percent reduction in the risk of hip fracture. *Lancet* (November 5, 1988): 1,046–1,049.

The authors conclude that within 10 years of menopause, in normal postmenopausal women whose calcium intake is below 1,000 milligrams, increasing intake to 1,400 milligrams reduces the rate of bone loss. *Journal of Clinical Nutrition* 117 (1987): 1,929–1,935.

This article reviews the role of calcium supplementation in the treatment of bone loss in postmenopausal women. It points out that calcium supplementation results in a significant slowing of bone loss, with no side effects, at a cost similar to that of some forms of hormone replacement therapy. *Pharmacoeconomics* 5 (1994): 1–4.

This article reviews the importance of copper, manganese, and zinc supplementation, in addition to calcium, for increasing mineral density in postmenopausal women. In a 2-year double-blind placebo-controlled trial including 200 postmenopausal women, the group taking calcium had no significant bone loss, but the group taking 1,000 milligrams of calcium, 15 milligrams of zinc, 2.5 milligrams of copper, and 5 milligrams of manganese experienced an *increase* in bone density. *Journal of the American College of Nutrition* 12 (1993): 384–389.

In this study of 3,000 elderly females, half were given 1,200 milligrams of calcium plus 800 international units of vitamin D, and half were given a placebo. The supplemented group had a 30 percent lower incidence of nonvertebral fractures and a 41 percent lower incidence of hip fractures compared with the placebo group. *Nutrition Reviews* 51 (1993): 183–185.

A study of 118 women who had recently gone through menopause showed that calcium supplementation alone was less effective than estrogen, progesterone, and calcium given together. However, calcium alone still resulted in a significant slowing of bone loss, and the authors believe that calcium supplementation should be encouraged to help prevent bone loss during the early part of menopause. *Annals of Internal Medicine* 120 (January 15, 1994): 97–103.

This double-blind, placebo-controlled trial included 137 women age 65 or older. Some subjects were supplemented with 1,000 milligrams a day of calcium citrate malate, or with the same amount of calcium plus 2.5 milligrams of copper, 5 milligrams of manganese, and 1.25 milligrams of zinc. In the placebo group, spinal bone density decreased after 2 years. The women who took the calcium with trace minerals experienced an increase in spinal bone density. *Geriatrics* 46 (July 1991): 67.

Calcium Intake and Absorption

Anthropologically speaking, humans were high consumers of calcium until the onset of the Agricultural Age, 10,000 years ago. Current calcium intake is one-quarter to one-third that of our evolutionary diet and, if we are genetically identical to the late Paleolithic Homo sapiens, we may be consuming a calcium-deficient diet our bodies cannot adjust to by physiologic mechanisms. Meta-analyses of calcium and bone mass studies demonstrate supplementation of 500 to 1,500 milligrams of calcium daily improves bone mass in adolescents, young adults, older men, and postmenopausal women. Calcium citrate malate has high bioavailability and thus has been the subject of calcium studies in these populations. The addition of trace minerals and vitamin D in separate trials has improved the effect of calcium citrate malate on bone density and shown a reduction of fracture risk. *Alternative Medicine Review* 4(2) (1999): 74–85.

In an article that considers the nature and current implications of Paleolithic nutrition, the authors determine that our early ancestors consumed approximately 1,600 milligrams of calcium per day. *New England Journal of Medicine* 312:5 (1985): 283–289.

In this article, the author reviews factors that influence calcium intake and absorption, and may therefore contribute to the development of osteoporosis. These include age; high phosphorus intake; and the use of drugs such as glucocorticoids (steroids), diuretics, tetracycline, and aluminum-containing antacids. Depending on age, two-thirds to three-fourths of U.S. females ingest less than the RDA; fully one-fourth ingest less than 300 milligrams. The author notes that a large percentage of patients with osteoporosis had a calcium imbalance with a calcium intake of 800 milligrams per day, and concluded that the RDA of 800 milligrams cannot be sufficient for the entire population. *American Journal of Clinical Nutrition* 36 (October 1982): 776–787.

Absorption of calcium is normally only 20 to 40 percent of intake. A vegetarian diet contains acids that may bind 360 milligrams of calcium per day. However, over 80 percent of these acids are fermented in the intestine so that much of the calcium may be released and become available for absorption. *American Journal of Clinical Nutrition* 35 (April 1982): 783–808.

Calcium absorption may be impaired in postmenopausal women owing to inadequate stomach acid. In this population, calcium citrate is better absorbed (45 percent) than calcium carbonate (5 percent) on an empty stomach. If taken with food, calcium carbonate absorption is essentially the same as it is in normal people (it's over 20 percent). *New England Journal of Medicine* 313 (July 11, 1985): 70–73.

Calcium malabsorption was discovered and correlated with rheumatoid arthritis activity in 20 women with this disease. Osteoporosis may result. *Annals of Rheumatoid Disease* 44 (September 1985): 585–588.

In this study, a group of women who were given 700 to 800 milligrams of calcium plus 375 international units of vitamin D experienced an increase in bone density. The other group of women took a balanced supplement consisting of calcium, vitamin D, and the RDA of 15 other vitamins and minerals. The latter group experienced a 2 to 3 times greater increase in bone density than the former group. *Nutrition Reports International* 31 (March 1985): 741–755.

Antacids as a Source of Calcium

Adverse effects of aluminum-containing antacids include high levels of calcium secreted in the urine, bone resorption, impairment of fluoride absorption, and phosphorus depletion—all of which may contribute to bone disease. *Gastroenterology* 76 (1979): 603–606.

Toxicity and Adverse Effects

In a study of 200 ulcer patients and 200 normal controls, the authors suggest that the slightly higher risk of kidney stone formation in ulcer patients (7 versus 1 percent) was due to milk-alkali syndrome. This occurs when patients drink 2 to 5 quarts of milk per day, in addition to taking antacids. *American Journal of Gastroenterology* 68 (1977): 367–371.

Chapter 22: Phosphorus

Overviews

This chapter discusses the uses of phosphorus in the body, including its role in the bone and its many soft-tissue functions. According to the Food and Nutrition Board, the average daily intake of phosphorus is 1,500 to 1,600 milligrams. Committee on Dietary Allowances, *Recommended Daily Allowances*, 9th ed. (Washington, D.C.: National Academy of Sciences, 1980), 133–134.

The author describes the uses of phosphorus in the body, and points out that although it is recommended that the intake of calcium and phosphorus be equal, in most diets the phosphorus intake exceeds the calcium intake. Corinne H. Robinson, *Normal and Therapeutic Nutrition*, 15th ed. (New York: Macmillan, 1977), 108–109.

Phosphorus/Calcium Balance

In this study, 34 men and women were tested for calcium and phosphorus intakes. It was found that the intakes for both minerals were higher for men than for women— 1,075 milligrams and 1,533 milligrams versus 695 milligrams and 1,095 milligrams. However, both groups were in negative balance. The authors discuss the contribution that high phosphorus intake makes to the eventual decrease in bone mass. They suggest that diets high in protein, soft drinks, and phosphorus additives are responsible for the undesirable calcium-to-phosphorus ratio. *American Journal of Clinical Nutrition* 40 (December 1984): 1368–1379.

In a survey of a large number of women, the frequency of skeletal fractures was increased by a factor of 2.3 in athletic women who consumed carbonated beverages. This relationship seems to apply to phosphate contained in carbonated soft drinks rather than dietary phosphorus. *Journal of Nutrition* 118 (1988): 657–660.

Chapter 23: Magnesium

Osteoporosis

This study revealed that almost 75 percent of the women who took 250 to 750 milligrams of magnesium daily for 2 years had bone density increases of 1 to 8 percent. *Medical Tribune* (July 22, 1993): 1.

Fibromyalgia and Chronic Fatigue

Leading health researchers are recommending magnesium malate (magnesium plus malic acid) supplements for the treatment of chronic fatigue. In particular, fibromyalgia pain may be reduced within 48 hours while fatigue may take 2 weeks. The therapeutic dose of 6 tablets generally contains 300 milligrams of magnesium and 1,200 milligrams of malic acid. *HealthWatch* 3 (Spring 1993): 1, 3.

In this study, 15 patients with fibromyalgia were treated with an oral dosage of 6 to 12 tablets of magnesium malate supplying 1,200 to 2,400 milligrams of malate and 300 to 600 milligrams of magnesium, respectively. Subjective improvement in symptoms occurred within 48 hours of supplementation. Subjective worsening of muscle pain occurred within 48 hours of placebo ingestion. *Journal of Nutritional Medicine* 3 (1992): 49–59.

Psychiatric Disorders

Of 41 unmedicated psychiatric patients, 11 women who attempted suicide had significantly lower cerebrospinal fluid levels of magnesium than nonsuicidal patients and controls. The authors hypothesize that magnesium may be required to maintain normal sero-tonergic (neurotransmitter) activity in the central nervous system. *Biological Psychiatry* 20 (February 1985): 163–171.

In this study, 165 boys who had been admitted to a psychiatric hospital were compared with normal boys. Patients with low magnesium blood levels had significantly more symptoms of depression, schizophrenia, and sleep disturbances. The authors concluded that low blood magnesium is associated with depressive and schizophrenic symptoms in children. *Biological Psychiatry* 19 (June 1984): 871–876.

The effects of vitamin B_6 and magnesium supplementation on 60 autistic children were tested in a double-blind trial. Neither supplement, when used alone, had any significant effect. A combination of the 2, however, resulted in significant improvement. *Biological Psychiatry* 20 (May 1985): 467–478.

When hair samples from 28 autistic children were taken, mean calcium and magnesium levels were found to be well below normal and significantly less than in controls. Although vitamin B_6 has also been found to be low in autistic children, B_6 supplementation when given without magnesium worsened the symptoms of some of the children in this study. *Orthomolecular Psychiatry* 13 (April–June 1984): 117–122.

Cardiovascular Disease

It is also noted that the need for protective substances found in cardioprotective diets such as antioxidants is greater when magnesium intake is insufficient. Some experts believe that the daily consumption of magnesium should be 6 mg/kg/day, which is equivalent to 420 milligrams/day for the average 70-kilogram individual. The NHANES I and the Atherosclerosis Risk in Communities (ARIC) show an inverse association between serum magnesium and the incidence of coronary heart disease in 10-year and 4- to 7-year follow-ups. *Magnesium Research* 12(1) (1999): 57–61.

Vascular disease underlies many of the complications of diabetes and includes coronary, cerebral, renal, peripheral, and retinal vascular abnormalities. Magnesium (Mg) and potassium (K) deficiencies occur frequently in diabetic patients. Because of the vasoconstrictive effects of hypomagnesemia and hypokalemia and the adverse effects of magnesium and potassium deficiency on carbohydrate metabolism we hypothesize that routine magnesium and potassium supplementation of all hypomagnesemic diabetics will ameliorate or prevent the ravages of diabetic vascular disease. *Medical Hypotheses* 55(3) (2000): 263–265.

Serum magnesium concentration (S-Mg) has been reported to be inversely associated with atherogenic lipid fractions and with blood glucose concentrations. In some studies on humans, oral magnesium supplementation has been found to improve the lipoprotein balance. Total S-Mg was measured in patients with non-insulin-dependent diabetes mellitus treated with the lipid-lowering drugs gemfibrozil and simvastatin. In conclusion, total S-Mg concentration decreased significantly during treatment with gemfibrozil and simvastatin in patients with NIDDM. During both drug regimens, changes in S-Mg status were inversely correlated to changes in plasma glucose concentrations. *Metabolism* 50(10) (2001): 1147–1151.

In this study, hypertensives had significantly less magnesium in their blood cells than did normal people. The authors point out that previous studies have shown magnesium supplementation to be an effective hypotensive agent in some types of blood pressure. *Proceedings of the National Academy of Science* 81 (October 1984): 6,511–6,515.

Previous studies have shown that magnesium is significantly lower in patients with angina. This study treated 15 patients who had 5- to 15-minute angina attacks with intravenous magnesium. During 41 occasions, the attacks ended within .5 to 2 minutes after treatment. Four patients who had daily attacks were treated daily for 5 days and had no further attacks. The authors contend that magnesium deficiency may be an important factor in the production of coronary vasospasm, which, in turn, can cause angina, *Magnesium* 3 (January–February 1984); 46–49.

In this study, 8 young men with untreated hypertension and abnormal blood vessels of the retina were found to have low levels of magnesium. When supplemented with 450 milligrams of magnesium for 3 months, the blood vessels returned to normal. *Magnesium* 3 (May–June 1984): 159–163.

A group of 71 insulin-treated diabetics all had low levels of magnesium. Those with the lowest levels had the severest degree of retinal disease. The author concluded that inadequate magnesium appears to be an additional risk factor in the development and progress of this complication. *Diabetes* 27 (1978): 1,075–1,077.

Pregnancy Complications
In a study of 534 women with threatening premature labor, the group of patients who received magnesium supplementation experienced a reduction in the proportion of prematurity and intrauterine growth retardation. The researchers concluded that a certain percentage of these conditions are due to magnesium deficiency and can be averted with supplementation. *Magnesium* 4 (January–February 1985): 20–28.

Menstrual Problems
In 50 individuals with primary dysmenorrhea, subjects were treated with magnesium. After a 6-month period, 21 of 25 women showed a reduction in symptoms, while only 4 reported no improvement. Magnesium therapy resulted in a reduction in pro-inflammatory prostaglandins (PGE 2) in menstrual blood to 45 percent of baseline compared with placebo at 90 percent at baseline. Magnesium's therapeutic benefit may be due to inhibition of the production of PGE2, as well as magnesium's direct muscle relaxant and vasodilatory effect. *Gynakologie* 111 (1989): 755–760.

Women who had primary dysmenorrhea received a dose of magnesium that contained 3 x 5 mmol of granulate orally on the day preceding menstruation and on the first and second day of the cycle for 6 cycles. On the second and third day, there was a definite therapeutic effect on both back pain and lower abdominal pain. There was a marked reduction in symptoms and in absences from work due to dysmenorrhea with magnesium. *Schweizerische Rundschau fur Medizin Praxis* 79(16) (1990): 491–494.

Diarrhea
After receiving radiation therapy, 20 cervical cancer patients developed diarrhea so severe that they required hospitalization. In the 10 patients who were treated with magnesium, diarrhea disappeared within 3 days. In the group that was treated conventionally, it took 2 to 6 weeks for symptoms to clear. Radiation caused decreases in blood levels of magnesium, and the authors suggest that pretreatment with magnesium might prevent this side effect. In addition, magnesium has been found to reduce diarrhea due to malnutrition, Crohn's disease, and other conditions. *Magnesium* 4 (January–February 1985): 16–19.

Drug Interactions
In this study, 12 bone marrow transplant patients who were treated with the drug cyclosporine experienced neurological symptoms. All patients had low magnesium levels at the onset of symptoms. These symptoms resolved or did not recur after magnesium levels were restored. The authors suggest that the neurotoxicity of this drug is due to magnesium depletion, and that supplementation would reduce the risk of these side effects. *Lancet* (November 17, 1984): 1,116–1,120.

Deficiencies
Magnesium deficiency results in thrombosis, and oral contraceptive use has been found to lower blood levels of magnesium. This offers a possible clue to the higher incidence of clotting disorders among women on oral contraceptives. *Medical World News* (September 13, 1974): 32.

A group of "Type A" behavior men and a group of "Type B" behavior men were given a stressful task. The results of the experiment led the authors to postulate that stress causes the release of magnesium from the cells, which is then excreted in the urine. Eventual magnesium depletion can increase the risk of hypertension, coronary vasospasm (angina), and damage to the heart. *Journal of the American College of Nutrition* 4 (April–June 1985): 165–172.

The levels of magnesium in the red blood cells of women with premenstrual tension (PMT) were significantly lower than those of the controls. This may be due to decreased intake absorption or increased excretion. Since PMT patients often complain of nervous tension, the magnesium may also be depleted because of stress. The author suggests that magnesium therapy may be beneficial to PMT patients with low red cell magnesium. *American Journal of Clinical Nutrition* 34 (November 1981): 2,364–2,366.

Chapter 24: Zinc

Overviews

Zinc is important in the physiology of insulin. Zinc pretreatment enhances the magnitude of the binding of insulin to the receptor, but simultaneously inhibits the degradation of insulin by the liver plasma membranes both in vivo and in vitro. Zinc modulates insulin's actions by stimulating lipogenesis in adipocytes in synergy with insulin. Zinc is a cofactor of over 200 enzymes, of which many involve food utilization. Zinc is involved in the general metabolism of protein, carbohydrate, and lipids. Zinc is a cofactor of key enzymes in glucose metabolism. Insulin resistance may be related to zinc deficiency by impairment of insulin secretion by the pancreas; interference in insulin-receptor binding; decreased insulin-receptor synthesis; and abnormal glucose carrier structure and/or translocation inside the cell. Increased urinary loss of zinc in diabetics may lead to zinc depletion. Diabetic patients may also malabsorb zinc and not be able to compensate for the excessive urinary loss. Zinc deficiency may account for impaired wound healing and decreased cell-mediated immunity and taste acuity in diabetic subjects. Zinc deficiency is also associated with oxidative stress. *Biological Trace Element Research* 81 (2001): 215–228.

Zinc is in high concentrations in ocular tissue, in particular the retina and choroid, and interacts with vitamin A and taurine. Suboptimal zinc status in North America may contribute to the development and progression of several chronic eye diseases, which include age-related macular degeneration. Excessive zinc intake can result in copper deficiency. Zinc deficiency has been suggested to occur in Parkinson's disease and may be specifically related to vision, olfactory, and taste loss in these patients. Zinc is also effective in blocking genes that encode for inflammatory cytokines and this strongly supports the supposition that adequate zinc nutrition may protect against many inflammatory diseases, including atherosclerosis. Zinc deficiency is also being linked to aging and age-related degenerative diseases, which manifest with an increase in the copper/zinc ratio and systemic oxidative stress in general. *Journal of the American College of Nutrition* 20(2) (2001): 106–118.

The authors discuss the possible symptoms of a marginal zinc deficiency in adults and children, including impaired wound healing, impaired growth, and loss of taste acuity. *Pediatric Clinics of North America* 30:3 (June 1983): 583–596.

This article reviews the possible causes of low zinc levels, including malabsorption syndromes and chronically debilitating diseases. The signs of chronic zinc deficiency include growth retardation, male hypogonadism, skin changes, poor appetite, mental lethargy, and delayed wound healing. Zinc has a wide variety of functions, including protection of the liver from carbon tetrachloride, a possible direct effect on free radicals, and the alleviation of the toxic effects of cadmium and lead. *Nutrition Reviews* 41:7 (July 1983): 206.

Growth, Pregnancy, and Development

Pregnant women with the lowest levels of zinc in their blood had more complications than did women with the highest levels of zinc. *American Journal of Clinical Nutrition* 40 (September 1984): 496–507.

This study found that pregnant women take in marginal amounts of zinc (8.6 milligrams per day) and copper (0.95 milligrams), resulting in poor body retention. Supplements containing 10 to 12 milligrams of zinc and 2 milligrams of copper combined with normal dietary intakes are sufficient to achieve positive balances during pregnancy. The authors point out that prenatal zinc and copper deficiencies in animals have been shown to cause birth defects. *American Journal of Clinical Nutrition* 42 (June 1985): 1,184–1,192.

Data shows that women with zinc malabsorption and/or low blood levels of zinc have an increased risk of having a malformed child. The authors point out that few prenatal supplements contain zinc. *American Journal of Clinical Nutrition* 38 (December 1983): 943–953.

The offspring of zinc-deficient monkeys were fed a diet deficient in zinc after they were weaned. They developed bone abnormalities similar to those found in rickets. *American Journal of Clinical Nutrition* 40 (December 1984): 1,203–1,212.

Recent U.S. studies indicate that zinc deficiency in infants and preschool children is not uncommon. Earliest signs of deficiency include slowing of physical growth, poor appetite, and diminished taste acuity. The authors suggest that calcium carbonate in hard tap water may interfere with zinc absorption or utilization. *American Journal of Clinical Nutrition* 37 (January 1983): 37–42.

Zinc levels in the sweat of dyslexic children were only 66 percent as high as those in controls. Since dyslexia tends to be a family trait, further studies on zinc levels and the effects of supplementation before conception, during pregnancy, and in childhood are urgently needed. *British Medical Journal* 296 (February 27, 1988): 607–609.

Taste, Vision, and Smell

There is strong evidence to support the connection between zinc depletion and the development of night blindness and loss of taste acuity. It is likely that impaired color discrimination and smell acuity may also develop. Other investigators have suggested that such impairments may be better indicators of zinc depletion than are the traditional blood tests, which are notoriously unreliable. *Annals of Internal Medicine* 99 (1983): 227–239.

The highest concentration of zinc in the human body is in the eye. It is well established that zinc is an essential component of many parts of the eye, including the retina, choroid, cornea, and lens. Zinc deficiency causes functional impairment in various parts of the eye, and there is a growing body of evidence that this deficiency is related to many conditions, such as night blindness, cataract formation, and optic neuritis. *Survey of Ophthalmology* 27:2 (September–October 1982): 114–122.

In a study of almost 5,000 people funded in part by the National Eye Institute, a mixture of 80 milligrams of zinc and 2 milligrams of copper reduced the risk by 11 percent. *Nutrition Week* 31(40) (2001): 7.

The authors found that zinc and copper levels were lower in patients with cataracts when compared with controls. Since zinc and copper are required for superoxide dismutase (SOD) to protect the lens from oxidation damage, diets chronically deficient in these nutrients may impair this important mechanism. *Nutrition Reports International* 37 (January 1988): 157–163.

The authors treated 12 chronic hemodialysis patients with zinc. Sensitivity to 4 taste qualities was significantly heightened, and the authors suggest that zinc replacement may be an effective therapy for loss of taste acuity in dialysis patients. *Kidney International* 24: Supplement 16 (December 1983): S315–S318.

Physical and Mental Stress

The data from this study supports other reports that injury results in zinc depletion. The average zinc levels in injured subjects in this study were significantly lower than those in controls for at least 4 days after hospital admission. *Nutrition Research* 5 (1985): 253–261.

Diabetics were found to have lower zinc levels than did controls. This may be related to several common complications of diabetes, including impaired immune function, low testosterone levels, slow healing of ulcers, and neurosensory changes. *Nutrition Research* 8 (1988): 889–897.

In an 8-week study, 18 patients with arterial or venous leg ulcers were treated with compresses of zinc oxide. In addition, 19 controls were treated with unmedicated compresses. Of the treated group, 83 percent improved, versus 42 percent of the untreated group. Four weeks after the end of the treatment, 61 percent of the zinc oxide-treated ulcers were healed, compared with 2 percent of the untreated group. The authors note that previous studies have shown that zinc given orally for 1 to 2 months improves the healing of similar ulcers in patients with low zinc levels. *British Journal of Dermatology* 111 (October 1984): 461–468.

The authors review the effectiveness of topical zinc applications in treating types I and II herpes virus lesions. Solutions of zinc have been shown to relieve pain, tingling, burning, and itching; to shorten healing time by 40 to 60 percent; and to reduce recurrence rates from 100 percent in controls to 0 to 14 percent in treated patients. For facial and upper body skin infections and genital infections, solutions can be applied as warm rinses, wet dressings, douches, or wet vaginal sponges. For oral lesions and colds due to nasal herpes, lozenges can be used. *Medical Hypotheses* 17 (June 1985): 157–165.

In a study of 20 "Type A" personalities and 19 "Type B" personalities, the "Type A" personalities had higher levels of zinc in their red blood cells and lower levels in their urine. After a 20-minute stressful task, urinary zinc was increased in both groups, but more so in the "Type A." "Type A" personalities appear to deplete zinc most rapidly in stressful situations. *Journal of the American College of Nutrition* 4 (April–June 1985): 165–172.

In a study of 9 healthy male runners, it was found that strenuous running led to significant losses of chromium and zinc. *Biological Trace Element Research* 6 (1984): 327–336.

The Immune System

In this study, 83 normal human subjects were given 660 milligrams of zinc sulfate daily for one month. When compared with 20 untreated controls, the zinc-supplemented group experienced significantly increased lymphocyte responses. This beneficial effect does not result from a correction of latent zinc deficiency. The authors note that the supplementation of an excess of zinc had no effect on serum copper. They suggest that since the treatment is so well documented, nontoxic, and inexpensive, their findings encourage additional studies in various conditions associated with immune deficiencies. *American Journal of Clinical Nutrition* 34 (1981): 88–93.

The author notes that zinc deficiencies have been reported in many malignant conditions, and that this is frequently associated with a high copper-to-zinc ratio. A significant survival advantage was demonstrated for patients with squamous cell lung cancer who had high zinc concentrations in their blood. *Progress in Clinical and Biological Research* 129 (1983): 1–33.

The authors studied 88 healthy people, ages 1 month to 85 years, and 72 people with Down syndrome, ages 10 days to 25 years. They found that biologically active thymic hormone (involved in immunity) decreased with age in normal subjects, and was low in most Down syndrome subjects, regardless of age. When zinc was added to samples of their blood plasma, thymic hormone activity increased to levels found in healthy young people. *Lancet* (May 5, 1984): 983–986.

The author proposes that zinc deficiency may be a factor in the development of AIDS (Acquired Immune Deficiency Syndrome). Zinc deficiency has been associated with acquired immune deficiency states of other types. Since semen contains a remarkable quantity of zinc, sexually overactive men will have a large loss of zinc. *Journal of the American Medical Association* 252 (September 21, 1984): 1,401–1,410.

People with AIDS had much lower zinc levels than did control subjects, and nearly undetectable thymulin. When zinc was added to blood samples, thymulin increased to the same levels as those found in controls. Some of the immune deficiency observed in AIDS may be the result of poor zinc status, and supplementation may correct some of the immune derangement. *Journal of the American Medical Association* 259 (February 12, 1988): 839–840.

Anorexia Nervosa
The authors studied 8 women with anorexia nervosa and 8 healthy women. Zinc levels after meals were significantly lower in anorexic women than in the controls. The authors hypothesize that food restriction may lead to reduced zinc levels, which, in turn, may result in impaired small intestinal metabolism and zinc absorption. *Lancet* (May 4, 1985): 1,041–1,042 (letter).

In this randomized double-blind placebo-controlled trial, 35 female anorexia nervosa patients received either 100 milligrams of zinc gluconate or a placebo. The rate of increase in body mass in the supplemented patients was twice that in the unsupplemented group. The authors conclude that zinc supplementation may improve the rate of weight gain in anorexia nervosa patients. *International Journal of Eating Disorders* 15 (1994): 251–255.

The Prostate Gland
Zinc inhibits the specific binding of androgens to the prostatic cytosol and nuclear androgen receptors. *Acta Endocrinologia* 105 (1984): 281–288.

Zinc supplementation reduced the size of the prostate and BPH (benign prostatic hypertrophy) symptomatology in the majority of patients. *Federation Proceedings* 35 (1976): 361.

In one study, 19 patients took 150 milligrams of zinc sulfate (supplying 34 milligrams of elemental zinc) for 2 months, followed by 11 to 23 milligrams of elemental zinc. All patients reported symptomatic improvement, and 14 out of 19 patients experienced shrinkage of the prostate. *Zinc and the Prostate*; presentation at the annual meeting of the American Medical Association, Chicago, 1974.

Lead and Cadmium Accumulation
In a study comparing hair mineral concentrations of normal and hypertensive women, researchers found that hypertensives had 5 times as much cadmium, 2.5 times as much lead, and almost 3 times as much zinc as did the controls. They suggest that enhanced dietary zinc might prevent the hypertensive effect of cadmium. *Bulletin of Environmental Contamination and Toxicology* 32 (May 1984): 525–532.

Behavioral Changes
Experimental monkeys were marginally deprived of zinc from conception and compared with controls. In the deprived monkeys, the amount and variety of problem behaviors were significantly less than in the controls (10 to 71 percent). These and other results suggest that syndromes of lethargy, apathy, and slowed activity are characteristic behavioral effects of marginal zinc deprivation in primates. *American Journal of Clinical Nutrition* 42 (1985): 1,229–1,239.

Osteoporosis
This article reviewed the importance of copper, manganese, and zinc supplementation, in addition to calcium, for increasing mineral density in postmenopausal women. In a 2-year double-blind placebo-controlled trial involving 200 postmenopausal women, the group taking 1,000 milligrams of calcium (as calcium citrate-malate) had a bone mineral density (BMD) of -.50 percent, compared with the placebo group, which had a BMD of -2.23 percent. This demonstrated that the calcium supplement clearly slowed bone loss. However, the group that received 1,000 milligrams of calcium along with 2.5 milligrams of copper, 5 milligrams of manganese, and 15 milligrams of zinc had a BMD of +1.28 percent, indicating an increase in BMD. *Journal of the American College of Nutrition* 12 (1993): 384–389.

Absorption

Normal subjects were given zinc after an overnight fast. The absorption ranged from 40 to 86 percent. Patients with a wide variety of diseases exhibit decreased zinc absorption. *American Journal of Clinical Nutrition* 34 (1981): 2,648–2,652.

Laboratory rabbits were given 3 different forms of zinc. Zinc sulfate and zinc pantothenate appeared to be absorbed and utilized similarly. Zinc orotate was absorbed more slowly than these 2. There were no significant differences in the zinc concentrations in the blood. *European Journal of Drug Metabolism and Pharmacokinetics* 7:3 (1982): 233–239.

Deficiencies

Some endurance athletes have a significant increase in carbohydrate intake and low amounts of protein and fat intake, which may lead to suboptimal zinc intake in as much as 90 percent of athletes. Mild zinc deficiency is difficult to evaluate due to lack of specific indicators of zinc status. Zinc deficiency can lead to anorexia, loss in body weight, fatigue, reduction in endurance, and an increased risk of osteoporosis. *Sports Medicine* 31(8) (2001): 577–582.

The authors surveyed 58 people of over 62 years of age and found that average zinc intake was only 7 milligrams—less than half the RDA. Lower taste acuity was also found in these patients, which is a symptom of zinc deficiency. These findings indicate that this population is at risk for zinc deficiency. *Journal of the American Dietetic Association* 82 (February 1983): 148–153.

The authors note that recent "advances" in food production and an increase in the consumption of highly refined foods have led to a reduction of zinc and other important nutrients in the modern diet. They further note that nutritional deficiency states for some of these trace elements have been reported in certain population groups. *British Journal of Nutrition* 48 (1982): 241–248.

Certain diuretics used to control hypertension cause increased zinc excretion, which may lead to zinc deficiency. Side effects of these drugs, such as impotence, may be linked to zinc depletion rather than to the drugs themselves. Diuretic therapy before or after myocardial infarction may contribute to a zinc deficiency, which might slow the healing of the heart. *South African Medical Journal* 64 (December 1983): 936–941.

Zinc levels were low and prolactin levels were high in 32 men with end-stage kidney disease who had been undergoing hemodialysis. Zinc has been shown to inhibit prolactin synthesis in vitro. Zinc deficiency may be the cause of high prolactin levels in these patients. *Lancet* (October 5, 1985): 750–751.

Zinc deficiency has been found in people with malabsorption syndromes such as Crohn's disease, celiac disease, short bowel syndrome, and jejunoileal bypass. Diarrhea is a symptom of zinc deficiency and can also cause zinc losses. Subtle signs of zinc deficiency such as loss of appetite, impaired night vision, and depressed immune and mental functions may appear in these patients. *Journal of the American College of Nutrition* 4 (January–March 1985): 49–64.

In this study, healthy men given 400 micrograms of folic acid daily excreted more zinc and had lower blood levels of zinc than did controls. The authors express concern that women treated with folic acid to reverse cervical dysplasia (see Chapter 16) could develop zinc deficiency. This may be a hazard, especially for users of oral contraceptives, which decrease folic acid and zinc. The authors recommend that people receiving folic acid supplements be monitored for zinc status. *Journal of the National Cancer Institute* 74 (January 1985): 263 (letter).

When blood samples from 450 pregnant women were tested, it was found that women with the lowest levels of zinc had significantly higher pregnancy complications, including infection and miscarriage, than did those with the highest zinc levels. *American Journal of Clinical Nutrition* 40 (September 1984): 496–507.

Skin Disorders

In this study, 3 patients with folliculitis had significant improvement with combination therapy of oral fusidic acid plus zinc sulfate. It is noted that zinc is also used in acrodermatitis enteropathica, acne vulgaris, alopecia areata, and leg ulcers. *ACTA Dermato-Venereologica* 72 (1992): 143–145.

Toxicity and Adverse Effects

A 57-year-old man who had been taking 450 milligrams of zinc a day for 2 years developed severe anemia, which appears to have been caused by impaired copper metabolism. *Annals of Internal Medicine* 103 (September 1985): 385–386.

In this study, 9 healthy young men were fed a high-protein diet that was supplemented with copper sulfate and various amounts of zinc. Based on the results of this study, the authors conclude that short-term daily intake of 18.5 milligrams of zinc results in increased copper excretion. *American Journal of Clinical Nutrition* 41 (February 1985): 285–292.

In a study of 25 men, the group that received 50 milligrams of zinc per day for 6 weeks did not have their blood levels of copper affected. Copper and zinc superoxide dismutase levels did decrease, which may suggest that zinc supplements decreased copper status. *American Journal of Clinical Nutrition* 40 (October 1984): 743–746.

The authors studied 11 men who were given 150 milligrams of zinc twice a day. None of the subjects showed evidence of untoward side effects, However, there was impairment of some immune functions, which returned to normal when supplements were stopped. There was also a significant decrease of HDLs and a slight increase in LDL levels. *Journal of the American Medical Association* 252 (September 21, 1984): 1,443–1,446.

The authors gave 23 healthy men 50 milligrams; of zinc per day for 6 weeks along with a diet marginal in copper. During this time, diastolic blood pressure decreased, and there was a tendency for cholesterol to decrease and HDL cholesterol to increase. *Nutrition Reports International* 32 (August 1985): 373–382.

Over 200 milligrams per day of zinc were given to 2 patients with Wilson's disease accompanied by severe neurological symptoms. After 2 years of the zinc treatment, liver copper content was reduced by 40 percent in one patient and 57 percent in the other. Their neurological symptoms almost completely disappeared. The authors note that there were no side effects in these patients nor in others taking zinc for up to 25 years. *British Medical Journal* 289 (August 4, 1984): 273–276.

Chapter 25: Iron

Fatigue and Behavioral Changes

Iron-deficient women experience cold sooner, but so do women with low to normal hemoglobin levels. Iron supplementation improves cold tolerance. This suggests that nonanemic women can be symptomatically iron-deficient, and that non-iron-deficient women may be experiencing other symptoms as well as cold intolerance, such as effects on attention span and learning, and minor sleep disturbances. *Journal of the American Medical Association* 260 (August 5, 1998): 607.

The authors suggest that iron-deficient nonanemic runners suffer from diminished endurance exercise performance, which can be prevented by oral iron therapy. *American Journal of Diseases of Children* 142 (February 1988): 165–169.

Adolescent runners with low iron levels run the risk of developing iron deficiency and anemia during the running season, and should be treated with iron supplementation. *Journal of Pediatrics* 114 (April 1989): 657–663.

In a group of 69 normal university students, iron status was significantly related to cognitive performance. *American Journal of Clinical Nutrition* 39 (1984): 105–113.

In a study of 78 iron-deficient children and 41 nonanemic children, it was found that the iron-deficient children responded to supplementation with significantly higher school achievement scores. *American Journal of Clinical Nutrition* 42 (1985): 1,221–1,228.

NHANES III found that in 5,300 children age 6 to 16 years, lower than average math scores were linked to iron deficiency, even if their deficiency was not severe enough to induce anemia. Iron-deficient children were more than twice as likely to have below-average math scores than children of normal iron status. It was most common in girls (8.7 percent) and its overall frequency was 3 percent. *Pediatrics* 107(6) (2001): 1381–1386.

The Immune System

Iron deficiency is one of the likeliest forms of single micronutrient deficiency to occur. Iron is one of the most important micronutrients in terms of its influence on immune system functions and on other aspects of host defense, including increased susceptibility to infection, reduced white blood cell counts, and impaired antibody production. *American Journal of Clinical Nutrition* (Supplement) 35:2 (February 1982): 442–449.

Angular Cheilosis

Of 156 cases of angular cheilosis observed in a dental practice, 19.2 percent were due to iron deficiency, and only 5.8 percent to vitamin B deficiencies. In 17 of the 30 iron-deficient patients, the condition was accompanied by smooth tongue and difficulty swallowing, which represents a premalignant condition called Plummer-Vinson syndrome. *Journal of Oral Medicine* 39 (October–December 1984): 199–206.

Salt Craving

A hypertensive 33-year-old woman had a salt craving that caused her to consume a half pound of salt per week. After treatment with large amounts of iron, her craving decreased dramatically. The authors note that pica, the compulsive consumption of particular substances, occurs in about 50 percent of iron-deficient patients, half of whom eat ice. Salt craving is recognized as a symptom of several conditions, but has not been previously reported in connection with iron deficiency. *American Journal of Kidney Diseases* 5 (January 1985): 67–68.

Low Intakes

The authors studied the diets of 74 female college students. Based on 4-day dietary records, they found that only 6 of the 74 met the RDA for iron. *Nutritional Reports International* 31 (February 1985): 281–285.

Iron deficiency is the most common single nutrient deficiency in the world. The authors note that even in the absence of anemia, iron deficiency may have detrimental effects on behavior and learning. *New England Journal of Medicine* 313 (November 7, 1985): 1,239–1,240.

The actual foods eaten by lacto-ovo vegetarian women were analyzed, and it was found that their average iron intake was 11 to 14 milligrams per day. These women had normal hemoglobin values, and were not considered to be anemic. However, they also did not appear to have enough iron stores to cope with heavy menstrual losses or pregnancy without possible jeopardy to their iron nutritional status. *Nutrition Report International* 27 (January 1983): 199–206.

Toxicity and Adverse Effects

Excess of pharmaceutical iron may cause toxicity and therapeutic doses may cause gastrointestinal side effects. Excess iron in primary and secondary hemochromatosis may lead to hepatic fibrosis, diabetes mellitus, and cardiac failure. An upper safe level of iron is 25 to 50 milligrams/day. Iron increases oxidative stress and free iron concentration. This process may cause damage to lipid membranes, proteins, and organs. Some studies suggest that the risk of atherosclerosis and acute myocardial infarction is related to body iron stores. Most recent, well-controlled studies support the hypothesis that iron stores are related to cardiovascular risk. Oxidative stress may also increase DNA damage and oxidative activation of precancerogens and support tumor cell growth. This is supported by numerous studies. High iron stores may present a health hazard. Evidence strongly supports not increasing iron intake beyond physiological requirements. To avoid iron deficiency symptoms do not exceed the RDI. *Annals of Nutrition & Metabolism* 45(3) (2001): 91–101.

Thirty-three studies were reviewed. Of the larger studies, approximately three-quarters supported the association of iron with colorectal cancer risk. Because iron is broadly supplemented in the American diet, the benefits of iron supplementation need to be measured against the long-term risks of increased iron exposure, one of which may be increased risk of colorectal cancer. *Nutrition Reviews* 59(5) (2001): 140–148.

This is a commentary on the role of iron in heart disease. A 3-year Finnish study of 1,391 men, ages 42 to 60, showed an increased risk in heart attack with serum ferritin levels of at least 200 micrograms per deciliter. Two follow-up studies found no link between serum ferritin and heart attack. No link between dietary iron intake and heart disease has been found. *Medical Tribune* (April 8, 1993): 7.

This study assessed the relation of serum iron, dietary iron, and the use of iron supplements to the risk of heart attack in thousands of patients. Although an association between serum iron levels and heart attack was found, there was no association found with dietary iron or iron supplements. The association of higher serum iron with heart attack was not explained by iron intake. *Epidemiology* 5 (1994): 243–246.

Chapter 26: Copper

Bone Density

This article reviewed the importance of copper, manganese, and zinc supplementation, in addition to calcium, for increasing mineral density in postmenopausal women. In a 2-year double-blind placebo-controlled trial involving 200 postmenopausal women, the group taking 1,000 milligrams of calcium (as calcium citrate-malate) had a bone mineral density (BMD) of -.50 percent, compared with the placebo group, which had a BMD of -2.23 percent. This demonstrated that the calcium supplement clearly slowed bone loss. However, the group that received 1,000 milligrams of calcium along with 2.5 milligrams of copper, 5 milligrams of manganese, and 15 milligrams of zinc had a BMD of +1.28 percent, indicating an *increase* in BMD. *Journal of the American College of Nutrition* 12 (1993): 384–389.

Immunity

Experimentally induced deficits or excesses of copper have each been reported to increase the severity of infection in laboratory animals. *American Journal of Clinical Nutrition* (Supplement) 35:2 (February 1982): 455.

Copper Compounds

Copper complexes of anti-arthritic drugs are more potent than the parent drugs, and are used to treat a wide range of degenerative diseases, such as rheumatoid arthritis, ankylosing spondylitis, and lupus erythematosus. *Inflammation* 2:3 (1977): 217–238.

Urinary copper was measured in 5 patients with chorea and in 22 controls. In 4 of the chorea patients, copper was markedly depressed. When copper supplements were given to a chorea patient, her symptoms began to lessen within 3 weeks, and she improved steadily over the next 3 months. When a placebo was substituted, her shoulder and arm jerking returned within 4 days. The authors suggest that copper deficiency could be an underlying abnormality in some patients with chorea. *Biological Psychiatry* 19 (December 1984): 1,677–1,684.

Cholesterol

Copper and other trace minerals have been shown to lower cholesterol in experimental animals and humans. A copper deficiency is associated with increased cholesterol levels, and the mean copper intake in United States diets is approximately half the RDA. Copper deficiency is suspected to occur in the United States population and abroad. *Federation Proceedings* 41 (September 1982): 2,807–2,812.

A healthy 29-year-old man was given a copper-depleting diet for 105 days. The total cholesterol in his blood plasma increased from 202 to 234 milligrams. In addition, 6 abnormal heartbeats were recorded near the end of depletion. When his copper was replenished over a period of 39 days, his cholesterol levels returned to normal. The authors conclude that diets inadequate in copper lead to high cholesterol and abnormal ECG patterns, and may be important in the development of ischemic heart disease. *Metabolism* 33 (December 1984): 1,112–1,118.

Pregnancy and Oral Contraceptive Use
This study found that pregnant women take in marginal amounts of zinc (8.6 milligrams per day) and copper (0.95 milligrams), resulting in poor body retention. Supplements containing 10 to 12 milligrams of zinc and 2 milligrams of copper combined with normal dietary intakes are sufficient to achieve positive balance during pregnancy. The authors point out that prenatal zinc and copper deficiencies in animals have been shown to cause birth defects. *American Journal of Clinical Nutrition* 42 (June 1985): 1,184–1,192.

In 259 pregnant women being screened for fetal abnormalities, the average blood copper level was lower in pregnancies that ended in spontaneous abortion and in which fetal abnormalities were discovered. The authors suggest that decreased copper levels in the mother may be associated with the development of spontaneous abortion and neural tube defects. *Clinical Chemistry* 30 (October 1984): 1,676–1,677.

Absorption and Depletion
Copper absorption was measured in patients with celiac disease (inability to digest the gluten in cereal grains) and in healthy controls. The controls absorbed 67 percent more copper than the celiac patients. The authors conclude that patients with intestinal disease have a reduced uptake of copper, zinc, and perhaps other minerals, and may have signs of deficiency. *Science of the Total Environment* 42 (March 15, 1985): 29–36.

A 36-year-old woman complained of difficulty walking and had other signs of copper deficiency, including anemia. After 3 weeks of copper therapy, her symptoms improved. She had been taking an antacid that contained aluminum, magnesium, sodium, and other oxides for 6 years. The authors conclude that use of antacids should be considered a risk factor for copper deficiency. *Nutrition Reviews* 42 (September 1984): 319–321.

Copper Toxicity From Tap Water
This article reports on a family in Vermont who acquired copper intoxication from drinking water from their faucet, indicating that tap water must be taken into consideration when determining copper intakes. *Pediatrics* 74:6 (1994): 1,103–1,106.

Chapter 27: Manganese
Overview
The author reviews the functions of manganese in the body, including normal bone growth and development, enzyme activation, normal lipid metabolism, reproduction, and nerve function. Corinne H. Robinson, *Normal and Therapeutic Nutrition*, 15th ed. (New York: Macmillan, 1977), 119–120.

Numerous studies have shown that MnSOD can be induced to protect against prooxidant insults resulting from cytokine treatment, ultraviolet light, irradiation, certain tumors, amyotrophic lateral sclerosis, and ischemia/reperfusion. In addition, overexpression of MnSOD has been shown to protect against pro-apoptotic stimuli as well as ischemic damage. Conversely, several studies have reported declines in MnSOD activity during diseases including cancer, aging, progeria, asthma, and transplant rejection. The precise biochemical/molecular mechanisms involved with this loss in activity are not well understood. *Free Radical Research* 34(4) (2001): 325–336.

Osteoporosis

This article reviewed the importance of copper, manganese, and zinc supplementation, in addition to calcium, for increasing mineral density in postmenopausal women. in a 2-year double-blind placebo-controlled trial involving 200 postmenopausal women, the group taking 3,000 milligrams of calcium (as calcium citrate-malate) had a bone mineral density (BMD) of -.50 percent, compared with the placebo group, which had a BMD of -2.23 percent. This demonstrated that the calcium supplement clearly slowed bone loss. However, the group that received 1,000 milligrams of calcium along with 2.5 milligrams of copper, 5 milligrams of manganese, and 15 milligrams of zinc had a BMD of +1.28 percent, indicating an *increase* in BMD. *Journal of the American College of Nutrition* 12 (1993): 384–389.

Birth Defects

A total of 61 infants and their mothers were tested for manganese levels. Infants with congenital malformations (including central nervous system defects, cleft lip and palate, and hermaphroditism) and their mothers both had much lower levels of manganese than did normal infants and their mothers. The authors conclude that low levels of manganese could be a factor in the development of birth defects. *American Journal of Clinical Nutrition* 41 (May 1985): 1,042–1,044.

Congenital dislocation of the hip is high in certain areas of France, Canada, and the United States. It may be due to manganese deficiency, which results from the practice of alkalinizing the soil, thereby impairing the absorption of manganese by plants. Further experimental work showed that a manganese-deficient diet leads to bone and joint malformation of the offspring. *South African Medical Journal* 63:12 (1983): 393.

Epilepsy

In this study, blood manganese levels were measured in 197 young patients with convulsive disorders and 120 children without neurologic problems. The blood manganese levels were significantly lower in patients with convulsive disorders when compared with controls. The researchers conclude that low manganese levels may heighten a tendency to seizures. They also note that rats fed manganese-deficient diets have an increased susceptibility to convulsions. *Biochemical Medicine* 33 (March–April 1985): 246–255.

The Immune System

Manganese stimulates microphage, phagocyte, granulocyte, and antibody activity. *American Journal of Clinical Nutrition* (Supplement) 35:2 (February 1982): 456.

Manganese deficiency reduces superoxide dismutase, a substance that prevents free radical damage. *Journal of Nutrition* 114 (1984): 1,438–1,446.

Glucose Tolerance

The offspring of manganese-deficient laboratory rats were maintained on a manganese-deficient diet. They experienced significantly greater hyperglycemia and lower blood insulin levels than did rats fed a diet sufficient in manganese. The authors concluded that manganese deficiency during prenatal and postnatal periods may result in an impaired ability to synthesize insulin. *Journal of Nutrition* 114 (August 1984): 1,438–1,446.

Guinea pigs born to manganese-deficient mothers and fed manganese-deficient diets had abnormal glucose tolerance. *Journal of Nutrition* 94 (1968): 89–94.

The authors report on an 18-year-old male who had been controlling his diabetes with an alfalfa extract, which is high in manganese. When the hospital allowed this man to use his extract, it was found that his blood sugar could be reduced from 648 milligrams per milliliter to 68 milligrams per milliliter within 2 hours. This was repeated on

12 occasions, with the same response. The authors suggest that the manganese contained in the extract was responsible for the blood sugar–lowering effect. *Lancet* (December 29, 1962): 1,318.

Toxicity

Toxicity to manganese may occur with environmental exposure such as mining. Toxicity may appear as delusional thinking and hyperactivity. Subsequently, symptoms similar to Parkinson's disease appear. *Environmental Research* 34 (1984): 242–249.

Chapter 28: Chromium

Glucose Tolerance/Diabetes

Insulin resistance may be a common etiology, at least in part, behind the pathobiological alterations of advancing age. Prevalent age-related disorders such as cardiovascular diseases, obesity, and cancer have been associated with impaired glucose/insulin metabolism and its consequences. Increasing the intake of antioxidants and/or substances recognized to enhance insulin sensitivity is a natural means of combating the glucose/insulin perturbations and free-radical damage. Accordingly, ingestion of niacin-bound chromium and natural antioxidants such as grape seed proanthocyanidin extract has been demonstrated to improve insulin sensitivity and/or ameliorate free-radical formation and reduce the signs/symptoms of chronic age-related disorders, including syndrome X. These natural strategies possess a highly favorable risk/benefit ratio. *Annals of the New York Academy of Sciences* 957 (2002): 250–259.

Chromium is an essential nutrient involved in the metabolism of glucose, insulin, and blood lipids. Suboptimal dietary intake of chromium is associated with increased risk factors associated with diabetes and cardiovascular diseases. Within the past five years, chromium has been shown to improve glucose and related variables in subjects with glucose intolerance and Type I, Type II, gestational, and steroid-induced diabetes. Chromium increases insulin binding to cells, insulin receptor number and activates insulin receptor kinase leading to increased insulin sensitivity. *Diabetes & Metabolism* 26(1) (2000): 22–27.

In this study, 5 hyperglycemic people were given 218 micrograms of chromium daily for 6 months. All of them had improved blood glucose control. They also had significant lowering of total serum-to-HDL cholesterol ratios, corresponding to halving their risk of coronary heart disease. *Nutrition Report International* 30 (October 1984): 911–918.

In this study, 16 healthy elderly volunteers were divided into three groups and given 200 micrograms of chromium, 100 milligrams of nicotinic acid, or 200 micrograms of chromium and 100 milligrams of nicotinic acid daily for 28 days. Only the chromium-nicotinate complex caused a 15 percent decrease in the glucose area integrated total, and a 7-percent decrease in fasting glucose. It is possible that the inability to respond to chromium supplementation may result from suboptimal levels of dietary nicotinic acid. *Metabolism* 36:9 (September 1987): 896–899.

In this study, 10 elderly people were supplemented with chromium. Four out of the ten experienced a disappearance of all abnormal features of the glucose tolerance test. The pattern of response in these individuals suggests the possibility that the nonresponders were suffering from such a severe chromium deficiency that a longer period of supplementation may have been required for them to show a response. *Metabolism* 17 (February 1968): 114–125.

Lean Body Mass and Decreased Body Fat

In this study, 42 football players were randomly given either 1.6 milligrams of chromium picolinate (200 micrograms of trivalent chromium) or a placebo for 42 days. In the group given chromium picolinate, lean body mass increased significantly after only 14 days and continued to increase until the end of the study. Total body weight decreased significantly by 2.63 pounds, and total body fat decreased from 15.8 percent to 12.2 percent—a loss of 22 percent of body fat. The results of this study confirm previous findings that chromium picolinate accelerates the development of lean body mass and concurrent loss of body fat. It may be a safe alternative to anabolic steroids. *International Journal of Biosocial and Medical Research* 11:2 (December 1989): 163–180.

High Cholesterol
Chromium picolinate was shown to significantly lower serum lipids including total cholesterol and LDL cholesterol, to raise HDL cholesterol, and to lower glucose in human subjects. It is an effective agent for the treatment of lipid disorders. *Western Journal of Medicine* 152 (1990): 41–45.

In this study, subjects were given 24 to 48 micrograms of GTF (organic) chromium, in the form of brewer's yeast, daily for 8 weeks. The treatment resulted in decreased levels of total cholesterol and increased levels of HDL cholesterol. The authors found it striking that treatment with organic chromium raised HDL cholesterol in physically active, relatively young adults with normal blood lipid levels, as well as in subjects with high blood lipid levels. They also noted that previous investigations have shown that GTF chromium influenced blood glucose levels, insulin response, and lipid levels. *Journal of the American College of Nutrition* 1 (1982): 263–274.

In this study, 200 micrograms of chromium plus 100 milligrams of niacin lowered serum cholesterol levels in patients with hypercholesterolemia. Supplementation for 4 months resulted in a further decrease in serum cholesterol. These results are similar to those seen with the administration of 2,000 milligrams of niacin. *Journal of Family Practice* 27 (December 1988): 603–606.

Psoriasis
This study examined the role of insulin resistance in psoriasis. Sores of psoriatic severity improved in response to chromium in patients with insulin resistance. Chromium supplementation may improve psoriasis and insulin resistance in these patients. *Journal of the American College of Nutrition* 12 (1993): 588/abstract 35.

Deficiencies
Marginal dietary chromium intake is widespread in the United States and other developed countries. In a double-blind study of 76 people, chromium or a placebo was given for three months. Chromium was used as well as absorbed by the subjects, as indicated by a significant improvement in the glucose tolerance of a number of subjects. *American Journal of Clinical Nutrition* 36 (December 1982): 1,184–1,193.

The majority of people eating typical Western diets consume less than the upper limit of the estimated safe and adequate daily dietary intake, which is set at 50 to 200 micrograms per day. Insufficient chromium intake is associated with signs and symptoms similar to those seen in diabetes and cardiovascular diseases. The efficacy of chromium in the general population relates to its prevention of deficiency or a reduction in the risk of chronic diseases. It is possible that doses above the estimated safe and adequate daily dietary intake are necessary for the treatment of certain chronic disease states. In a study performed in China, the use of 1,000 micrograms of chromium was highly effective in relieving many of the symptomatic manifestations of Type II diabetes mellitus, including a return of the HbA1C levels into the normal range. Most recent evidence strongly supports the conclusion that there is little fear of toxic reactions from chromium consumption. In addition to Type II diabetes mellitus, chromium supplementation may be useful to direct overall weight decrements specifically toward fat loss with the retention of lean body mass and to ameliorate many manifestations of aging. *Current Opinion in Clinical Nutrition and Metabolic Care* 1(6) (1998): 509–512.

In a study of 9 healthy male runners, the authors found that strenuous running led to significant losses of chromium, presumably because of its increased use in glucose metabolism. *Biological Trace Element Research* 6 (1984): 327–336.

Chapter 29: Selenium

Cancer

The authors review the anticancer properties of selenium in humans and experimental animals. Dietary selenium intake is inversely correlated with death from leukemia and cancers of the breast, ovary, lung, colon, rectum, and prostate. Selenium should be considered not only as a preventive, but also as a therapeutic agent in cancer treatment, and may act additively or synergistically with drug and X-ray treatments. *Journal of Agricultural Food Chemistry* 32 (May–June 1984): 436–442.

Many animal studies demonstrate a cancer-protective effect of selenium. Human epidemiological studies suggest that cancer risk is reduced in people living in high-selenium areas, in people with high-selenium food supplies, and in people with higher blood levels of selenium. *Seminars in Oncology* 10 (September 1983): 305–310.

In a study of over 10,000 people, the average selenium level of 111 subjects who subsequently developed cancer was lower than that of the 210 matched controls. Also, the risk of cancer was twice as high for people in the lowest quintile of selenium levels. Selenium supplementation in animals reduces the frequency of chemically induced cancers and inhibits the growth of transplanted tumors. *Lancet* (July 16, 1983): 130–134.

A population of over 8,000 with low selenium levels was followed for 6 years. Cancer was subsequently diagnosed in 128 people who had significantly lower selenium levels than the controls. The authors suggest that selenium may act by reducing the mutagenicity of carcinogens, by affecting carcinogen metabolism, or by protecting against oxidative damage. *American Journal of Epidemiology* 120 (September 1984): 342–349.

The authors studied 12,000 people in Finland, 51 of whom died of cancer during the following 4 years. They found that selenium levels were significantly lower in cancer patients than in controls, and that the difference was greater in smokers than in nonsmokers. The risk of cancer mortality in people with the lowest selenium levels was nearly 6 times greater than that of the controls. For people with both low selenium levels and low vitamin E levels, the risk of death from cancer was more than 11 times that of people who had higher levels of both these nutrients. The data suggests that dietary selenium deficiency is associated with an increased risk of fatal cancer, that low vitamin E intake may enhance this effect, and that decreased vitamin A intake contributes to the risk of lung cancer among smoking men with low selenium intake. *British Medical Journal* 290 (February 9, 1985): 417–420.

This study showed that vitamin E enhances selenium's ability to inhibit the development of breast cancer in laboratory rats treated with a potent carcinogen. In general, the chemopreventive effect of selenium is manifested in the form of lower tumor incidence, a reduction in the size of tumors, and a longer latency period. *Cancer Research* 43 (November 1983): 5,335–5,341.

The combined effect of selenium and vitamin A on breast cancer development in rats was studied. This investigation provided evidence that vitamin A increases the protective effect of selenium. The authors suggest that the results warrant further study. *Cancer Research* 41 (April 1981): 1,413–1,416.

Several geographic studies have suggested that states or countries with higher selenium levels in the soil and in locally grown foods experience lower death rates from cancer. The author of this review article found that the results of such studies indicate a decreased mortality from cancer of the lung, colon, rectum, bladder, esophagus, pancreas, breast, ovary, and cervix. Lower selenium levels have been found in patients with various types of cancer, as well as lower levels of vitamins E and A and beta-carotene. The author emphasizes the need to consider several nutrients in diet and cancer studies, instead of focusing on just one nutrient per study. He also points out that current selenium trials are limited to 200 micrograms per day, which may not be the optimum amount needed to prevent cancer. *Federation Proceedings* 44 (June 1985): 2,584–2,589.

In a study of 1,458 healthy adults in 24 regions of China, low blood selenium levels were associated with higher deaths from cancer of the stomach, esophagus, liver, and other sites. The authors expect that selenium supplementation will reduce cancer incidence. *Biological Trace Element Research* 7 (January–February 1985): 21–29.

This letter to the editor reviews the research concerning selenium and other antioxidants in protecting the skin from the damages of ultraviolet radiation. In an animal study, selenomethionine was effective in protecting them against UV radiation-induced skin cancer. Selenium retarded the onset and number of lesions and reduced inflammation, blistering, and pigmentation. The author notes that he has given as much as 600 micrograms to patients without any toxic side effects. He recommends daily doses of 3 grams of vitamin C, 800 international units of vitamin E, and 200 micrograms of selenium to protect against excessive UV radiation. *Canadian Medical Association Journal* 147 (September 15, 1992): 839–840.

Patients over a 4-year period who suffered from interstitial lymphedema due to irradiation of the head and neck area for advanced squamous cell carcinoma of the head and neck; subjects had received simultaneous radiochemotherapy with carboplatin. When lymphedema was present, 200 micrograms of sodium selenite was given, 3 times daily, by mouth for a period of 8 weeks. After supplementation with sodium selenite, there was an observable reduction in edema in 18 of 30 patients. There was subjective improvement in breathing capacity, as seen by patients' own responses after 8 weeks of treatment. This study showed that sodium selenite appeared to reduce the severity of interstitial lymphedema due to irradiation of the head and neck area. *Trace Elements and Electrolytes* 19(1) (2002): 33–37.

It has been found by researchers that selenium intakes of approximately 2 times the Recommended Dietary Allowance or more can have positive health benefits. Selenium may be antitumorigenic in two ways: 1) It is an essential nutrient in antioxidant enzymes; and 2) it may help directly inhibit tumorigenesis. *Nutrition and Cancer* 40(1) (2001): 6–11.

Cardiovascular Disease
The authors studied over 8,000 people in Finland. During a follow-up period of 7 years, 367 of these people had heart attacks or died of heart disease. Their mean serum selenium levels were lower than those of the controls. Those with the lowest selenium levels had a 6- to 7-fold increase in the risk of death from heart disease. *Lancet* (July 24, 1982): 175–179.

Skin Conditions
In a study of patients with acne, those given 400 micrograms per day of selenium and 25 international units per day of vitamin E showed improvement in their condition. In patients not treated, there was a marked worsening of the acne. A few patients who were previously treated with zinc and tetracycline experienced complete healing of the acne when given the supplements. In addition, 3 patients with seborrheic dermatitis also improved with this treatment. *Acta Dermatologica Venerealogica* 64 (1984): 9–14.

Autoimmune Diseases
The authors measured the selenium levels of 87 rheumatoid arthritis patients. Low selenium levels were found in all patients, with lowest levels in those with the most severe disease. Although selenium deficiency is probably not a primary etiological factor in rheumatoid arthritis, patients with low selenium levels may develop more severe disease. Selenium supplementation might have some therapeutic benefit in rheumatoid arthritis. *Scandinavian Journal of Rheumatology* 14 (April–June 1985): 97–101.

In this study, 7 rheumatoid arthritis patients who no longer responded to conventional treatment were given 350 micrograms of selenium and 400 international units of vitamin E daily. Ten to fourteen days later, their normal treatment was resumed. In 4 patients, joint pain disappeared. In the remaining 3 patients, joint pain was diminished and mobility was markedly increased. *Biological Trace Element Research* 7 (May–June 1985): 195–198.

Female patients with autoimmune thyroiditis and elevated plasma thyroid peroxidase antibodies and/or thyroid antibodies received sodium selenite (liquid solution)—200 micrograms per day or placebo for 3 months. Thyroid peroxidase antibodies (TPOAB) concentrations decreased significantly in the selenium selenite group compared to no change in the placebo group. A subgroup analysis of patients with extremely high concentrations of TPOAB revealed a 40 percent decrease in antibody concentrations in the selenium group and a 10 percent increase in the placebo group. A significant number of patients in the selenium group had completely normalized TPOAB levels only. Ultrasound of the thyroid showed normalized thyroid in these patients. Evaluation of subjective well-being revealed significant improvement in the selenium group only. *Journal of Clinical Endocrinology and Metabolism* 87 (2002): 1687–1691.

Immunity

Selenium is needed for a fully functioning immune system. In studies with mice, the offspring of selenium-deficient mice have had impaired immune responses, and selenium supplements have enhanced the effects of vaccines. When a modest excess of selenium was given to dogs, it stimulated their immune systems. This effect was greatest when they were fed diets high in polyunsaturated fats. *American Journal of Clinical Nutrition* (Supplement) 35:2 (1982): 452–453.

Muscular Dystrophy

The author notes that it is well known that muscular dystrophy in cattle and sheep is a selenium-deficiency disease preventable by supplementation. In this study of 24 patients with muscular dystrophy, serum selenium levels were lower for patients than for controls. Patients who were more severely disabled had lower selenium levels than did patients with mild symptoms. One patient received selenium therapy and experienced considerable functional improvement. The authors suggest that muscular dystrophy may be a selenium-deficiency disease. A long-term study is being undertaken. *Acta Medica Scandinavica* 211 (1982): 493–499.

The Elderly

In a double-blind study involving 30 elderly people, half received 1,720 micrograms of sodium selenate, 45 micrograms of organic selenium, and 400 milligrams of vitamin E. The other half received a placebo. After 2 months, the supplemented group showed obvious improvement in mental well-being when compared with controls. They showed significant improvement in fatigue, anorexia, depression, anxiety, emotional stability, hostility, mental alertness, motivation and initiative, self-care, and interest in the environment. There were no adverse effects after one year of treatment. *Biological Trace Element Research* 7 (April–May 1985): 161–168.

Absorption and Deficiencies

According to this study, selenium levels were significantly greater in humans with selenomethionine than with a selenite supplement. *American Journal of Clinical Nutrition* 42 (1985): 439–448.

In this study, 46 alcoholics were compared with 45 nonalcoholic individuals. Alcoholics had low blood selenium levels, especially if their livers were diseased. The authors conclude that inadequate selenium intake is likely in alcoholics. Impaired absorption, increased requirements, or altered metabolism of selenium may also be factors. Selenium deficiency, by reducing glutathione peroxidase activity, may contribute to liver damage in alcoholics. *American Journal of Clinical Nutrition* 42 (July 1985): 147–151.

In this study, 30 young women were given 150 micrograms of sodium selenate per day, 600 milligrams of vitamin C per day, or both. After 4 weeks, selenium levels were increased by 34 percent in the women taking selenium only, by 29 percent in those taking vitamin C only, and by 63 percent in those taking both. The authors conclude that vitamin C improves the bioavailability of dietary selenium. *Human Nutrition. Clinical Nutrition* 39C (May–June 1985): 221–226.

Blood selenium levels were measured in 16 patients with celiac disease and in 32 healthy controls. Selenium levels in plasma, leukocytes, and whole blood were significantly lower in celiac patients than in the controls. The authors hypothesize that gluten-free diets might be deficient in selenium, or that selenium may be poorly absorbed by celiac patients. Decreased selenium levels in these individuals may explain the increased incidence of cancers of the gastrointestinal tract and other parts of the body that has been reported in celiac patients. *British Medical Journal* 288 (June 23, 1984): 1,862–1,863.

The authors studied 86 Texas oil refinery workers. Selenium levels were significantly lower in industrial workers than in controls. Their glutathione peroxidase levels were also lower. The authors conclude that lower selenium was not due to dietary inadequacy, but may have been due to exposure to environmental oxidants that may affect selenium status. *Nutrition Research* 3 (1983): 805–817.

There is a continuing but controversial interest in the use of hair as a diagnostic tool for the assessment of trace element status. The authors of this paper studied blood and hair selenium before, during, and after selenium supplementation. Selenium supplementation for 6 weeks caused no increase in plasma selenium levels, but did cause an increase in selenium levels in new hair growth. There was a significant decline in hair selenium levels during the final 6 weeks after the selenium supplement was withdrawn. There was no correlation between hair and blood selenium levels. *Nutrition Research* 4 (1984): 577–582.

Toxicity

The authors report that the average daily selenium intake in an area that was high in selenium but free of toxicity was 750 micrograms. The authors indicate that the chronically toxic dose of dietary selenium is likely to be near 5 milligrams (5,000 micrograms) per day. The chronically toxic dose of sodium selenate is estimated to be lower, in the range of 1 milligram per day. *American Journal of Clinical Nutrition* 37 (May 1983): 872.

The authors review numerous data on the toxicity of selenium. Various studies have shown no adverse effects from the long-term consumption of 500 micrograms, 350 micrograms, or 600 micrograms daily. Selenium intake in China is reported to be 750 micrograms per day with no signs of toxicity. Toxicity for selenium, extrapolated from animal studies, may occur in humans ingesting 1,000 to 2,000 micrograms per day. The Food and Nutrition Board has stated that toxicity occurs in humans ingesting 2,400 to 3,000 micrograms daily. Based on these data, they point out the board's claim that the safe upper limit of 200 micrograms per day is a conservative one and has definite implications for chemoprevention studies based on supplementation. *Seminars in Oncology* 10:3 (1983): 311–319.

Chapter 30: Iodine

Overview

The author reviews the functions of iodine, its dietary sources, and geographical regions of high incidence of iodine deficiency. Corinne H. Robinson, *Normal and Therapeutic Nutrition*, 15th ed. (New York: Macmillan, 1977), 115–116.

The Thyroid Gland

Iodine in the form of sodium iodide can be used to treat goiter and hyperthyroidism. A severe iodine deficiency can cause hypothyroidism. *The Merck Manual*, 14th ed. (Rahway, N.J.: Merck Sharp and Dohme Research Laboratories, 1982), 997–1,012.

Hearing

Children in an area of China with endemic iodine deficiency had a lower hearing level than did children in an area without endemic iodine deficiency. After 3 years of iodine supplementation, thyroid function tests and hearing levels became normal. The authors suggest that hearing loss is one of the iodine deficiency disorders that are now being identified based on a broader understanding of iodine deficiency states. *Lancet* (September 7, 1985): 518–520.

Nuclear Accidents

A nuclear reactor accident could pose a hazard to the public because of the release of radioactive iodine, which could damage the thyroid and ultimately lead to thyroid cancer. In the event of such an accident, a single dose of 300 milligrams of potassium iodide would block the uptake of radioactive iodine by the thyroid, and so may be advisable in high-risk individuals. *Lancet* (February 1983): 451.

It is believed that predistribution of potassium iodide tablets to households near nuclear power plants may be worthwhile as a preventive measure in the event of a nuclear accident. *Public Health Reports* 98 (April 1983): 123–126.

Chapter 31: Potassium

Overview

The author reviews the uses of potassium in the body, good dietary sources, and the causes and symptoms of deficiency. Corinne H. Robinson, *Normal and Therapeutic Nutrition*, 15th ed. (New York: Macmillan, 1977), 130–131.

Cardiovascular Disease

Blood Pressure

The authors studied the relationship between dietary nutrients and blood pressure in over 10,000 people. The 10 percent of the group with the highest blood pressure tended to have decreased intakes of calcium, potassium, vitamin A, and vitamin C. *Science* 224 (June 29, 1984): 1,392–1,398.

Only 2 percent of vegetarians have been found to have high blood pressure, as compared with 26 percent of nonvegetarians. Vegetarians with the highest potassium excretion, indicating a high intake, had the lowest blood pressure. *American Journal of Clinical Nutrition* 37 (May 1983): 755–762.

The authors of this article studied 12 subjects with mild hypertension. Some subjects responded to sodium restriction while others responded to potassium supplementation. The authors conclude that individuals respond differently to changes in sodium or potassium intake. *Lancet* (April 7, 1984): 757–761.

Hypertensive Kidney Damage

Salt-sensitive rats fed a high-salt diet developed hypertension and related symptoms. When potassium was added to their diet, blood pressure was unchanged, but there was less damage to the kidneys. The authors suggest that potassium exerts a protective effect and that blacks in the United States, who have a low potassium intake and a high rate of hypertensive kidney failure, might benefit from tripling their potassium intake. *Hypertension* (Supplement) 6 (March–April 1984): 1,170–1,176.

Bioavailability and Retention

Since many potassium chloride supplements are distasteful, many physicians tell their patients to consume large amounts of potassium-rich foods, usually in the form of fruit. The authors measured the potassium levels in various fruits and concluded that the retention of potassium in these foods is poor. The authors conclude that potassium chloride supplements must continue to be the mainstays for potassium repletion. *New England Journal of Medicine* 313 (August 29, 1985): 582–583.

Increasing potassium and decreasing sodium in diets could benefit people with hypertension, those who are overweight, and some diabetics. The authors suggest several approaches to achieving a more favorable sodium-to-potassium ratio in the diet: preserving potassium through steaming rather than boiling foods; adding modest amounts of potassium chloride salt substitute to cooking water, and adding less salt. *Lancet* (February 12, 1983): 362–363.

Chapter 32: Boron

A study examined the effects of boron on 12 women, ages 48 to 82. Daily supplementation of 3 milligrams of boron markedly reduced their urinary excretion of calcium and magnesium. It also markedly elevated the serum concentration of estradiol and testosterone, suggesting an endocrine mechanism. These findings suggest that supplementation of a low-boron diet induces changes in postmenopausal women consistent with the prevention of calcium loss and bone demineralization. Boron may be an important nutritional factor determining the incidence of osteoporosis. *FASEB Journal* 1 (1987): 394–397.

This review presents the concept that bone health doesn't depend only on estrogen and calcium, but on a wide range of other nutrients, including vitamins B_6, C, D, and K; folic acid; and magnesium, manganese, boron, zinc, copper, strontium, and silicon. The typical Western diet, high in sugar and refined foods, appears to be deficient in many of these nutrients. The requirement for certain nutrients may be increased by genetic factors or by metabolic changes that occur during menopause. Supplementation with a balanced combination of appropriate micronutrients may prove to be a useful adjunct to calcium and estrogen therapy. *Journal of the American Osteopathic Association* 4(2) (December 1988): 2–5.

Animal and human research suggests that boron enhances the utilization of vitamin D_3, and enhances and mimics some of the effects of estrogen therapy in postmenopausal women to positively affect mental alertness, psychomotor skills, and the cognitive processes of attention and memory. Experiments with humans show that people consuming about .25 milligram per day respond positively to boron supplementation, suggesting that boron intake should be higher than this. Based on both human and animal experimental data, humans may have a boron requirement between .5 and 1.0 milligram a day. *Journal of the American College of Nutrition* 15 (October 1996): 520 (abstract 27).

Analytical evidence reveals lower boron concentrations in femur heads, bones, and synovial fluid in people with arthritis than in those without this disorder. Moreover, bones of patients using boron supplements are much harder to cut than bones of unsupplemented people. Epidemiologic evidence reveals that in areas of the world where boron intakes are 1.0 milligram or less per day, the estimated incidence of arthritis ranges from 20 to 70 percent, versus the 0 percent to 10 percent incidence in areas where intakes are 3 to 10 milligrams per day. In a double-blind placebo-controlled trial, 50 percent of patients receiving 6 milligrams of boron a day experienced a significant improvement in their osteoarthritis symptoms, versus only a 10 percent improvement in those receiving the placebo. *Environmental Health Perspectives* 102 (November 1994): S83–S85.

In a double-blind study, patients with osteoarthritis were randomly assigned to receive boron (6 milligrams per day as sodium tetraborate decahydrate) or a placebo for 8 weeks. Of those receiving boron, 50 percent improved, compared with 10 percent of those given placebo. When the 5 subjects who dropped out of the study were excluded from the analysis, 71 percent of those in the boron group improved, compared with 12.5 percent of those in the placebo group. No side effects were seen and there were no significant changes in common laboratory parameters. These results suggest boron supplementation may be helpful for individuals with OA whose diets are likely to be low in boron. There is no evidence that populations with a high intake of boron (such as the French) have an increased incidence of hormone-related cancers. *Journal of Applied Nutrition* 46 (1994): 81–85 and *Journal of Nutritional Medicine* 1 (1990): 127–132.

Boron is especially effective in cases of vitamin D, magnesium, and potassium deficiency. Vitamin K is essential for the activation of osteocalcin. Vitamin C is an important stimulus for osteoblast-derived proteins. Increasing the recommended amounts (US RDA 1989), adequate intakes (US DRI 1997), or assumed normal intakes of mentioned food components may lead to a considerable reduction or even prevention of bone loss, especially in late postmenopausal women and the elderly. *Critical Reviews in Food Science and Nutrition* 41(4) (May 2001): 225–249.

Chapter 33: Coenzyme Q₁₀

Overviews

This review of human and animal studies and reports documents the beneficial effects of CoQ for ischemic heart disease, congestive heart failure, toxin-induced cardiotoxicity, angina pectoris, arrhythmia, and hypertension. The authors found that the most intriguing property of CoQ is its potential to protect and preserve ischemic myocardium during surgery. *Medical Clinics of North America* 72 (January 1988): 243–257.

CoQ is capable of stabilizing cell membranes and preventing depletion of metabolites necessary for creating ATP. It may also help inhibit free radical formation. K. Folkers and Y. Yamamura, eds., *Biomedical and Clinical Aspects of Coenzyme Q*, vol. 3 (Amsterdam: Elsevier/North Holland Biomedical Press, 1981), 159–168.

This article reviews the biochemistry and use of coenzyme Q10. Double-blind studies have confirmed the efficacy of CoQ as an adjunctive treatment in heart failure. *Clinical Investigator* 71 (1993): S116–S123.

This study evaluated the effects of CoQ in the prevention of LDL oxidation. Doses of CoQ ranged from 100 to 300 milligrams. The results of the study demonstrated that CoQ is incorporated into plasma and all lipoproteins, increasing their resistance to oxidation. *Biochimica Et Biophysica ACTA* 1126 (1993): 247–254.

Cardiovascular Disease

Angina

In a placebo-controlled trial of subjects with chronic stable angina, the group receiving CoQ was able to exercise significantly longer than the control group. K. Folkers and Y. Yamamura, eds., *Biomedical and Clinical Aspects of Coenzyme Q*, vol. 4 (Amsterdam: Elsevier Science Publ. BV, 1984), 291–301.

In a double-blind random crossover study of 12 patients with chronic stable angina, exercise time increased significantly in the CoQ-treated group. *American Journal of Cardiology* 56 (1985): 247–251.

In a double-blind crossover study of patients with chronic stable angina, CoQ was found to be as effective as drug therapy in reducing abnormal EKGs during exercise. K. Folkers and Y. Yamamura, eds., *Biomedical and Clinical Aspects of Coenzyme Q*, vol. 5 (Amsterdam: Elsevier Science Publ. BV, 1985), 385–394.

Congestive Heart Failure

Approximately 31 reports from Japan have described the beneficial effects of CoQ in small numbers of patients with various forms of congestive heart failure. G. Lenaz, ed., *Coenzyme Q Biochemistry, Bioenergetics, and Clinical Applications of Ubiquitone* (New York: Wiley-Interscience 1985), 479–507.

At the Seventh International Symposium on the biomedical and clinical aspects of CoQ in Copenhagen, Dr. Karl Folkers reviewed more than 35 years of research. On the basis of this research, he concluded that heart failure is caused by a dominant deficiency of

CoQ, and that its clinical use is definitely positive to the health and well-being of the patient. *Clinical Investigator* 71 (1993): S51–54.

This study evaluated the use of CoQ at a dose of 50 milligrams per day in 1,715 patients with chronic congestive heart failure. Patients were stabilized on standard therapy for 3 months. In just 4 weeks, CoQ resulted in improvements in shortness of breath at rest, exertional dyspnea, palpitations, cyanosis, hepatomegaly, pulmonary rates, ankle edema, heart rate, and systolic and diastolic blood pressure. The authors conclude that CoQ treatment led to an improvement in the signs and symptoms and quality of life in these patients. *Clinical Investigator* 71 (1993): S129–S133.

This study evaluated the effect of CoQ supplementation on 2,500 patients with heart failure. Patients received 50 to 150 mg of CoQ, with the majority receiving 100 milligrams. After 3 months, there was improvement in: cyanosis, 81 percent; edema, 76.9 percent; pulmonary rates, 78.4 percent; palpitations, 75.7 percent; sweating, 82.4 percent; arrhythmia, 62 percent; insomnia, 60.2 percent; vertigo, 73 percent; and nocturia, 50.7 percent. *Clinical Investigator* 71 (1993): S145–S149.

This study evaluated 641 patients with heart failure in a double-blind trial. Patients received CoQ at a dose of 2 milligrams per kilogram per day (e.g., 140 milligrams of CoQ for a 154-pound man). Episodes of pulmonary edema or cardiac asthma were significantly reduced with CoQ supplementation. Results suggest that CoQ therapy, along with conventional therapy, reduces hospitalization for worsening of heart failure and the incidence of serious complications in patients with congestive heart failure. *Clinical Investigator* 71 (1993): S134–S136.

Cardiomyopathy

In 77 men and 49 women with cardiomyopathy, survival at 6 months varied from 50 to 78 percent, and at 12 months, from 35 to 65 percent. The subjects who were between 19 and 80 years of age were observed over a 6-year period while receiving 33.3 milligrams of coenzyme Q_{10} 3 times daily. The mean coenzyme Q_{10} blood level upon entry was 0.85 microgram/milliliter, which was significantly lower than the mean level of 1.07 microgram/milliliter in 54 control subjects. The mean ejection fraction was 41 percent at control and increased to 59 percent at 6 months. A significant improvement in the ejection fraction occurred in 71 percent of the subjects at 3 months and in 16 percent at 6 months, totaling 87 percent. There was a significant second delayed improvement seen in 25 percent of the patients. Only 13 percent showed no improvement. A total of 106 of 122 patients with at least 1 follow-up or who died before follow-up (87 percent in all) improved by I or II New York Heart Association classes. Two patients complained of minor itching, but otherwise there were no adverse side effects in 350 patient-years of treatment for patients taking coenzyme Q_{10} daily for up to 6 years. Of 9 published cardiomyopathy studies, survival at 6 months varied from 50 to 78 percent, and at 12 months, from 35 to 65 percent. The positive results in class II were the most encouraging. All of the subjects appeared to become asymptomatic after coenzyme Q_{10} administration, with the longest time a patient was treated being 6 years. Seventy-one percent of the patients in this study responded within 3 months, and 16 percent of the subjects responded within 6 months, which may suggest that 100 milligrams of coenzyme Q_{10} is too low. *American Journal of Cardioliology* 65 (1990): 521–523.

Heart Surgery

This randomized study indicates that administering CoQ before surgery improves postsurgical cardiac output. *Thoracic Surgery* 33 (1982): 145–151.

When CoQ was given to patients prior to coronary bypass surgery, the CoQ group had less damage to the heart muscle. K. Folkers and Y. Yamamura, eds., *Biomedical and Clinical Aspects of Coenzyme Q*, vol. 4 (Amsterdam: Elsevier Science Publ. BV, 1984), 333–342.

The investigators reviewed the research on the use of CoQ for high-risk cardiac surgery patients who have a natural or clinically induced coenzyme Q_{10} deficiency. The results support the use of oral CoQ in high-risk heart surgery patients. *Clinical Investigator* 71 (1993): S155–S161.

Arrhythmia

In one of several studies using CoQ in patients with arrhythmia, the results suggest that 20 to 25 percent of patients experience improvement. *Tohoku Journal of Experimental Medicine* 141 (Supplement, 1983): 453–463.

Coenzyme Q_{10} was found to be of therapeutic value in patients experiencing arrhythmia as a side effect of psychotropic drugs. Lenaz, G., ed., *Coenzyme Q* (New York: John Wiley & Sons, 1985), 479–505.

Hypertension

In this small double-blind controlled study of subjects with essential hypertension, the group that received CoQ showed a decline in both systolic and diastolic blood pressure after 12 weeks. K. Folkers and Y. Yamamura, eds., *Biomedical and Clinical Aspects of Coenzyme Q*, vol. 5 (Amsterdam: Elsevier Science Publ. BV, 1986), 337–343.

In this study, 10 patients with hypertension were treated with 100 milligrams of CoQ for 10 weeks. At the end of the trial, CoQ had significantly decreased both systolic and diastolic blood pressure and total serum cholesterol levels, with a small increase in HDL cholesterol. CoQ's beneficial effects on cholesterol and hypertension are significant. *Current Therapeutic Research* 51 (1992): 668–672.

A study of 83 men and women with hypertension found that 60 milligrams of CoQ_{10} twice daily significantly dropped systolic blood pressure as compared to placebo. *Southern Medical Journal* 94(11) (2001): 1112–1117.

Mitral Valve Prolapse

This study evaluated the use of CoQ in patients with mitral valve prolapse, chronic fatigue, or hypertension. CoQ supplementation reduced high blood pressure in 80 percent of the patients with hypertension, and improved diastolic function in all patients. A reduction in myocardial thickness in 53 percent of hypertensives and 36 percent of the combined prolapse and fatigue group also occurred. *Clinical Investigator* 71 (1993): S140–S144.

This study examined the use of CoQ in children, ages 6 to 16, with mitral valve prolapse. The normal Frank-Starling mechanism was recovered due to CoQ supplementation, which may improve disturbed bioenergetic function at a molecular level. Researchers used 3 to 3.4 milligrams per kilogram per day, with no adverse side effects noted. *Clinical Investigator* 71 (1993): S150–S154.

High Cholesterol

Statins are effective drugs for lowering cholesterol. The 6 statin drugs approved by the U.S. Food and Drug Administration (FDA) were introduced between 1987 and 1997. Published data suggest that statins can cause myopathies and rhabdomyolysis with renal failure, and in May 2000, the FDA warned about liver failure with regard to statin drugs. Estimates suggest that the drugs may cause liver and muscle injury in up to 1 percent of users, which equals 130,000 individuals with liver and muscle toxicity problems in the United States. Statins have been associated with the increased incidence of cataracts, neoplasia, peripheral neuropathies and some psychiatric disturbances. It has been estimated that as many as 26 million Americans qualify for long-term cholesterol-lowering therapy. Pharmaceutical companies have filed for over-the-counter status for their statin drugs, which has been rejected by the FDA at present. In 2000, sales of cholesterol-reducing agents topped $9 billion—up almost 25 percent from the previous year. Overall, sales of cholesterol- and triglyceride-reducing drugs reached $15.9 billion. The cardioprotective, cytoprotective, and neuroprotective potential of coenzyme Q_{10} has been well researched and discussed. Deficiencies of coenzyme Q_{10} are believed, at least in part, to be involved in some of the side effects of statin drugs. Animal and human data suggest that statin drugs impair energy metabolism. The author recommends from the accumulated evidence that coenzyme Q_{10} therapy should be given during statin therapy. Package inserts and marketing do not mention the statins–coenzyme Q_{10} link. It is noted that two U.S. patents, filed in January and February of 1989 and granted in 1990, describe a method for counteracting statin-associated myopathy and potential liver damage by concurrent administration of the statins with coenzyme Q_{10}. Both of these patents were assigned to Merck & Co. For more than 12 years, the producers of statins did not act upon this information and failed to reveal the statins–coenzyme Q_{10} relation to millions of statin users and to the medical community. It is noted that drug manufacturers spend twice as much on advertising to promote their products compared with research and development. *Biomedicine & Pharmacotherapy* 56 (2002): 56–59.

Ischemia
Compared with controls, animal hearts pretreated with CoQ had significantly less depletion of ATP and reduced mitochondrial oxygen utilization following induced ischemia. Coenzyme Q_{10} protects against ischemia. K. Folkers and Y. Yamamura, eds., *Biomedical and Clinical Aspects of Coenzyme Q*, vol. 2 (Amsterdam: Elsevier/North Holland Biomedical Press, 1980), 409–425.

Cancer and AIDS
The researchers report reduction in Adriamycin's toxic effect on the heart in cancer patients who received CoQ prior to chemotherapy treatment. K. Folkers and Y. Yamamura, eds., *Biomedical and Clinical Aspects of Coenzyme Q*, vol. 3 (Amsterdam: Elsevier/North Holland Biomedical Press, 1981), 339–412.

Dr. Knud Lockwood, M.D., an oncologist from Denmark, described his successful treatment of 32 breast cancer patients who were treated with conventional therapy and were at high risk for recurrence. He used high-dose CoQ therapy (90 to 390 milligrams), and after 24 months, all were still alive when at least 6 deaths would have been expected. Six of the 32 patients showed partial tumor regression, and 2 had complete tumor regression. *Biochemical and Biophysical Research Communications* 199 (March 30, 1994):1,504–1,508.

In this report, AIDS showed a striking clinical response to high-dose CoQ therapy. Also, 8 new case histories of cancer patients, plus 2 previously reported cases, showed survival periods of 5 to 15 years. *Biochemical and Biophysical Research Communications* 192(1) (April 15, 1993): 241–245.

Chronic Fatigue and Immune Dysfunction
In this study, compared with healthy controls, a group of female patients, ages 28 to 43, who had had CFIDS for 2 to 5 years, had lower tissue levels of CoQ. Levels were further decreased after exercise. Supplementation with 100 milligrams of CoQ for 90 days resulted in 100 percent improvement in exercise tolerance; 85 percent improvement in postexercise fatigue; and 90 percent improvement in overall clinical symptoms. Coenzyme Q_{10} presented at the American College of Nutrition Annual Meeting, 1996, San Francisco.

Other Uses
A double-blind study was conducted with patients who had progressive muscular dystrophies and neurogenic atrophies, including Duchenne, Becker, limb-girdle dystrophies, myotonic dystrophy, and Welander disease. After a three-month trial using CoQ, improved physical well-being was observed. The results indicate that the subjects' impaired my-

ocardial function and impaired skeletal muscle function may be associated, and that both may be improved with CoQ therapy. *Proceedings of the National Academy of Science* 32 (July 1985): 4,513–4,516.

Parkinson's disease (PD) is a degenerative neurological disorder for which no treatment has been shown to slow the progression. Subjects with early received placebo or coenzyme Q_{10} at dosages of 300, 600, or 1,200 milligrams/day. The subjects underwent evaluation with the Unified Parkinson's Disease Rating Scale (UPDRS) at the screening, baseline, and 1-, 4-, 8-, 12-, and 16-month visits. They were followed up for 16 months or until disability requiring treatment with levodopa had developed. The adjusted mean total UPDRS changes were +11.99 for the placebo group, +8.81 for the 300-milligrams/day group, +10.82 for the 600-milligrams/day group, and +6.69 for the 1,200-milligrams/day group. A prespecified, secondary analysis was the comparison of each treatment group with the placebo group, and the difference between the 1,200-milligrams/day and placebo groups was significant (P=.04). Coenzyme Q_{10} was safe and well tolerated at dosages of up to 1,200 milligrams/day. Less disability developed in subjects assigned to coenzyme Q_{10} than in those assigned to placebo, and the benefit was greatest in subjects receiving the highest dosage. Coenzyme Q_{10} appears to slow the progressive deterioration of function in PD, but these results need to be confirmed in a larger study. *Archive of Neurology* 59(10) (October 2002): 1541–1550.

CoQ markedly improved the course of treatment for periodontal disease in both double-blind and open trials. In one study, 100 percent of patients receiving CoQ improved, compared with 30 percent of the placebo group. *Communications in Chemistry, Pathology, and Pharmacology* 14 (1976): 715.

The benefits of CoQ supplementation for patients recovering from surgery for severe periodontal disease were dramatic. *Research Communication in Chemistry, Pathology, and Pharmacology* 12 (1975): 111.

In this study, 39 stable diabetics received CoQ. Fasting blood sugar was reduced by at least 80 percent in 12, and by at least 30 percent in another 12, while ketone levels fell in 13. *Journal of Vitaminology* 12 (1966): 293.

Toxicity and Adverse Effects

Mice given CoQ orally, subcutaneously, intramuscularly, or intravenously showed no evidence of toxicity. *Applied Pharmacology* 6 (1972): 769–779.

Up to 600 milligrams per day of CoQ were given to rabbits. No toxic effects were observed. *Applied Pharmacology* 6 (1972): 781–786.

Chapter 34: Essential Fatty Acids

Overview

This article reviews the therapeutic effects of diet and nutrients on dermatological disorders. Topics covered include fish oil, evening primrose oil, and Chinese herbal teas for atopic dermatitis; vitamins and wound healing; vitamins A and D for psoriasis; and antioxidants, vitamins, and skin cancer. *Journal of the American Academy of Dermatology* 29 (1993): 447–461.

Omega-3 Fatty Acids (EPA, DHA, and Fish Oil)

Cardiovascular Disease

The author of this overview of EPA and the multiple ways in which it protects against heart disease concludes that EPA may be even more effective than aspirin in this regard. *Annals of Internal Medicine* 107 (1987): 890–899.

This article reviews the many benefits of fish oil in relation to cardiovascular disease. The author suggests that a modest intake of fish oil will prove to be a safer, more efficacious alternative to mass prophylaxis with aspirin. *Lancet* (May 14, 1988): 1,081–1,083.

In this controlled study of patients with exercise-induced angina, those given EPA for 4 weeks lowered their triglycerides and blood pressure. Half of the men did not experience chest pain during exercise, as compared with the placebo group. *American Journal of Medicine* 84 (January 1988): 45–52.

This is an analysis of 31 placebo-controlled trials evaluating the role of fish oil on blood pressure in 1,356 patients. There was a statistically significant dose-response effect observed in relation to the effects of EPA and DHA on blood pressure. The hypotensive effect of fish oil may be strongest in hypertensive subjects and those with clinical atherosclerotic disease or hypercholesterolemia. *Circulation* 88 (August 1993): 523–533.

The results of this analysis demonstrate that restenosis after coronary angioplasty is reduced by fish oil supplementation. The benefit is dose dependent, with doses ranging from 3,000 to 6,484 milligrams. *Archives of Internal Medicine* 153 (July 12, 1993): 1,595–1,601.

This is an extensive review on the role of fish oil in cardiovascular disease. Fish oils have been shown to: reduce triglycerides; reduce platelet reactivity; decrease blood pressure; reduce the use of nitroglycerin in patients with angina pectoris; reduce cardiac arrhythmias; and reduce LDL cholesterol. The increased risk of bleeding in patients taking fish oil is low and is less than with aspirin intake. *Drugs* 47 (1994): 405–424.

This article reviews the role of fibrinogen in cerebrovascular disease. Elevated fibrinogen levels result in generation of atherosclerosis. Fish oil supplementation has resulted in significant reductions in fibrinogen levels. In crossover trials, both serum triglycerides and fibrinogen levels were significantly reduced for up to 48 months in patients with hyperlipidemia who received EPA. *Heart Disease and Stroke* 2 (November–December 1993): 503–506.

In evaluating 84,688 female nurses enrolled in the Nurses' Health Study who were between 34 and 59 years of age and free from cardiovascular disease and cancer in 1980, subjects completed questionnaires in 1980, 1984, 1986, 1990, and 1994. During the 16 years of follow-up, there were 1,513 cases of coronary heart disease, of which 484 were coronary heart disease deaths and 1,029 were nonfatal myocardial infarctions. Compared with women who rarely ate fish at <1 per month, those who had higher fish intake had a lower risk of coronary heart disease. Women with a higher intake of omega-3 fatty acids had a lower risk of coronary heart disease. For both fish and omega-3 fatty acid intake, there was an inverse association that appeared to be stronger for coronary heart disease deaths than for myocardial infarction, with a relative risk for fish consumption >5 times per week of 0.55 versus 0.73, respectively. *Journal of the American Medical Association* 287(14) (2002): 1815–1821.

In a double-blind, placebo-controlled trial of 223 patients, 1.5 grams/day of omega-3 fatty acids appeared to reduce the progression/increased regression of established coronary artery disease, as assessed by angiography. The mechanism of action appears to be only with omega-3 fatty acids and not with other unsaturated fatty acids. Omega-3 fatty acids appear to reduce inflammatory mediators. Seven grams/day of omega-3 fatty acids, but not omega-6 or omega-9 fatty acids, for 4 weeks further reduced inflammatory mediators. *Lipids* 36(Suppl) (2001): S99–S102.

Omega-3 fatty acids can prevent heart disease. They prevent arrythmias (ventricular tachycardia and fibrillation), have anti-inflammatory properties, are antithrombotic, inhibit atherosclerosis, and reduce the risk of primary cardiac arrest. *American Journal of Clinical Nutrition* 71(suppl) (2000): 171S–175S.

Marine n-3 fatty acids, in particular DHA, may protect against heart disease by reducing circulating levels of C-reactive protein (CRP), a bio-marker of inflammation. There is an association of high levels of CRP and an increased risk of heart attack in healthy individuals. High CRP may also signal the risk of heart attack in persons who already have heart disease. *American Journal of Cardiology* 88 (2001): 1139–1142.

The cardioprotective effects of DHA and EPA may be due to reductions in malignant ventricular arrhythmias; increases in heart rate variability; antithrombotic effects, such as reduced blood platelet reactivity, moderately long bleeding times, and reduced plasma viscosity; lipid lowering, which includes fasting triglycerides and VLDL levels, with a moderate rise in HDL cholesterol; improved endothelial function by enhancing nitric oxide–dependent and nitric oxide–independent vasodilation; inhibition of atherosclerosis and inflammation through the inhibition of smooth-muscle cell proliferation, altered eicosanoid synthesis and reduced expression of cell adhesion molecules; and suppressed production of inflammatory cytokines, such as interleukins and tumor necrosis factor, and mitogens. It is noted that many patients with vascular disease rarely eat fish. Patients should be advised to increase fish intake to 3 servings per week. Fish oil supplements taken with meals or functional food sources, which include liquid egg enriched in omega-3 polyunsaturated fatty acids, can serve as alternative dietary sources. "Clinical Nutrition: 4. Omega-3 Fatty Acids in Cardiovascular Care," Holub, B.J., *CMAJ* 166(5) (March 5, 2002): 608–615.

At a recent conference sponsored by the American College of Cardiology, researchers discussed the results from the Diet and Reinfarction Trial involving 2,033 men from England and Wales who survived a myocardial infarction and were randomized to eat fish 2 or more times per week, reduce fat intake, or boost consumption of cereal fiber. Results showed that during 2 years of follow-up, those who were urged to eat more fish and thereby increase their omega-3 fatty acid intake from 0.6 to 2.4 grams/week had a reduced risk of all-cause mortality by 29 percent, which is identical to what one sees with statin medications. If fish oil were a drug, most drug representatives would have these data in front of them. *Family Practice News* (April 15, 2002): 9.

An expert panel came up with the following conclusions regarding marine sources of omega-3 fatty acids and coronary heart disease. These results were published at the 34th Annual Scientific Meeting of the European Society for Clinical Investigation and include: 1) consumption of 1 to 2 fish meals per week is associated with reduced coronary, heart disease mortality; 2) those who have had a myocardial infarction can reduce their risk of total, cardiovascular, coronary and sudden death by taking 1 gram/day of ethylesters of omega-3 polyunsaturated fatty acids, mainly as eicosapentaenoic acid (EPA) and docosahexaenoic acid (DHA), which is irrespective of fish intake or simultaneous intake of other drugs; 3) patients who have had coronary artery bypass surgery with venous grafts may reduce graft occlusion rates by the administration of 4 grams/day of omega-3 polyunsaturated fatty acids; 4) following heart transplantation, 4 grams/day of omega-3 polyunsaturated fatty acids may prevent the development of hypertension; 5) patients with dyslipidemia and/or postprandial hyperlipidemia may reduce their coronary risk by taking 1 to 4 grams/day of marine omega-3 polyunsaturated fatty acids; 6) there is accumulating evidence that the daily intake of up to 1 energy percent of nutrients from plant omega-3 polyunsaturated fatty acids, such as alpha-linolenic acid, may decrease the risk of myocardial infarction and death of patients with coronary heart disease. *Lipids* 36(Suppl) (2001): S127–S129.

Three fish oil capsules daily in conjunction with low-dose aspirin were found to reduce the tendency to arterial thrombosis in patients who were being treated for atherosclerotic disease. Those receiving aspirin and fish oil experienced a reduced likelihood of developing symptoms of atherosclerotic disease, including cardiac arrest, heart attack, and stroke, compared with those taking only aspirin. In the Physician's Health Study, aspirin was associated with a slight but significantly increased risk of strokes. *Family Practice News* (December 1, 1992): 9.

Rheumatoid Arthritis and Other Inflammatory Conditions
In this study, 64 patients with rheumatoid arthritis taking NSAIDS were given 10 MaxEPA or placebo capsules daily for 12 months. There was a significant reduction in NSAIDS use in patients after 3 months of taking MaxEPA. The authors conclude that MaxEPA may be a useful therapy in patients with mild rheumatoid arthritis or in those who cannot tolerate NSAIDS. *British Journal of Rheumatology* 32 (1993): 982–989.

This article reviews the role of fish oil in inflammatory conditions such as rheumatoid arthritis, Raynaud's phenomenon, systemic lupus erythematosus, psoriasis, psoriatic arthritis, gout, and osteoarthritis. The results of the study have shown modest clinical benefits. It may be a safer alternative than NAIDS in some patients. *Seminars in Arthritis and Rheumatism* 21 (June 1992): 368–375.

In this study, 49 patients with RA completed a 24-week prospective double-blind randomized study of dietary supplementation with 27 milligrams per kilogram of EPA (18 milligrams per kilogram of DHA), 54 milligrams per kilogram of EPA (36 milligrams per kilogram of DHA), or olive oil capsules (6.8 grams of oleic acid). A total of 5 of 45 clinical measures were significantly changed from baseline in the olive oil group; 8 of 45 in the low-dose fish oil group; and 21 of 45 in the high-dose fish oil group. The authors conclude that clinical benefits of fish oil supplementation are more commonly observed at higher doses for time intervals that are longer than previously studied. The use of olive oil also requires further investigation. *Arthritis and Rheumatism* 33 (June 1990): 810–815.

Numerous studies have demonstrated that fish oil supplements result in significant improvement in Crohn's disease and ulcerative colitis. The doses used ranged from 3 to 4 grams of EPA (16 to 24 capsules of fish oil) to 2.7 grams EPA + 1.8 grams of DHA (15 capsules of fish oil). Patient tolerance was best achieved with enteric-coated fish oil capsules. It was compared to a common fish oil preparation and it was found that the enteric-coated supplement showed the best incorporation into cell membranes and had no side effects. It is very difficult to get excellent patient compliance with non-enteric–coated fish oil supplements when high doses are used due to gastrointestinal side effects. *American Journal of Clinical Nutrition* 71(suppl) (2000): 339S–342S.

Vitamin C and E have shown benefit in osteoarthritis. Selenium, which has shown benefit, is a component of the antioxidant enzyme glutathione peroxidase. Omega-3 polyunsaturated fatty acids have been shown to oppose the inflammatory effects of omega-6 polyunsaturated fatty acids. Gamma-linolenic acid is a precursor of prostaglandin E1, which may account for its ability to ameliorate arthritic symptoms. Fish oil supplements rich in omega-3 polyunsaturated fatty acids have shown benefit in rheumatoid arthritis, possibly by suppressing the immune system and cytokine production. Green-lipped mussel and vegetable oils, such as olive oil and evening primrose oil, may have indirect anti-inflammatory actions. *British Journal of Nutrition* 85 (2001): 251–269.

The use of EPA and DHA may lead to striking improvements in critically ill patients. It is particularly therapeutic in acute and chronic disorders where inappropriate activation of the immune system occurs, such as rheumatoid arthritis, systemic lupus erythematosus, and Crohn's disease. Studies have also shown that EPA and DHA may prevent relapse of disease and may slow the progression of certain types of kidney disease such as glomerulonephritis. Constant consumption of omega-3 fatty acids could suppress the autoreactive (or hyperreactive) T cells and may explain why in some populations there is a decreased incidence of inflammatory and autoimmune disease. The consumption of omega-3 fatty acids can even be made to the general healthy population not only to prevent atherosclerosis but to reduce the risk of autoimmunity. *Israeli Medical Association Journal* 4(1) (2002): 34–38.

Skin Conditions

In this study, 10 capsules of EPA were given to patients with atopic dermatitis for 12 weeks. Compared with controls, the EPA significantly reduced symptoms, particularly of itch and scale. Higher doses and longer treatment might have resulted in further improvement. *British Journal of Dermatology* 117 (1987): 463–469.

A double-blind randomized controlled study of psoriasis patients was conducted for 8 weeks. The group that received EPA had a significant lessening of symptoms, and tended to have less of their body surface affected. *Lancet* (February 20, 1988): 378–380.

Supplementing the diet of patients with psoriasis with fish oil has been reported to alleviate skin lesions with moderate to excellent results in inflammatory skin disorders such as psoriasis. It's antiproliferative effects result in a reduction of epidermal scaly lesions. The metabolites from these oils attenuate inflammatory and proliferative cutaneous disorders and may serve as less toxic in vivo montherapies or as adjuncts to standard therapeutic regimens for the management of inflammatory skin disorders. *American Journal of Clinical Nutrition* 71(suppl) (2000): 361S–366S.

Reduced conversion of linoleic acid to gamma-linolenic acid (GLA) occurs in patients with atopic ezcema. These patients have higher levels of linoleic acid in blood, milk, and adipose tissue but lower levels of the metabolites such as GLA. In most studies, administration of GLA has been found to improve the clinically assessed skin condition and skin roughness. Atopic eczema may be a minor inherited abnormality of EFA metabolism. *American Journal of Clinical Nutrition* 71(suppl) (2000): 367S–372S.

Cancer

In an animal study of advanced breast cancer, omega-3 fatty acid-rich diets prolonged survival and slowed tumor growth. This may have implications for the use of omega-3 diets at the time of diagnosis or surgical therapy for Stage II disease. *American Journal of Clinical Nutrition* 45 (1987): 859.

In a double-blind randomized crossover trial, 12 volunteers not at risk for colon cancer were given fish oil supplements or a corn oil placebo. A reduction in mucosal enzyme (ornithine decarboxylase) was seen with fish oil supplementation. Increased levels of this enzyme may be a risk factor for colon cancer in patients with familial polyps. *Gastroenterology* 105 (1993): 1,317–1,322.

Dysmenorhea

In this study, 42 adolescent girls with dysmenorrhea (painful menstruation) were randomly assigned to 2 groups. Group 1 received 1,080 milligrams of EPA, 720 milligrams of DHA, and 1.5 milligrams of vitamin E. Group 2 received a placebo. At the end of 2 months, the supplemented group experienced a marked reduction in Cox Menstrual Symptom Scale, suggesting that omega-3 fatty acid supplementation has a beneficial effect on symptoms of dysmenorrhea in adolescents. *American Journal of Obstetrics and Gynecology* 174 (1996): 1,335–1,338.

Kidney Disease

In an animal study, EPA supplements prevented the deterioration of kidney function in mice with kidney disease. *Prostaglandins, Leukotrienes, and Medicine* 22 (1986): 323–334.

Results from this study show that EPA produces potentially beneficial effects on blood fats, platelets, and blood pressure, and so may help protect against cardiovascular disease in high-risk dialysis patients. *Nephronology Research* (1986): 196–202.

Men and women with a history of urinary stones were given a highly purified EPA preparation of omega-3 fatty acids at 600 milligrams orally immediately after each meal, totaling 1,800 milligrams per day. After 3 months in 26 hypercalciuric patients, calcium excretion was reduced in 17 subjects. After 18 months, urinary magnesium and phosphorus were significantly reduced, and urea nitrogen and uric acid showed a tendency toward reduction. Urinary calcium was reduced 3 months after EPA administration, but at 18 months, there was no further reduction. In the hyperlipidemic subjects, the reduction in total cholesterol, triglycerides, and phospholipids was significant. This study shows that EPA can protect against stone formation when given for long periods of time. *European Urology* 39 (2001): 580–585.

The Respiratory System

The first NHANES found higher forced respiratory volume (better lung function) in those with higher fish oil consumption in asthmatic and other subjects with impaired lung function. Fish consumption and omega-3 fatty acids are protective against emphysema and chronic bronchitis and may protect children against asthma. EPA or GLA given to animals appears to protect their lungs against various toxins. More research is needed to further elucidate the role of essential fatty acids in lung disease. *American Journal of Clinical Nutrition* 71(suppl) (2000): 393S–396S.

Hyperactivity (ADHD)
Boys with ADHD have clinical and biochemical signs of essential fatty acid deficiency. Overall academic achievement and mathematical ability was found to be significantly better in boys with high n-3 fatty acid concentrations compared to those with low concentrations. Dark adaptation improved in 5 dyslexic patients after DHA-rich fish oil (480 milligrams DHA per day) supplementation and movement skills improved in 15 dyspraxic children after 4 months of supplementation of DHA-rich fish oil plus evening primrose and thyme oil (480 milligrams DHA + 96 milligrams gamma-linolenic acid + 80 milligrams vitamin E and 24 milligrams of thyme oil). Individuals with dyslexia and dyspraxia have poor conversion of essential fatty acids as do those with ADHD. A subclinical DHA deficiency may be responsible for the abnormal behavior of these children. *American Journal of Clinical Nutrition* 71(suppl) (2000): 327S–330S.

Aerobic Exercise
In this study, 34 hyperlipidemic subjects were randomly assigned to one of 4 groups: fish oil and exercise; aerobic exercise; fish oil; or corn oil. The aerobic exercise improved the effects of fish oil on LDL cholesterol and apo-B, and improved fitness and body composition. *Medicine and Science in Sports and Exercise* 21 (1989): 498–505.

Omega-6 Fatty Acids (GLA)
Overview
This is an extensive review on the biochemistry of GLA and potential benefits in diseases such as diabetes, skin disorders (e.g., atopic eczema), reproduction, breast pain, PMS, inflammatory and autoimmune disorders, cardiovascular disease, and viral infections. A major source of GLA is evening primrose oil. The author argues that since high-dose fish oil may lower GLA levels, it should be given with GLA. *Progress in Lipid Research* 31 (1992): 163–194.

In studying 1,012 women there was an increasing trend in the odds ratios seen with increasing dietary intake of omega-6 polyunsaturated fatty acids and the risk of allergic rhinoconjunctivitis. There was a positive association between dietary intake of omega-6 polyunsaturated fatty acids and seasonal allergic rhinoconjunctivitis symptoms in spring with a dose-response relationship. Margarine contains approximately 10 to 20 times more omega-6 polyunsaturated fatty acids than butter. It is noted that in the former East Germany, the prevalence of hay fever was significantly higher among children whose parents reported increased consumption of margarine and decreased consumption of butter after German unification. High levels of transfatty acids were positively correlated with the prevalence of allergic rhinoconjunctivitis in a study from Europe. *Annals of Epidemiology* 11(1) (2001): 59–64.

Cardiovascular Disease
A mixture of EPA and GLA have synergistic activities. Blood platelet aggregation is inhibited more strongly with a mixture of these essential fatty acids than by either compound alone. *JPN Kokai Tokkyo Koho* (July 1986).

GLA as evening primrose oil has a cholesterol-lowering effect on rats. *Annals of Nutrition and Metabolism* 301 (1986): 289–299.

GLA weakened the cardiovascular responses to chronic stress in animals with a genetic predisposition to hypertension. These findings suggest that GLA may be useful in preventing hypertension in high-risk individuals. *Lipids* 20 (1985): 573–577.

Evening primrose oil offers the angina patient relief when given for a relatively short period of time. *Abstract Book, International Prostaglandin Conference,* Washington, D.C. (May 1979): 10.

Rheumatoid Arthritis and Other Inflammatory Conditions

In this study, patients with rheumatoid arthritis and with gastrointestinal lesions from nonsteroidal anti-inflammatory drugs (NSAIDS) were supplemented daily with 6 grams of evening primrose oil (EPO) supplying 540 milligrams of GLA or a placebo in a double-blind controlled trial. EPO significantly reduced morning stiffness in 3 months. Pain and articular index were reduced in 6 months with the olive oil placebo. In both groups, 23 percent were able to reduce NSAIDS. The authors note other studies that have shown better effects with EPO with regard to reducing or eliminating NSAIDS. They suggest that olive oil should not be used as a placebo, and should be investigated for its own therapeutic effect. The authors feel they can recommend EPO for use in mild RA. *British Journal of Rheumatology* 30 (1991): 370–372.

This randomized double-blind controlled study compared daily supplementation of 1,400 milligrams of GLA from borage seed oil to a cotton seed oil placebo in patients with RA. GLA resulted in a significant reduction of signs and symptoms. The placebo group had no change. This was a very high-dose GLA study with no adverse effects noted in any subjects. *Annals of Internal Medicine* 119 (November 1, 1993): 867–873.

Inflammation was suppressed in rats who were exposed to a potent inflammatory agent by the administration of evening primrose oil. Chronic proliferative adjuvant arthritis was also suppressed. *Progressive Lipid Research* 20 (1987): 885–888.

EPA and GLA were given to rats in which acute inflammation was induced. GLA significantly suppressed the cellular phase of inflammation. EPA suppressed the fluid phase. *Arthritis and Rheumatism Journal* 31 (December 1988): 1,543–1,551.

Observations of adults with atopic eczema and normal controls suggest that atopic eczema is associated with abnormal metabolism of essential fatty acids. Treatment with oral evening primrose oil partially corrected the abnormality. *British Journal of Dermatology* 11 (1984): 643–648.

In a controlled study on the effect of evening primrose oil on atopic eczema, the treatment group had a statistically significant improvement in the severity of symptoms and percentage of body surface affected. *British Journal of Dermatology* 117 (1987): 11–19.

Cancer

Evening primrose oil has caused a highly significant inhibition of cancer growth without affecting normal cells. It is likely that GLA bypasses the block in the metabolic pathway of cancer cells that prevents them from producing an immunoactivating substance. The regression of cancer through such proposed normalization offers preliminary hope for a new effective and harmless approach to the treatment of cancer. *S.A. Medical Journal* 62 (October 2, 1982): 505.

Recent studies suggest that GLA may unblock the metabolic defect in cancer cells involving a substance that is responsible for the conversion of linoleic acid to gamma linoleic acid. This may explain some of its anticancer properties. *Medical Hypotheses* 12 (1983): 195–201.

In a study of breast cancer in rats, evening primrose oil inhibited the growth of the tumors. *Journal of Nutrition, Growth, and Cancer* 2 (1985): 41.

The cells of 2 types of human esophageal cancers were treated with GLA. After 7 days, the cells died. *S.A. Medical Journal* 62 (October 30, 1982): 681–683.

Malignant liver cells reverted back to normal when GLA was added to the cell culture. *S.A. Medical Journal* 62 (1982): 683.

Premenstrual Syndrome

In a double-blind crossover study, patients received either evening primrose oil or a placebo for 2 menstrual cycles, and then a placebo for a further 2 cycles. Overall improvement in the treated group was 60 percent, compared with 40 percent for the placebo. The greatest results were for irritability and depression. *Journal of Reproductive Medicine* 28 (1983): 465–468.

In this study, 30 patients with severe PMS received evening primrose oil twice a day, or a placebo. After 4 menstrual cycles, the treated group showed decreased menstrual symptoms compared with the placebo group. *Journal of Reproductive Medicine* 39 (1985): 149–153.

Diabetes
Seven noninsulin-dependent diabetics were given 4 grams of evening primrose oil, 2.4 grams of sardine oil, and 200 milligrams of vitamin E for 4 weeks. Fasting plasma glucose, hemoglobin A1C, total cholesterol, body weight, and percentage of body fat decreased significantly. These results suggest that these supplements are useful in improving abnormal lipid parameters in diabetic patients. *Prostaglandins, Leukotrienes and Essential Fatty Acids* 49 (1993): 569–571.

Obesity
Researchers have observed that the more linoleic acid in the fat tissue, the less obese the person. This may be of particular significance in those with a family history of obesity. *2nd International Congress on Essential Fatty Acids, Prostaglandins, and Leukotrienes* (March 1985).

In this study, obese subjects received a daily supplement of evening primrose oil. After 6 to 8 weeks, half of those who were more than 10 percent overweight noted a reduction in appetite and had lost weight without dieting. The higher the dose of primrose oil, the greater the weight loss. *IRCS Journal of Medical Science* 7 (1979): 52.

Chapter 35: Flavonoids
Overviews
These are 3 excellent reviews of all aspects of known plant flavonoid modulation of the immune system, cancer, and inflammatory cell function. They cover many topics, including T-lymphocytes, B-lymphocytes, natural killer cells, interferon, macrophages, monocytes, mast cells, basophils, neutrophils, eosinophils, and platelets. *Human Nutrition—A Comprehensive Treatise*, vol. 8, Nutrition and Immunology, ed. David M. Klurfeld (New York: Plenum Press, 1993), 239–266. J. B. Harborne, ed., *The Flavonoids: Advances in Research Since 1986*. (London: Chapman & Hall, 1993), 619–652. *Biochemical Pharmacology* 43 (1992): 1,167–1,179.

The total dietary intakes of 10,054 men and women were examined and those with higher quercetin intakes had lower mortality from ischemic heart disease. Men with higher quercetin intakes had a lower lung cancer incidence. Asthma incidence was lower at higher quercetin. A trend toward a reduction in risk of Type II diabetes was associated with higher quercetin. (The risk of some chronic diseases may be lower at higher dietary flavonoid intakes.) *American Journal of Clinical Nutrition* 76(3) (2002): 560–568.

Fruits and vegetables protect against cancer by so far not well-characterized mechanisms. One likely explanation for this effect is that dietary plants contain substances able to control basic cellular processes such as the endogenous defense against oxidative stress. Onion extract and quercetin were able to increase the intracellular concentration of glutathione by approximately 50 percent. Our data strongly suggest that flavonoids are important in the regulation of the intracellular glutathione levels. *Free Radical Biology & Medicine* 32(5) (2002): 386–393.

Cancer and Viruses
Selected naturally occurring flavonoids (amentoflavone, scutellarein, and quercetin) had a concentration-dependent effect on inhibiting the reverse transcriptases of several viral and cancer cell lines. *Antiviral Research* 12 (1989): 99–110.

This study demonstrates the synergistic effect of vitamin C and two plant flavonoids on squamous cell carcinoma. Exposure of these cancer cells to ascorbic acid and either fisitin or quercetin resulted in 61 percent and 45 percent inhibition, respectively. Ascorbic acid may amplify the cancer growth inhibitory effect of flavonoids. *Anticancer Drugs* 4 (February 1993): 91–96.

The citrus flavonoids nobilitin and tangeretin markedly inhibited the growth of human squamous carcinoma cell-lines. *Cancer Letters* 56 (1991): 147–152.

A popular herbal medicine in Japan known as *Sho-saiko-to* has been used in the treatment of various chronic liver diseases. This study demonstrated that this herbal medicine inhibits the proliferation of a human hepatocellular carcinoma cell line and cholangiocarcinoma cell line. In fact, the combination of herbs in this medicine more strongly inhibited these cell lines than did any one of its major ingredients. *Cancer Research* 54 (January 15, 1994): 448–454.

Four flavonoids—baicalein, quercetin, quercitagentin, and myricetin—were found to be potent inhibitors of reverse transcriptases from Rauscher murine leukemia virus (RLV) and human immunodeficiency virus (HIV). Each of these flavonoids almost completely inhibited the activity of RLV. HIV reverse transcriptase was inhibited by these flavonoids 100 percent, 100 percent, 90 percent, and 70 percent, respectively. *European Journal of Biochemistry* 190 (1990): 469–476.

The ability of baicalin, a flavonoid purified from the Chinese medicinal herb *Scutellaria baicaleniss georgi*, to inhibit human T-cell leukemia virus type 1 (HTLV-1) was examined. Baicalin produced concentration-dependent inhibition of HTLV-1 replication in infected T- and B-cells. It also inhibited reverse transcriptase activity in the infected cells. These results suggest that baicalin may be a potential therapeutic agent against HTLV-1 associated T-cell disease. *The Journal of Infectious Diseases* 165 (1992): 433–437.

This study illustrates the variable spectrum of antiviral activity of several naturally occurring flavonoids against certain viruses. The viruses used in this study included herpes simplex virus Type I, polio virus Type I, parainfluenza virus Type III, and respiratory syncytial virus. For example, quercetin caused a concentration-dependent reduction in the infectivity of each virus and reduced intracellular replication. On the other hand, catechin inhibited only the infectivity of specific viruses. *Journal of Medical Virology* 15 (1985): 71–79.

Among 87 chemically defined tannins and related compounds, several were found to significantly inhibit both the cytopathic effect of HIV and the expression of HIV antigen in HTLV-I. *Antiviral Research* 18 (1992): 91–103.

The suppression of proliferation-stimulating activity, induced by environmental estrogen, by flavonoids, such as daidzein, genistein, quercetin, and luteolin, was studied and it was found that these flavonoids suppressed the induction of the proliferation-stimulating activity of environmental estrogens. The suppressive effect of flavonoids suggests that these compounds have anti-estrogenic and anticancer activities. *Bioscience, Biotechnology and Biochemistry* 66(7) (2002): 1479–1487.

Quercetin has been shown to induce growth inhibition in certain cancer cell types. In the present study we have pursued the mechanism of growth inhibition in human breast cancer cells. Quercetin induced significant apoptosis in breast cancer cells in addition to cell cycle arrest, and the induction of apoptosis. The present data, therefore, demonstrate that a flavonoid quercetin induces growth inhibition in the human breast carcinoma cell line through at least 2 different mechanisms; by inhibiting cell cycle progression through transient M phase accumulation and subsequent G2 arrest and by inducing apoptosis. *International Journal of Oncology* 19(4) (2001): 837–844.

In the present study, we evaluated the individual and combined effects of environmental estrogens and flavonoids on the proliferation of human breast carcinoma cells. Quercetin and luteolin exhibited cell proliferation–inhibiting activity. We also found that flavonoids were able to inhibit the proliferation-stimulating activity in breast cancer cells by environmental estrogens. *In Vitro Cellular & Developmental Biology Animal* 37(5) (May 2001): 275–282.

A number of quercetin's actions make it a potential anticancer agent, including cell cycle regulation, interaction with Type II estrogen binding sites, and tyrosine kinase inhibition. Quercetin appears to be associated with little toxicity when administered orally or intravenously. Much in vitro and some preliminary animal and human data indicate quercetin inhibits tumor growth. More research is needed to elucidate the absorption of oral doses and the magnitude of the anticancer effect. *Alternative Medicine Review* 5(3) (2000): 196–208.

Quercetin is a flavonoid well-known to inhibit growth and heat shock protein (HSP) synthesis of cancer cells. It was compared to sunphenon (a flavonoid) concerning effects on cancer cells. Effects were compared on a human carcinoma cell line. The heat shock reduced the cell viability of the quercetin-treated cells only. Quercetin appears to be more useful than sunphenon in combined therapy with hyperthermia for cancer. *Experimental Molecular Pathology* 66(1) (Apr 1999): 66–75.

When quercetin was added to the cultures of ovarian cancer cells followed later by genistein, synergism was observed in growth inhibition. The synergistic action of quercetin and genistein may be of interest in clinical treatment of human ovarian carcinoma. *Oncology Research* 9(11–12) (1997): 597–602.

Intraperitoneal administration of quercetin, apigenin, and the anti-estrogen tamoxifen were given to mice at the same time as the injection of cancer cells. Quercetin and apigenin significantly potentiated the inhibitory effect of a nontoxic dose of cisplatin. When tested for the ability to inhibit lung colonization, quercetin, apigenin, and tamoxifen significantly decreased the number of cancer colonies in the lungs, with quercetin and apigenin being more effective than tamoxifen. In conclusion, quercetin and apigenin inhibit melanoma growth and invasive and metastatic potential; therefore, they may constitute a valuable tool in the combination therapy of metastatic melanoma. *International Journal of Cancer* 87(4) (2000): 595–600.

A Phase I clinical trial with quercetin was conducted. Quercetin has antiproliferative activity in vitro and is known to inhibit signal transduction targets including tyrosine kinases, protein kinase C, and phosphatidyl inositol-3 kinase. Quercetin was administered by short IV infusion. The authors make specific recommendations for Phase II trials. In 9 of 11 patients, lymphocyte protein tyrosine phosphorylation was inhibited following administration of quercetin at 1 hour, which persisted to 16 hours. In one patient with ovarian cancer refractory to cisplatin, following 2 courses of quercetin (420 milligrams/m2), the CA 125 had fallen from 295 to 55 units/milliliters, and in another patient with hepatoma, the serum alpha-fetoprotein fell. Quercetin can be safely administered by IV bolus and evidence of antitumor activity was seen. *Clinical Cancer Research* 2(4) (1996): 659–668.

Phytoestrogens
This letter to the editor comments on potential explanations as to why Japanese women have less severe menopausal symptoms than Westerners. The excretion of flavonoids (i.e., genistein, daidzein) was as much as 100 to a 1,000 times higher than in American and Finnish women. Flavonoid excretion was associated with intakes of soy products such as tofu, miso, aburage, atuage, koridofu, soy beans, and boiled beans. This high level of flavonoid phytoestrogen intake may partly explain why hot flashes and other menopausal symptoms are reduced in Japanese women. *Lancet* 339 (May 16, 1992): 1,233.

Other Uses
In a controlled study, the authors found that 35 percent more vitamin C was absorbed when it was given with a citrus bioflavonoid extract than when it was given alone. They note that processing removes much of the bioflavonoids from frozen or reconstituted fruit juice. *American Journal of Clinical Nutrition* 48 (September 1988): 601–604.

Bioflavonoids scavenge free radicals. They also have an antibiotic-like action because of their influence on cell permeability. *Biochemical Pharmacology* 32:7 (1983): 1,141–1,148.

Experimental animals were given a drug to induce capillary fragility. Bioflavonoids were able to prevent this condition. *Farmaco Edizione Scientifica* 38:11 (1983): 67–72.

Bioflavonoids were effective in reducing cholesterol levels in the blood and liver in experimental animals. *Indian Journal of Experimental Biology* 19 (August 1981): 787–789.

Patients suffering from chronic venous insufficiency were treated with a combination of drugs containing bioflavonoids, which proved more effective in repairing tissue damage and alleviating symptoms. *Clinica Therapeutica* 108 (January 31, 1984): 91–98.

Bioflavonoids were shown to have pharmacological properties that may prove useful in the treatment of some connective tissue disorders, including rheumatoid arthritis. *Scandinavian Journal of Rheumatism* 12 (1983): 39–42.

Many bioflavonoids have anti-inflammatory effects that are considered to be superior to that of corticosteroids because of their low toxicity. Bioflavonoids are also useful for correcting capillary permeability and fragility. *Agents and Actions* 12:3 (1982): 298–302.

In this study, 13 out of 30 bioflavonoids tested inhibited the enzyme responsible for cataract formation. Animal studies have suggested that bioflavonoids may be useful in the prevention of cataracts in diabetics. *Biochemical Pharmacology* 31:23 (1982): 3,807–3,822.

In this study, 2 bioflavonoids were shown to inhibit cataract formation in humans. *Biochemical Pharmacology* 32:13 (1983): 1,995–1,998.

Pycnogenol, a naturally occurring plant flavonoid, significantly inhibited foam cell production by oxidized low-density lipoproteins (LDLs). *The International Conference on Pycnogenol Research*, Bordeaux, France (October 4–6, 1990).

In this study, 90 milligrams of pycnogenol were given daily to 110 persons with varicose veins. Of these subjects, 77 percent demonstrated improvement, and of those who complained of calf cramps, 93 percent had an improvement of symptoms. *Zeitschrift fur Allgemeinmedizin* 51 (June 30, 1975): 839.

Reviews on Pycnogenol research are contained in Richard A. Passwater, *The New Superantioxidant—Plus* (New Canaan, CT: Keats Publishing, 1992).

Six patients with systemic lupus erythematosus were treated with conventional medicine and Pycnogenol. Five other patients received the medication and a placebo. Pycnogenol reduced inflammation associated with lupus. *Phytotherapy Research* 15(8) (2001): 698–704.

Patients were treated with Pycnogenol or placebo at 50 milligrams, 3 times daily, for 2 months. A beneficial effect was shown on the progression of the retinopathy in the Pycnogenol group. With the placebo treatment, retinopathy progressed during the trial and the visual acuity decreased. With the Pycnogenol-supplemented patients, there was no deterioration in retinal function, and a significant recovery of visual acuity was noted. Fluorangiography showed an improvement in retinol vascularization and a reduction in endothelial permeability and leakage with Pycnogenol supplementation only. Pycnogenol may work by its antioxidant scavenging, anti-inflammatory and capillary protective benefits. Pycnogenol may bind to blood vessel wall proteins and mucopolysaccharides and produce a "sealing" effect, which reduces capillary permeability and edema formation. *Phytotherapy Research* 15 (2001): 219–223.

Chapter 36: Other Nutrients
Alpha-Lipoic Acid
Overview
An extensive monograph highlighting the research for ALA with respect to diabetic neuropathy, AIDS-related neuropathy, glaucoma, heart disease, Alzheimer's, and more. *Alternative Medicine Review* 3(4) (August 1998): 308–311.

Diabetes

Alpha-lipoic acid can effectively treat diabetic neuropathy. It enhances insulin function, required for energy production in the mitochondria, and may reduce glucose levels. The researchers reviewed the use of ALA in treating diabetes and concluded that its greatest benefit might be in preventing the progression of the disease to its full-blown state, owing to the ability of ALA to protect nerves from free-radical damage and improve insulin sensitivity. *Envionmental Toxicology and Pharmacology* 10 (2001): 167–172.

This article reviews numerous studies using ALA orally and intravenously to treat diabetic neuropathy. In a 2-year study involving Type I diabetic patients, compared with placebo, lipoic acid at 600 or 1,200 milligrams/day was found to improve neurological symptoms. In a 7-month trial involving Type II diabetic patients receiving lipoic acid at 600 milligrams/day intravenously followed by 1,800 milligrams/day orally for 6 months, there was improvement in neuropathic symptoms. ALA given at 800 milligrams/day orally for 4 months to Type II diabetic patients demonstrated modest improvements in the variability of heart rate in the group receiving lipoic acid. *Environmental Toxicology and Pharmacology* 10 (2001): 167–172.

Alzheimer's Disease

Subjects with Alzheimer's disease were given 600 milligrams of alpha-lipoic acid per day in addition to an acetylcholinesterase inhibitor (Aricept, Exelon) for an average period of 337 days. There was stabilization of cognitive function shown by constant scores in the Mini-Mental State Examination (MMSE) and Alzheimer's Disease Assessment Scale (ADAScog). The authors believe that alpha-lipoic acid may be a "neuroprotective" agent and that placebo-controlled, double-blind trials are warranted. *Gerontology and Geriatrics* 32 (2001): 275–282.

Garlic

Overviews

Allium vegetables have been shown to have beneficial effects against several diseases, including cancer. Garlic, onions, leeks, and chives have been reported to protect against stomach, colorectal, and other forms of cancer. The protective effect appears to be related to the presence of organosulfur compounds and mainly allyl derivatives, which inhibit carcinogenesis. Organosulfur compounds modulate the activity of several metabolizing enzymes that activate or detoxify carcinogens and inhibit the formation of DNA adducts in several target tissues. Antiproliferative activity has been described in several tumor cell lines, which is possibly mediated by induction of apoptosis and alterations of the cell cycle. *Environmental Health Perspectives* 109(9) (September 2001): 893–902.

Chemical constituents of garlic and their variations on the methods of isolation have been discussed in the present review. Effect of garlic and its constituents against various human and plant pathogenic and saprophytic microorganisms has also been reviewed. *Indian Journal of Experimental Biology* 39(4) (2001): 310–322.

Although there are many garlic supplements commercially available, they fall into 1 of 4 categories, i.e., dehydrated garlic powder, garlic oil, garlic oil macerate, and aged garlic extract (AGE). Garlic and garlic supplements are consumed in many cultures for their hypolipidemic, antiplatelet, and procirculatory effects. In addition to these proclaimed beneficial effects, some garlic preparations also appear to possess hepatoprotective, immune-enhancing, anticancer, and chemopreventive activities. *Journal of Nutrition* 131(3s) (2001): 955S–962S.

Cardiovascular Disease

Previous studies using garlic have found alterations on a number of cardiovascular disease (CVD) risk factors including blood pressure, plasma viscosity, platelet activity, and serum lipid levels. The latest clinical research suggests that consumption of garlic powder does not play a significant role in lowering plasma lipid levels when in conjunction with a low-fat, low-cholesterol diet. Additional well-controlled, long-term studies that explore dosage and preparation type are necessary to confirm the efficacy of garlic in lowering cholesterol levels and to fully understand garlic's potential role in CVD. *Nutrition Reviews* 59(7) (2001): 236–241.

New data have increased the interest in garlic and its role in normalization and treatment of cardiovascular disease risk factors. Recent studies have shown the complex composition of garlic, containing many compounds, that present potential positive effects in the field of health. It can be summarized that garlic can normalize plasma lipid, check lipid peroxidation, stimulate fibrinolytic activity, inhibit platelet aggregation, smooth the thickening and structural changes of the artery wall related to aging and atherosclerosis, and decrease blood pressure. However, some other studies do not support these benefits. The positive effects found have promoted many study projects; nevertheless, the extract liability and the lack of result consensus call for a moderate consumption of garlic and garlic extracts. It is necessary for the application of some norms in the production and consumption of this functional food in order to guarantee its use in adequate form and doses. *Archivos Latinoamericanos de Nutricion* 50(3) (2000): 219–229.

Reports of cardiovascular-related effects were limited to randomized controlled trials lasting at least 4 weeks. From 1,798 pertinent records, 45 randomized trials and 73 additional studies reporting adverse events were identified. Compared with placebo, garlic preparations may lead to small reductions in the total cholesterol level at 1 month and 3 months but not 6 months. Changes in low-density lipoprotein levels and triglyceride levels paralleled total cholesterol level results; no statistically significant changes in high-density lipoprotein levels were observed. Trials also reported significant reductions in platelet aggregation and mixed effects on blood pressure outcomes. Trials suggest possible small short-term benefits of garlic on some lipid and antiplatelet factors. Conclusions regarding clinical significance are limited by the marginal quality and short duration of many trials and by the unpredictable release and inadequate definition of active constituents in study preparations. *Archives of Internal Medicine* 161(6) (2000): 813–824.

This is a review article on the health benefits of garlic. Garlic has been shown to reduce cholesterol in human trials. It also reduces the susceptibility of LDL to oxidation. At the Fourth International Congress on Phytotherapy in Munich, Germany, September 1992, Dr. Jorg Grunwald concluded that the 3 main cardiovascular effects of garlic are: reduction of free radicals; reduction of oxidation of lipoproteins, particularly LDL; and inhibition of infiltration of lipids into the vascular wall. It is noted that Kwai garlic is made from Chinese garlic and is a licensed drug for the treatment of atherosclerosis in Germany. Kwai is noted to reduce LDL cholesterol, increase HDL cholesterol, and improve peripheral blood flow. *British Journal of Clinical Practice* 47 (March/April 1993): 64–65.

Males ages 18 to 35 with cholesterol levels of 160 to 250 were given 10 grams of raw garlic daily for 2 months. Cholesterol levels decreased significantly in all subjects. *Indian Journal of Physiology and Pharmacology* 23:3 (July–September 1979): 211.

Using a MEDLINE search, the studies revealed that patients treated with garlic consistently showed a greater decrease in total cholesterol levels when compared with the effects of a placebo. Analysis showed that half to a full clove of garlic (or the equivalent) resulted in a 9 percent reduction in serum cholesterol levels. *Annals of Internal Medicine* 119 (October 1, 1993): 599–605.

In this randomized double-blind trial, 10 volunteers took Kwai garlic or a placebo. After 2 weeks, blood samples revealed that lipoprotein susceptibility to oxidation was lowered by the garlic supplement by 34 percent. The authors note previous garlic studies demonstrating beneficial effects on serum lipids, platelet function, fibrinolysis, and blood pressure. *Lipids* 28 (1993): 465–477.

Infections and Immunity

A fresh extract of garlic was given orally to human volunteers. Within 30 minutes to an hour after administration, anticandidal and anticryptococcal activities were detected in the subjects' blood. *Antimicrobial Agents and Chemotherapy* 23:5 (May 1983): 700–702.

The effect of garlic juice on the growth and respiration of *staphylococcus, E. coli,* and *C. albicans* was studied. *Candida albicans* proved to be the most sensitive organism of the 3 examined. *Acta Microbiology Polonica* 5:22 (1973): 51–62.

Of 16 cases of cryptococcal meningitis given garlic therapy, 6 were cured and 5 improved, giving an effective rate of 68 to 75 percent. Preliminary studies show that garlic may kill fungi directly and improve the patients' immunologic function. The author points out that garlic is also cheap and plentiful, and causes no major side effects. *Chinese Medicine Journal* 93:2 (1980): 123–126.

Cancer

This study supports prior research that showed that garlic inhibits tumor formation in chemically induced cancers. In rats exposed to mammary carcinogen, raw garlic powder and garlic extract reduced DMBA-DNA adducts (biochemical markers) of breast cancer by an average of 40 percent. A commercial deodorized garlic powder reduced adducts by 64 percent, and a commercial high-sulfur garlic powder reduced adducts by 56 percent. *Carcinogenesis* 14 (1993): 1,627–1,631.

Animal and in vitro studies provide evidence of an anticarcinogenic effect of active ingredients in garlic. This review of the epidemiologic literature on garlic consumption addresses cancers of the stomach, colon, head and neck, lung, breast, and prostate. An indication of publication bias was observed. Evidence from available studies nevertheless suggests a preventive effect of garlic consumption in stomach and colorectal cancers. The study limitations indicate the need for more definitive research and improved nutritional epidemiologic analyses of dietary data. *Journal of Nutrition* 131(3s) (2001): 1032S–1040S.

Glutathione and N-Acetylcysteine (NAC)

Overviews

Oral and intravenous N-acetyleysteine is an antidote for acetaminophen (Tylenol) toxicity. NAC shows promise in the treatment of chronic bronchitis and immune system disorders; as a cancer preventive agent; and in the treatment of diseases including acute pulmonary oxygen toxicity, septicemia, and endotoxin shock. NAC supports glutathione biosynthesis. *Toxicology Letters* 553 (1992): abstract W4-01. See also *Pharmacy Therapy* 60 (1993): 91–120.

Glutathione is important for the detoxification of free radicals, toxic oxygen radicals, thiol-disulfate exchange, and storage and transfer of cysteine. It is very important in organs that are exposed to toxins, such as the liver, kidney, lung, and intestine. *Pharmacological Therapy* 52 (1991): 287–305.

This comprehensive review article discusses the effects of glutathione and ascorbic acid in reducing oxidative stress. The administration of glutathione and vitamin C in patients experiencing high levels of oxidative stress from diseases such as aging, cancer, atherosclerosis, viral infections (including AIDS), stroke, myocardial infarction, and arthritis may be of clinical benefit. *Biochemical Pharmacology* 44 (1992): 1,905–1,915.

Infection and Immunity

This article reviews the role of glutathione, NAC, and vitamin C supplementation in HIV infection and AIDS, with specific focus on the fact that glutathione is frequently deficient in these individuals. Glutathione is the main intracellular defense against oxidative stress, and is decreased in the plasma, lung fluid, and T-lymphocytes in individuals with AIDS. NAC and other glutathione-replenishing substances can inhibit oxidative stress and HIV transcription or replication. *Lancet* 339 (April 11, 1992): 909–912. See also *Lancet* 339 (June 27, 1992): 1,603–1,604.

The intracellular concentration of glutathione was correlated with the absolute CD4 lymphocyte counts. The concentration of glutathione and mononuclear cells was significantly lower in patients with more advanced immunodeficiency. A single dose of NAC increased the concentration of cysteine in the plasma and mononuclear cells of HIV-infected patients. *AIDS* 6 (1992): 815–819.

An adequate supply of cysteine is important for maintaining the oxidant/antioxidant balance of the immune system. Since glutathione deficiency is prevalent in AIDS patients and important for lymphocyte function, NAC may be important in the treatment of HIV-infected patients. Anecdotal observations have reported that AIDS patients improve substantially on NAC. It is possible that NAC intervention in early-stage patients may help prevent progression of the disease. *Immunology Today* 13 (1992): 211–214.

This study reviewed the synergistic effects of NAC and vitamin C on HIV suppression. NAC caused approximately a 2-fold inhibition of HIV reverse transcriptase activity and had a synergistic effect when tested simultaneously with ascorbic acid. These results support the potent antiviral effects of ascorbic acid and suggest its synergistic effect with compounds such as NAC. *American Journal of Clinical Nutrition* 54 (1991): S1,231–S1,235.

NAC suppresses HIV expression in chronically infected monocytic cells. It has been shown that HIV seropositive patients treated with NAC for 4 months show a normalization in plasma cysteine and a reduction in tumor necrosis factor. The expected decline in CD4 helper cells is diminished. *Toxicology Letters* 54 (1992): SW4–L5.

Cancer

This review article discusses glutathione deficiency in association with aging and increased cancer risk. It is believed that glutathione is important in the detoxification of a wide variety of carcinogens and free radicals, and in the maintenance of normal immune function. *Experimental Gerontology* 27 (1992): 615–626.

Several studies have demonstrated that sulfur-containing compounds such as glutathione appear to optimize the effectiveness of cisplatin, a potent anticancer drug, in the treatment of ovarian cancer. This combined treatment demonstrated a superiority over conventional cisplatin treatment as follows: 21 out of 21 stage I or stage II patients, and 9 out of 11 stage III patients had no evidence of ovarian cancer. All patients with early disease were alive after a median follow-up of 18 months. In the advanced stage group, 10 out of 11 patients were alive after a median follow-up of 22 months. Glutathione also appears to protect against kidney toxicity of cisplatin. *Cancer Treatment and Reviews* 18 (1991): 253–259.

This article reviews the importance of total parenteral nutrition with L-glutamine and glutathione in cancer patients. Glutathione is important because it helps to protect the gut mucosa from methotrexate, which may damage the gastrointestinal tract. *Physician Assistant Practice* 12 (Summer 1993): 14–16.

Glutathione has been shown to have cancer prevention activity in experimental models. This study evaluated the use of vitamin E, beta-carotene, glutathione, and vitamin C alone or in combination in preventing DMBA-induced cancer in the hamster buccal pouch. The authors conclude that the mixture of antioxidants produced a significant synergistic chemoprevention of oral cancer. *Nutrition and Cancer* 20 (1993): 145–151.

NAC prevented chemotherapy-induced hair loss when administered intravenously or applied topically to animals. *Cancer Investigation* 10 (1992): 271–276.

Detoxification

NAC given within 12 hours of carbon tetrachloride exposure may decrease the severity of liver and kidney damage. Oral NAC is available and may be of benefit in carbon tetrachloride exposure. *American Family Physician* (October, 1992): 1,199–1,207.

Sperm Motility
In this study, 11 infertile men with dyspermia received glutathione at 600 milligrams per day intramuscularly for 2 months. This treatment significantly boosted sperm motility patterns and reduced atypical sperm. *Archives of Andrology* 29 (1992): 65–68.

This placebo-controlled double-blind study evaluated the use of 600 milligrams daily of injected glutathione over a 2-month period. The patients had dyspermia associated with unilateral varicocele or a germ-free genital tract inflammation. Glutathione significantly improved sperm motility and sperm morphology *Human Reproduction* 10 (1993): 1,057–1,062.

Cataracts and Aging
This extensive review article discusses the role of antioxidant nutrients in defending the lens of the eye from oxidative stress. Recent work suggests that supplementing the diet with vitamins C and E decreases the risk of cataract by 50 percent. Keeping high concentrations of glutathione in the lens may also protect against oxidative stress. Abraham Spector, *Oxidative Stress: Oxidants and Antioxidants* (New York: Columbia University, 1991), 529–558.

Cardiovascular Disease
NAC ingested at doses of 1.2 grams per day for 6 weeks showed a significant decrease in lipoprotein(a) concentrations of approximately 7 percent. *Journal of Internal Medicine* 230 (1991): 519–526.

This study examines the importance of glutathione and glutathione-dependent enzymes in the cellular defense against oxidized low-density lipoproteins. *Journal of Lipid Research* 43 (1993): 479–490.

Pulmonary Disease
Several studies have demonstrated that the inhalation of NAC (i.e., Mucomyst) is efficacious in controlling chronic bronchitis. *European Respiratory Reviews* 2 (1992): 5–8.

Parkinson's Disease
There is a reduced level of glutathione in the brains of Parkinson's patients. This may result in oxidative stress that may lead to or be derived from mitochondrial damage. *Annals of Neurology* 32 (1992): S111–S115. See also *Annals of Neurology* 32 (1992): 804–812.

Surgical Complications
Oxidative stress may participate in creating surgical complications of cardiopulmonary bypass procedures. Antioxidants (e.g., glutathione peroxidase, NAC, and superoxide dismutase) may afford protection in cardiovascular surgery. *Klinische Wochenschrift* 69 (1991): 1,066–1,072.

L-Carnitine
Overview
This excellent review article discusses the metabolism and function of L-carnitine in humans and its therapeutic applications. *Annual Review of Nutrition* 6 (1986): 41–46.

Sports Nutrition
This article reviews the use of carnitine as an ergogenic aid. For example, in long-distance runners and sprinters, it has been found that L-carnitine supplementation at 2 grams per day over 6 months can increase muscle L-carnitine levels. There were reduced lactate and pyruvate levels in an L-carnitine-supplemented group when 2 grams were given one hour before progressive incremental cycle ergometry exercise to maximal heart rate, exhaustion, or dyspnea. In another study, 5 grams of L-carnitine given for 5 days resulted in

a small but significant decrease in heart rate during cycle ergometry. *International Journal of Sports Nutrition* 2 (1992): 185–190.

Several studies have examined the role of L-carnitine in athletic performance. Findings have indicated that trained subjects have greater muscle L-carnitine levels than do their untrained counterparts, and that the performance time of submaximal exercise (80 percent VO2max) is greatly increased by L-carnitine loading. This study examined the effect of L-carnitine loading (4 grams per day), given over a period of 2 weeks, on the aerobic and anaerobic performance of 6 long-distance runners. It was concluded that as a consequence of L-carnitine loading, VO2max is slightly but significantly raised. *European Journal of Applied Physiology* 54 (1985): 131–135.

In this double-blind crossover trial on 10 moderately trained young men, 2 grams of L-carnitine or a placebo were administered orally. Treatment with L-carnitine significantly increased both maximal oxygen uptake and power output. Carbon dioxide production, pulmonary ventilation, and plasma lactate were reduced. Under these experimental conditions, L-carnitine favored aerobic processes, resulting in a more efficient performance. *European Journal of Applied Physiology* 61 (1990): 486–490.

Chronic Fatigue Syndrome

Patients with Chronic Fatigue Syndrome appear to be deficient in acyl-carnitine. This deficiency may result in an energy deficit and an intramitochondrial condition in skeletal muscle, possibly resulting in fatigue, myalgia, muscle weakness, and post-exertional malaise. Patients who recovered from general fatigue had their levels of acyl-carnitine increased to normal. *Clinical Infectious Diseases* 18 (1994): S62–S67.

Cardiovascular Disease

L-propionyl carnitine has been shown to improve the heart's mechanical recovery and other parameters after ischemia-reperfusion. It may act as an energy substrate, directly as an antioxidant, and as a mild iron-chelating agent. When compared with D-propionyl carnitine, the L-form has a wider variety of benefits. *Archives of Biochemistry and Biophysics* 296 (August 1, 1992): 394–401.

In humans, supplementation with L-carnitine at a dose of 300 milligrams, 3 times a day, for 12 weeks significantly improved the exercise tolerance of patients with angina. In patients with chronic congestive heart failure, 55 percent improved with supplementation. The results suggest that L-carnitine is a useful therapeutic agent in conjunction with other pharmacologic therapy. *Japanese Circulation Journal* 56 (January 1992): 86–94.

This crossover study evaluated the use of propionyl carnitine supplementation on typical stable effort angina at 500 milligrams, 3 times a day, for 30 days, compared with a placebo. Subjects were 18 males, ages 37 to 70. The authors conclude from the results that propionyl carnitine appears to have an anti-ischemic effect. *Cardiovascular Drugs and Therapy* 4 (1990): 481–486.

The mortality from cardiomyopathy with traditional therapies is over 50 percent. The use of L-carnitine shows promise, since it plays a very important role in cardiac function, and the data suggest that some patients are responsive to L-carnitine treatment. *Journal of Child Neurology* 10(Supp 2) (1995): 45–51.

L-carnitine is able to transport this long-chain fatty acid into the mitochondrial matrix, where beta-oxidation and energy production occur. Carnitine can also remove compounds that are toxic to metabolic pathways. Supplementation with carnitine has been shown to reverse cardiomyopathy in patients with systemic carnitine deficiency. Carnitine may be valuable in both chronic and acute ischemic syndromes, peripheral vascular disease, congestive heart failure, cardiac arrhythmias, and anthracycline-induced cardiotoxicity, and possibly other cardiovascular conditions. *Clinical Therapeutics* 13(1) (1991): 2–21.

In evaluating patients with a diagnosis of recent myocardial infarction, 81 patients were randomly assigned to an oral dose of L-carnitine at 4 grams/day for 12 months, in addition to pharmacological treatment, while the other subjects received standard treatment. At 12 months, compared with controls, the L-carnitine-treated subjects showed improvement in heart rate, systolic arterial pressure, and diastolic arterial pressure; a reduction in anginal attacks, rhythm disorders, and clinical signs of impaired myocardial contractility; and a definite improvement in lipid profiles. There was a lower mortality rate in the treated group, at 1.2 percent compared with the control group at 12.5 percent. The authors recommend L-carnitine as an effective treatment in post-infarction ischemic cardiopathy, which may improve the clinical outcome of this condition. *Drugs Under Experimental and Clinical Research* 18(8) (1992): 355–365.

Hemodialysis

Some dialysis patients have abnormalities in carnitine metabolism, resulting in skeletal myopathy, cardiomyopathy, arrhythmias, and plasma lipid abnormalities. Muscle cramps, cardiac arrhythmias, and hypotension may also be related to carnitine metabolism. Given that oral carnitine tablets are the least expensive preparation, the authors believe that the time is ready for routine administration of L-carnitine in hemodialysis. They recommend 660 to 990 milligrams daily or 2 to 3 grams just prior to hemodialysis. *Seminars in Dialysis* 5 (April-June 1992): 94–98.

Alzheimer's Disease

In a randomized double-blind trial, patients received 2 grams of acetyl-L-carnitine or a placebo. The patients receiving acetyl-L-carnitine showed a consistently reduced rate of progression that was statistically significant for the Blessed Dementia Scale and for 3 neuropsychological tests. The 2-gram dose used in this study contained 1.6 grams of carnitine—about 5 to 10 times the average U.S. daily intake. *Neurology* 41 (November 1991): 1,726–1,732.

Antioxidant Powers

This article discusses new information that acetyl-L-carnitine may have direct antioxidant activity, as well as the ability to repair other antioxidants that have already been used to quench free radicals. *American Heart Journal* 123 (June 1992): 1,726–1,727.

Weight Reduction

This review article on chromium reports the possible synergistic effect of chromium picolinate, L-carnitine, and a high-fiber supplement on weight reduction. *The Nutrition Report* 11 (June 1993): 41, 46.

HIV Infection and AIDS

Patients with AIDS are at risk for developing carnitine deficiency for many reasons, including decreased appetite, dysphagia, prolonged or recurrent gastrointestinal infections, cancer, and drug use. The authors conclude that carnitine supplementation may be important to help supply fatty acids as energy to the muscle, and to maintain immunocompetence in HIV-infected individuals. *AIDS* 6 (1992): 203–205.

Melatonin

Insomnia/Sleep Problems

Doses of melatonin (0.1 to 10 milligrams) or a placebo were given to 20 volunteers to assess its effects. All melatonin doses significantly increased sleep duration, as well as self-reported sleepiness and fatigue, relative to the placebo. *Proceedings of the National Academy of Science* 91 (1994): 1,824–1,828.

Volunteers received melatonin (0.3 or 1.0 milligrams) or a placebo at 6, 8, or 9 P.M. Latencies to sleep onset, to stage 2 sleep, and to rapid eye movement (REM) sleep were measured. Either dose given at any of the 3 time points decreased sleep onset latency and latency to stage 2 sleep. Neither melatonin dose induced hangover effects. *Clinical Pharmacologic Therapy* 57 (1995): 552–558.

The combined circadian and hypnotic effects of melatonin suggest a synergistic action in the treatment of sleep disorders related to the inappropriate timing of sleep and wakefulness. Adjuvant melatonin may also improve sleep disruption caused by drugs known to alter normal melatonin production (e.g., beta-blockers and benzodiazepines). *Journal of Pineal Research* 15 (1993): 1–12.

Volunteers who had their sleep-wake schedules delayed 2 hours on Friday and Saturday to simulate a delayed weekend sleep pattern received 6 milligrams of melatonin or placebo on Sunday late afternoon. On Sunday, melatonin administration increased the sleepiness throughout the evening and reduced sleep-onset latency at bedtime. On Monday morning, subjective sleepiness was reduced in those who took melatonin. A single dose of melatonin reversed this weekend drift and mild phase-delay effect on the endogenous circadian rhythm. *Journal of Sleep Research* 24(3) (2001): 272–281.

Subjects participated in two 6-day laboratory sessions mimicking graveyard shift work. Results showed 1.8 milligrams increased sleep time more in those who showed difficulty in sleeping during the day. Melatonin had no effect on alertness on the multiple sleep latency test, or on performance and mood during the night shift. There were no hangover effects from melatonin administration. These data suggest that melatonin can help night workers obtain more sleep during the day. *Journal of Sleep Research* 10 (2001): 181–192.

Jet Lag

In this study, 15 subjects took either 8 milligrams of melatonin or a placebo on the day of a return flight from North America to France, and continued dosage for 3 consecutive days. On day 8, self-rating significantly discriminated between melatonin and a placebo for global treatment efficacy, morning fatigue, and evening sleepiness. *Biology and Psychiatry* 32 (1992): 705–711.

This double-blind placebo-controlled study investigated the efficacy of and optimal time for taking melatonin in 52 international cabin crew members assigned to 3 groups. The early melatonin group used 5 milligrams, starting 3 days prior to arrival and ending 5 days after the return home. The late melatonin group used a placebo for 3 days, and then took 5 milligrams of melatonin for 5 days. The third group used a placebo only. The late melatonin group experienced the best recovery and improvements in mood, jet lag, and sleepiness. The late melatonin group also reported significantly less jet lag and sleep disturbance 6 days after arrival when compared with the placebo group, and had a significantly faster recovery of energy and alertness when compared with the early melatonin group. *Biology and Psychiatry* 33 (1993): 526–530.

Aging

Transplantation of the pineal glands of younger mice to older mice extended the life span and enlarged the thymus glands of the older mice within 5 months. In a series of experiments, when old mice were given melatonin in their nighttime water, they experienced cataract-free eyes; improved digestion; increased strength, energy, and muscle tone; a thick, shiny coat of fur; and sexual interest and capacity until the end of their lives, as well as behavior of mice half their age. Their life span was increased to the human equivalent of adding 25 extra years. The aged mice not receiving the melatonin developed all the signs and symptoms of old age. Walter Pierpaoli and William Regelson, *Melatonin Miracle* (New York: Simon & Schuster, 1995).

Antioxidant Powers

Melatonin scavenges and neutralizes the hydroxyl radical 5 times more effectively than does glutathione, and is twice as effective in deactivating the peroxyl radical as vitamin E. It stimulates glutathione peroxidase activity and inhibits nitric oxide synthase, thereby reducing the production of the highly toxic hydroxyl and nitric oxide free radicals. *Journal of Pineal Research* 18 (1995): 1–11.

Hormone-Related Problems

Follicular fluid samples were obtained from the largest pre-ovulatory follicle of 120 women undergoing *in vitro* fertilization, and were examined for melatonin levels. The concentrations of melatonin and progesterone during the autumn and winter (dark) months were significantly higher than those of the spring and summer (light) months. By contrast, estradiol concentration was significantly lower during the dark months than during the light months. There was a positive correlation between follicular fluid melatonin and progesterone concentration, and a negative relationship between melatonin and estradiol. The results of this study suggest that melatonin may be involved in the regulation of steroidogenesis by the human ovaries. *Human Reproduction* 10 (1995): 50–55.

There is evidence that pineal melatonin is an anti-aging hormone, and that menopause is associated with a substantial decline in melatonin secretion and an increased rate of pineal calcification. Animal data indicates that pineal melatonin is involved in the regulation of calcium and phosphorus metabolism by stimulating the activity of the parathyroid glands, by inhibiting calcitonin release, and by inhibiting prostaglandin synthesis. The researchers propose that the fall of melatonin during the early stage of menopause may be an important contributory factor in the development of post-menopausal osteoporosis. Plasma melatonin levels measured in early menopause could be used as an indicator or marker for osteoporosis. Light therapy or administration of melatonin (2.5 milligrams), or of other agents that induce a sustained release of melatonin, could be useful agents in the prophylaxis and treatment of postmenopausal osteoporosis. *International Journal of Neuroscience* 62 (1992): 215–225.

Cardiovascular Disease

Patients with coronary heart disease have increased nocturnal noradrenaline. Melatonin suppresses sympathetic activity, and its insufficiency may play a role in these elevated levels. It was determined in this study that patients with coronary heart disease have significantly lower levels of melatonin than healthy controls. Impaired nocturnal secretion of melatonin was shown to be associated with coronary heart disease. *Lancet* 345 (1995): 1,408.

Cancer

In this study, 10 milligrams per day of melatonin were given to 63 metastatic lung cancer patients. The survival at one year was significantly higher in patients treated with melatonin than in patients who were treated only with supportive care. *Oncology* 49 (1992): 336–339.

In this phase II study, 14 women with metastatic breast cancer who had disease progression despite tamoxifen therapy were given 20 milligrams per day of melatonin, along with tamoxifen therapy, for approximately 8 months. A partial response was achieved in 4 out of the 14 patients—a 28.5-percent response rate. Patients on melatonin experienced a relief of anxiety and a reduction of insulin-like growth factor (a growth factor for breast cancer) *British Journal of Cancer* 71 (1995): 854–856.

In this study, 14 patients with inoperable hepatocellular carcinoma (HCC) were given 50 milligrams per day of melatonin with interleukin-2 (IL-2). Over a 7-month period, tumor regression occurred in 5 out of the 14 patients (36 percent)—there was 1 complete response, and 4 partial responses. In addition, 6 patients had stable disease and 3 patients progressed. *European Journal of Cancer* 30A (1994): 167–170.

In this study, 22 patients with progressing metastatic renal cell carcinoma entered a phase II trial on the effect of a long-term regimen (12 months) with interferon and melatonin (10 milligrams per day). There were 7 remissions (33 percent): 3 complete, involving lung and soft tissue, and 4 partial, with a median duration at the time of 16 months. In addition, 9 patients achieved stable disease, and 5 progressed. Toxicity was mild, and side effects (fever, chills, arthralgias, myalgias) occurred rarely. *Cancer* 73 (1994): 3,015 ? 019.

In this study, 14 patients with metastatic gastric cancer received IL-2 with 50 milligrams per day of melatonin. Tumor regression was obtained in 3 out of 14 patients (21 percent). There was 1 complete response and 2 partial responses, with a median duration of over 13 months. The disease stabilized in 6 out of 14 patients (43 percent), and progressed in the remaining 5 (36 percent). Survival was significantly longer in patients with response or stable disease than in those with progression disease. Toxicity was low in all cases. *Tumori* 79 (1993): 401–404.

In vitro and in vivo, melatonin can protect healthy cells from radiation-induced and chemotherapeutic drug-induced toxicity and reduce cancer cachexia and improve the quality of life in these patients with a wide variety of cancers. Melatonin appears to work with conventional approaches at dose ranges of 10 to 50 milligrams every evening for 3 to 5 weeks. It is suggested that melatonin acts synergistically with these chemotherapeutic agents to enhance their antitumor effects. The presence of melatonin has been shown to prolong disease progression-free and overall 1-year survival as well. Melatonin in combination with radical or adjuvant radiation therapy for untreatable glioblastoma increased the 1-year survival rate substantially compared with radiotherapy alone. Melatonin has been shown to reduce hypotension, myelotoxicity, and lymphocytopenia that is associated with toxic therapeutic agents. Patients appear to have a better performance status and less anxiety than those without melatonin. *Journal of Clinical Oncology* 20(10) (2002): 2575–2601.

Melatonin is protective against cellular damage caused by carcinogens. Melatonin has been shown to reduce cancer initiation and inhibit the growth of established tumors. These antioxidants and melatonin may be used in the treatment or co-treatment of several stages of cancer. *International Journal of Biochemistry Cellular Biology* 33 (2001): 735–753.

Other Effects

This is a report on 2 case studies with frequent severe headaches who took 9 milligrams of melatonin in conjunction with Verapamil. Headaches significantly improved and patients remained headache-free for the duration of the observation. *Cephalalgia* 21 (2001): 993–995.

This study evaluated premenopausal, perimenopausal, and postmenopausal women. One group received 3 milligrams of melatonin and the other group received a placebo at bedtime. All the females who took melatonin with low baseline levels of melatonin results showed a significant increase in levels of thyroid hormones. Within 6 months of treatment, melatonin resulted in a significant reduction of luteotropic hormone in the women who were between 43 and 49 years of age and a reduction in follicle-stimulating hormone in those with low baseline melatonin levels. Most of the melatonin-treated individuals reported a general improvement in mood and a significant reduction in depression. This study showed a recovery of pituitary and thyroid functions in melatonin-treated women toward more youthful patterns. *Experimental Gerontology* 36 (2001): 297–310.

DHEA
Overview

This extensive article on DHEA reviews the published studies and personal communications of researchers. Topics covered include: studies on DHEA relieving gout, psoriasis, and congestive heart failure; animal studies demonstrating anticancer effects; protection against heart disease in men with higher DHEA levels; animal studies demonstrating reversal of diabetes, weight loss, alleviation of stress, and restoration of memory by encouragement of neurite growth; beneficial effects on elderly subjects receiving flu vaccines; and beneficial effects on sleep and joint soreness in humans. There is one report of liver damage in rats given very high doses of DHEA that far exceed the normal levels occurring in the animal even at a young age. *The Sciences* (September–October 1995): 26–31.

Aging

In this study, 13 men and 17 women of ages 40 to 70 were given 50 milligrams per day of DHEA in a randomized placebo-controlled crossover trial. DHEA and DS serum levels were restored to those found in young adults within 2 weeks of DHEA replacement, and were sustained throughout the 3 months of the study. A 2-fold increase in serum levels of androgens was observed in women, with only a small rise in androstenedione in men. Levels of sex hormone–binding, globulin, estrone, or estradiol in either gender were unchanged. IGF-1 levels increased significantly in both groups, and were associated with a remarkable increase in perceived physical and psychological well-being for men (67%) and women (84%). These observations, together with the absence of side effects, constitute the first demonstration of novel effects of DHEA replacement in age-advanced men and women. *Journal of Clinical Endocrinology and Metabolism* 78 (June 1994): 1,360–1,367.

DHEA in appropriate replacement doses appears to have remedial effects with respect to its ability to induce anabolic growth factor, increase muscle strength and lean body mass, activate immune function, and enhance quality of life in aging men and women, with no significant adverse effects. Further studies are needed to confirm and extend our current results, particularly the gender differences. *Annals of the New York Academy of Sciences* 774 (1995): 128–142.

Older subjects in an open-label trial received 50 milligrams of DHEA for 3 months. A significant increase was found in lean body mass and a significant decrease in fat mass, of which most occurred on the trunk, while bone mineral density in the lumbar spine increased in both men and women. Only minor side effects, which included an initial drop in HDL cholesterol of 5 milligrams/daily, which did not persist, and facial hair and acne, occurred in some females. *Endocrinology* 53(5) (2000): 561–568.

Postmenopausal women who were divided into 2 groups and all underwent hormonal evaluation before and at the third and sixth month of therapy with DHEA at 50 milligrams/day orally, as well as a growth hormone-releasing hormone (GHRH) at 1 microgram/kilogram before and at the sixth month of treatment. Steroids that are derived from DHEA metabolism, including estrone, estradiol, androstenedione, testosterone, DHEA sulfate (DHEAS), and osteocalcin, were increased in the plasma after DHEA supplementation. DHEA also increased levels of growth hormone and insulinlike growth factor-1 (IGF-1). This study showed that DHEA had similar effects as estrogen-progestin replacement therapy on the GHRH-growth hormone–IGF-1 axis. DHEA should be considered as an effective hormonal replacement treatment. This study showed that DHEA significantly affected several endocrine parameters in early and late postmenopausal women, independent of weight. *Fertility and Sterility* 76(2) (2001): 241–248.

Erectile Dysfunction

Patients recruited from an impotence clinic received either an oral dose of 50 milligrams of DHEA or a placebo once daily for 6 months. The DHEA treatment was associated with a higher mean score for the International Index of Erectile Function (IIEF). There was no effect of DHEA on mean serum levels of prostate-specific antigen, prolactin, testosterone, and mean prostate volume, and the mean postvoid residual urine volume. *Urology* 53 (1999): 590–595.

Mean serum levels of DHEA sulfate (DHEAS) in patients with erectile dysfunction were lower than in healthy volunteers until 60 years of age. After 60 years of age, the results became inverted, and a higher mean DHEAS level was found in the erectile dysfunction group than in the control group, but the difference was not statistically significant. DHEAS is produced in the liver from the adrenal steroid DHEA and circulates in the blood in men in relatively large amounts. Serum levels of DHEA and DHEAS peak at approximately 20 years of age and decline thereafter. By 60, the levels are about one-third of those of young men. This study supports the hypothesis that younger men with lower DHEAS and DHEAS-dependent erectile dysfunction may receive benefit from being treated with DHEA. *Urology* 55 (2000): 755–758.

Immune Function
Human volunteers above age 65 were given DHEAS and the influenza vaccine, resulting in a 4-fold increase in response to the vaccine, compared with the response of the group that did not receive DHEAS. However, when DHEAS was administered along with the tetanus vaccine, it did not improve immune response. *Annals of the New York Academy of Sciences* 774 (1995): 232–248.

Cardiovascular Disease
Studies on humans and animals have suggested that DHEAS has an antiatherogenic effect. DHEAS levels are significantly decreased in insulin-dependent diabetes mellitus patients, who are at high risk for atherosclerosis. It appears that these depressed DHEAS levels are a result of chronic insulin administration therapy. DHEAS, then, may provide a novel way to follow up and improve the outcome of patients with this form of diabetes. *Minerva Endocrinologia* 19 (1994): 113–119.

A double-blind placebo-controlled study was conducted that assessed the effects of DHEA administration on plasma plasminogen activator inhibitor Type I (PAI-1) and tissue plasminogen activator antigen (tPA). In this study, 18 men received 50 milligrams of DHEA and 16 men received a placebo daily for 12 days. Androstenedione and estrone levels significantly increased, while PAI-1 and tPA levels significantly decreased. Reductions of PAI-1 and tPA are associated with a blood-thinning effect by enhancing fibrinolytic (the breakdown of fibrinogen) potential. *American Journal of Medical Science* 311 (May 1996): 205–210.

Diabetes
In this study, 50 milligrams per day of DHEA were given to 11 postmenopausal women a placebo-controlled, randomized, blinded, crossover trial. DHEAS, DHEA, testosterone, and free testosterone increased up to twice the premenopausal levels in the group receiving the DHEA. Fasting triglycerides declined, and T-lymphocytes insulin-binding and degradation increased. Since 50 milligrams per day give supraphysiologic androgen levels, 25 milligrams per day may be more appropriate. *Fertility and Sterility* 63 (1995): 1,027–1,031.

Lupus
In this study, 10 female patients with systemic lupus erythematosus (SLE) were given 200 milligrams per day of DHEA for 3 to 6 months. Indices for overall SLE activity, including the SLE Disease Activity Index score and physician's overall assessment, were improved. DHEA was well tolerated. The only frequently noted side effect was mild dermatitis. *Arthritis and Rheumatism* 37 (1994): 1,305–1,310.

General References
I have drawn on several reference works for much of the background information presented in this book. Although they are geared primarily toward the professional, the average reader may also find them of interest.

Bland, Jeffrey. *The Justification for Vitamin Supplementation*. Bellevue, WA: Northwest Diagnostic Services, 1981.

Murray, M., and J. Pizzorno. *Encyclopedia of Natural Medicine*, 2nd Edition. Rocklin, CA: Prima Publishing, 1998.

The National Research Council. *Recommended Dietary Allowances,* 10th ed. Washington, D.C.: National Academy of Sciences, 1989.

Robinson, Corinne H. *Normal and Therapeutic Nutrition,* 15th ed. New York: Macmillan, 1977.

Werbach, M. *Nutritional Influences on Illness,* 2nd Edition. Tarzana, CA: Third Line Press, 1993.

Dietary Reference Intakes for Thiamin, Riboflavin, Niacin, Vitamin B_6, Folate, Vitamin B_{12}, Pantothenic Acid, Biotin, and Choline (1999). A Report of the Standing Committee on the Scientific Evaluation of Dietary Reference Intakes and its Panel on Folate, Other B Vitamins, and Choline and Subcommittee on Upper Reference Levels of Nutrients, Food and Nutrition Board, Institute of Medicine. National Academies Press, Washington, D.C. Free read online at: search.nap.edu/napcgi/ napsearch.cgi?term=dietary+reference+intakes

Dietary Reference Intakes for Vitamin C, Vitamin E, Selenium, and Carotenoids. Panel on Dietary Antioxidants and Related Compounds, Subcommittees on Upper Reference Levels of Nutrients and Interpretation and Uses of DRIs, Standing Committee on the Scientific Evaluation of Dietary Reference Intakes, Food and Nutrition Board. National Academies Press, 2000, Washington, D.C. Free read online at: search.nap.edu/ napcgi/napsearch.cgi?term=dietary+reference+intakes

Dietary Reference Intakes for Calcium, Phosphorus, Magnesium, Vitamin D, and Fluoride. Standing Committee on the Scientific Evaluation of Dietary Reference Intakes, Food and Nutrition Board, Institute of Medicine. National Academies Press, 1999, Washington, D.C. Free read online at: search.nap.edu/napcgi/napsearch.cgi?term= dietary+reference+intakes

Dietary Reference Intakes for Vitamin A, Vitamin K, Arsenic, Boron, Chromium, Copper, Iodine, Iron, Manganese, Molybdenum, Nickel, Silicon, Vanadium, and Zinc. Panel on Micronutrients, Subcommittees on Upper Reference Levels of Nutrients and of Interpretation and Use of Dietary Reference Intakes, and the Standing Committee on the Scientific Evaluation of Dietary Reference Intakes. National Academies Press, 2002, Washington, D.C. Free read online at: search.nap.edu/napcgi/napsearch.cgi? term=dietary+reference+intakes

Dietary Reference Intakes: Proposed Definition and Plan for Review of Dietary Antioxidants and Related Compounds. Standing Committee on the Scientific Evaluation of Dietary Reference Intakes, Institute of Medicine. National Academies Press, 1998, Washington, D.C. Free read online at: search.nap.edu/napcgi/napsearch.cgi?term= dietary+reference+intakes

Index